THERAPY IN THE REAL WORLD

Therapy in the Real World

Effective Treatments for Challenging Problems

Nancy Boyd-Franklin
Elizabeth N. Cleek
Matt Wofsy
Brian Mundy

THE GUILFORD PRESS
New York   London

© 2013 The Guilford Press
A Division of Guilford Publications, Inc.
370 Seventh Avenue, Suite 1200, New York, NY 10001
www.guilford.com

Paperback edition 2016

Printed in the United States of America

This book is printed on acid-free paper.

Last digit is print number: 9 8 7 6 5

The authors have checked with sources believed to be reliable in their efforts
to provide information that is complete and generally in accord with the standards of practice that are accepted at the time of publication. However, in view
of the possibility of human error or changes in behavioral, mental health, or
medical sciences, neither the authors, nor the editor and publisher, nor any
other party who has been involved in the preparation or publication of this
work warrants that the information contained herein is in every respect accurate or complete, and they are not responsible for any errors or omissions or the
results obtained from the use of such information. Readers are encouraged to
confirm the information contained in this book with other sources.

Library of Congress Cataloging-in-Publication Data

Boyd-Franklin, Nancy.
  Therapy in the real world : effective treatments for challenging problems /
Nancy Boyd-Franklin, Elizabeth N. Cleek, Matt Wofsy, Brian Mundy.
    pages cm
  Includes bibliographical references and index.
  ISBN 978-1-4625-1028-3 (hardback : acid-free paper)
  ISBN 978-1-4625-2605-5 (paperback : acid-free paper)
    1. Psychotherapy—Practice. 2. Counseling psychology—Practice.
3. Psychotherapists—Professional ethics. I. Cleek, Elizabeth N.
II. Wofsy, Matt. III. Mundy, Brian. IV. Title.
  RC480.5.B69 2013
  616.89′14—dc23
                                                                2013008653

To Dr. Peter Campanelli
in recognition of his vision and leadership at the
Institute for Community Living,
his outstanding contribution to our field,
and his ongoing support of all of us
and of this book project

About the Authors

Nancy Boyd-Franklin, PhD, is a Distinguished Professor (Professor II) in the Graduate School of Applied and Professional Psychology at Rutgers, The State University of New Jersey. She has received awards for her outstanding contributions from many professional organizations, including the American Family Therapy Academy, the Association of Black Psychologists, the American Psychological Association (Divisions 45 and 43), the Association of Black Social Workers, and the American Psychiatric Association. She is the author or editor of five books—*Black Families in Therapy: Understanding the African American Experience* (1989, 2003); *Children, Families, and HIV/AIDS: Psychosocial and Therapeutic Issues* (coeditor with Gloria L. Steiner and Mary G. Boland; 1995); *Reaching Out in Family Therapy: Home-Based, School, and Community Interventions* (with Brenna Hafer Bry; 2000); and *Boys into Men: Raising Our African American Teenage Sons* (with A. J. Franklin and Pamela Toussaint; 2001)—as well as numerous professional articles and chapters.

Elizabeth N. Cleek, PsyD, is a Vice President at the Institute for Community Living, Inc., in New York City, where she oversees the Program Design, Evaluation, and Systems Implementation and Central Access departments. Dr. Cleek's work focuses on developing and supporting systems wherein best-practice and evidence-based work can be implemented. She has led and coauthored numerous successful grant- and proposal-related initiatives for innovative programming, one of which was awarded a Science and Service Award from the Substance Abuse and Mental Health Services Administration. Dr. Cleek also co-led the development of an award-winning agency Clinical Risk Assessment and

Intervention system, including the creation of tools, procedural guidelines, and systemic interventions. She has written and presented with colleagues on the use of technology to support implementation of best-practice work, the development and implementation of health-related interventions for people with serious mental illness, and multisystems work with families.

Matt Wofsy, LCSW, is Director of Evidence-Based Treatment and Practice Innovation at the Institute for Community Living, where he is responsible for the identification, dissemination, and implementation of best practices throughout a large behavioral health care agency. He has extensive training experience in the area of adapting evidence-based practices to diverse clinical settings and has presented his work at several statewide and national conferences. Mr. Wofsy is the recipient of the 2011 Exemplary Mid-Career Social Work Leader Award from the New York City chapter of the National Association of Social Workers. He is coauthor of the 2012 article "The Family Empowerment Program: An Interdisciplinary Approach to Working with Multi-Stressed Urban Families," which appeared in *Family Process*; is Adjunct Professor at the New York University Silver School of Social Work; and maintains a private practice in New York City.

Brian Mundy, LCSW, is a Clinical and Evaluation Specialist at the Institute for Community Living, where he primarily supports clinicians and service providers with making evidence-based practices live and breathe in their work with clients. He is the recipient of the 2012 Emerging Social Work Leader Award from the New York City chapter of the National Association of Social Workers, and he has coauthored articles on the role of intimacy in recovery, acceptance and commitment therapy, and multisystemic work with families. Mr. Mundy is Adjunct Professor at Long Island University and maintains a private clinical practice.

Preface

This book represents an amazing journey for all of us. It is the product of our collective desire to create a clinical resource that all of us wish we had when we were starting our professional careers in the mental health field. As experienced clinicians, and as teachers, supervisors, program planners, and developers, we are well aware that many new clinicians from some of the best schools feel unprepared to address the challenges they face in the real world of clinical work. This awareness motivated us to write a book that can benefit experienced as well as beginning clinicians by providing a carefully considered synthesis of evidence-based practices, other respected clinical scholarship, and the challenges that arise in everyday clinical practice.

The book is a core textbook for clinical training and practice in psychology, social work, marriage and family therapy, counseling, psychiatry, nursing, and a wide range of other health and human service professions. The cutting-edge knowledge presented here is also meant to be a valuable resource for clinicians who have been in practice for many years but who may be overwhelmed by the ever-expanding array of proven treatments. It provides a road map to guide these clinicians in addressing the real-world issues that they face.

We have written this book with the goal of offering vivid, practical guidance and tools that will help clinicians address the needs of their clients, while caring for themselves and avoiding burnout. For beginning and experienced therapists in clinics, agencies, schools, hospitals, and private practices, here is the opportunity to weave effective intervention strategies into their work. In addition, the book's chapters distill the complex and disparate theories and best practices that exist in the mental health field today. Those teaching new clinicians in all mental health disciplines will find this to be the comprehensive textbook they have been searching for to inspire their students.

We are four people from different positions, backgrounds, and perspectives, grappling with training clinicians and supporting and maintaining clinical excellence in real-world mental health settings. Our journey together began in 2003 when Dr. Peter C. Campanelli, the visionary leader and CEO of the Institute for Community Living (ICL) in New York, brought Nancy Boyd-Franklin to the agency as a consultant. This led to an exciting collaboration among the four of us for over a decade as we struggled to provide clinical consultations and to develop trainings for staff in the new era of evidence-based practice.

Nancy Boyd-Franklin is an African American clinical scholar with a deep commitment to training clinicians to provide culturally competent treatment to clients in the real world. She is a family therapist who has developed the multisystems model that has guided clinicians for generations in their treatment of African American and other ethnic-minority families. For 40 years, she has provided clinical interventions, supervision, training, and teaching for therapists from all of the mental health disciplines. As a Distinguished Professor (Professor II) at Rutgers University in the Graduate School of Applied and Professional Psychology, she has shared the school's commitment to training doctoral students to provide services to underserved communities. The process of consulting to ICL, collaborating with her three coauthors, and writing this book has forced her to grapple with the changing mental health field in which clinicians struggle to incorporate evidence-based practices with other respected models in the field. This book represents a marriage of her earlier work—on multicultural interventions, the treatment of African American and other ethnic-minority families, family therapy, group treatment, and the multisystems model, and her long-term commitment to providing supervision and training as a lifeline for clinicians and an antidote to burnout—with current ever-evolving evidence-based practices. This book will help clinicians to make this marriage in their own work. Dr. Boyd-Franklin is committed to helping clinicians to see that they do not have to abandon their original training and theoretical orientations as they expand and grow, incorporate new ideas, and continue the process of lifelong learning.

Elizabeth N. Cleek entered the field in the mid-1990s with a passion for understanding the policies, systems, and structures that could be put in place to better support children, adults, and families impacted by poverty, homelessness, and mental illness. She has a particular interest in understanding how we can build and facilitate resiliencies. She has worked at ICL since 2001, leading a department tasked with ensuring the agency continues to identify, implement, and evaluate empirically supported best-practice programs, and to develop program models that rely on these practices and principles in order to support individuals and families experiencing or impacted by homelessness, mental illness, substance abuse, and co-occurring health conditions. Dr. Cleek has worked to create systems and structures within which best practices can be implemented to understand service needs from the perspective of the client and staff, and to support programs in their work of bringing best-practice care to fruition.

Matt Wofsy entered the field in the early 1990s with a commitment to working with high-risk children and families. He has amassed a considerable amount of clinical experience working in diverse mental health settings, and applies this experience in supporting the implementation of evidence-based practice principles throughout a large behavioral health care system—teaching master's-level students at New York University and working clinically in private practice. As his interests have evolved to include mindfulness applications as well as substance abuse, he has learned the importance of continuously mining the field of behavioral research to inform everyday practice.

Brian Mundy's initial background was in web design production, where the focus was on efficient, rapid development of high-quality learning content across multiple platforms by an ever-changing staff. After working in that industry for many years, he changed careers and became a social worker. Since then, he has been compassionately transporting his earlier experience to develop competency modeling strategies through training, clinical support, and agency culture designed to create a uniform, high-quality standard of care across a large urban social service agency. His feet are firmly planted in both the clinical and evaluation worlds, with an evolving appreciation of the complexities and nuances of translating research to practice and vice versa.

We set out to write this book prompted by the disconnect we all saw between the exciting ideas espoused in journal articles and conference presentations and the realities faced by highly skilled and well-intentioned treatment providers. We constantly were confronted with the question of how to translate evidence-based practice to private and public settings—where clinicians were struggling with complex cases, productivity demands, paperwork requirements, managed care, and tightening budgets—in a way that feels meaningful and authentic and is sustainable. Throughout our work, we have also struggled with the question of how to incorporate other respected clinical models (e.g., family therapy, multicultural approaches, multisystemic interventions, and crisis intervention) from our earlier training into our current work. Each chapter in this book is an attempt to answer these questions clearly and concisely.

Finally, it is our hope that this book will empower clinicians by reigniting the passion that led them to this field.

Acknowledgments

We gratefully acknowledge the Institute for Community Living (ICL); its leadership, particularly Dr. Peter C. Campanelli and Stella V. Pappas, whose extraordinary vision laid the foundation for these ideas to germinate and come to fruition; its staff, for their ongoing dedication, collaboration, and participation in brainstorming sessions to think through best-practice strategies for implementation and who make this work come alive on a day-to-day basis; and the persons it serves, an extraordinary group of individuals who demonstrate resiliency, perseverance, and a dedication to ongoing growth that never ceases to amaze.

We also wish to give our sincere thanks to Jim Nageotte, Senior Editor at The Guilford Press, who has been an amazing support to us throughout the entire publication process, and to Jane Keislar and Anna Nelson, who have helped in the final phases of this journey. Throughout this entire process, Hazel Staloff has provided exceptional editing, and her input has been invaluable in the preparation of this book; she has encouraged us from start to finish. Special thanks also to Bonnie Gordic, who also provided excellent editing and helped with the final stages of the book. We would also like to thank Destinay Erbie, a student from the School of Social Work at Rutgers University, who assisted with the preparation of the references.

Nancy Boyd-Franklin: I would like to give thanks to God for the opportunity to write this book and to work with this terrific team of coauthors. My special thanks to my husband and soul mate, Dr. A. J. Franklin, who has given me so much love and support throughout our years together. I also want to thank all of the children of my heart: Deidre, Remi, Jay, Tunde and his wife, Debbie, and my wonderful grandchildren, Kyra, Kayla, Kaylan, Jelani, Ajahni, and Adia, who bring such joy to my life. A special thanks to my brother, Randy Boyd, who read numerous drafts and gave very creative comments. To my mother, Regina Boyd, who proofread every one of my earlier books: I honor her memory and feel certain that she was looking down from heaven during the preparation of this book. I would also like to give a very personal thank-you to my "sister friends": Rosemary Allwood, JoAnn Tatum, Paulette Hines, Janis Sanchez Hucles, Brenna Bry, and Shalonda Kelly, who have always given me so much encouragement and emotional and spiritual support.

Elizabeth N. Cleek: The list of acknowledgments is long: First and last, to my husband Andy, who daily helps me reach one bar higher in all things personal and professional, and to my incredible children who make each day brighter with their beatific smiles, questions, thoughts, and glee. To my parents, Ellie and Charlie Miller, who continue to provide a wellspring of encouragement and support, and who exemplified that two-career-parent families are possible. Also to Marc and Ayelet Miller and the Miller family: Amanda Miller-Burg and Jordan Burg; Angela, John, and Katie Cleek; Sandi Bartel and David Polsky; and the entirety of my family and chosen family, all of whom help to create the "village" we all need. I also wish to thank Dr. Sandra T. Azar, a teacher and mentor, who encouraged me to think critically, to follow the logical progression in understanding research and its next steps, and to keep moving the process one step further; and the incredible staffs of the PDESI and CA departments—your thoughts and ideas continue to drive the work further each day. Finally, a huge thank-you to my coauthors, particularly Nancy Boyd-Franklin, who joined us at ICL as a consultant and without whom this book would not have been written.

Matt Wofsy: I would personally like to acknowledge my family, particularly my beautiful wife, Carrie, and our amazing daughter, whose love and support fortify my commitment and belief in the power of family every day. I also thank my parents, Jackie and Irwin Wofsy, whose love, compassion, and belief in me have fostered a commitment to this work and an ongoing curiosity that drives me daily; my sister, brother-in-law, and nieces, for providing me with an ongoing sense of belonging, family, and community; the many colleagues I have collaborated with over the years, whose dedication and commitment to excellence inspires me to do this work each day; and the clients I have worked with, whose trust and willingness to allow me to participate in their journey has been nothing less than a privilege.

Brian Mundy: I first thank the three people who have most helped me to learn, love, and grow during the writing of this book: my partner, Susannah Flicker, and two children, Ezra and Amelia. I would also like to acknowledge my supervisors Bernice Brief and Matt Wofsy, whose clinical guidance and support during the writing of this book was invaluable. I would like to express enormous gratitude to clients past and present for their willingness to collaborate with me in their own growing process—it is truly an honor to grow with you. Lastly, thank-you to my parents, Jack and Eileen Mundy, whose support went a long way in helping me switch careers to a path that I find so fulfilling and meaningful.

Contents

PART III. SYSTEMS INTERVENTIONS: FAMILY, MULTISYSTEMS, AND GROUP TREATMENT

PART IV. RISK ASSESSMENT AND CRISIS INTERVENTION

PART V. CHALLENGES OF CLINICAL WORK, CLINICIAN SELF-CARE, SUPERVISION, AND TRAINING

PART I

Therapy in the Real World

CHAPTER 1

Overview of the Book

Introduction

Clinical work in the real world is challenging and demanding, and it can also be extremely fulfilling. Clinicians must continuously navigate an ever-evolving web of theory, research, and technique. Yet they do this while they are caught between the demands of organizational policies, managed care, and multisystemic barriers. Many therapists have told us they are so overwhelmed by these constant realities that they often do not experience the most rewarding aspects of their work. This book offers clinicians the opportunity to re-energize their clinical practice through the infusion of effective strategies. It presents a concise framework that can help therapists to navigate systemic issues as well as the flood of new therapies and developing trends, so they can become more effective at relieving the suffering and addressing the needs of their clients.

We have repeatedly encountered therapists and counselors who are committed to doing a good job in their clinical work, but are hampered by the disconnect they feel between their training and the often overwhelming demands they experience in the world of service delivery. Many clinicians treating poor clients in public agencies, whether in urban or rural communities, may find themselves unprepared for the cultural diversity and the challenging life circumstances of the clients and families they treat; while many of those in private practice struggle with the ongoing and increasing pressures of managed care.

This book offers a lifeline for clinicians coping with the realities of real-world practice. It validates therapists for the meaningful work that they do and for the difference that they make in their clients' lives. In addition, the following chapters distill the complex and disparate theories and best practices that exist in the mental health field today and provide clinicians with a unified and accessible approach to healing. Therapists struggling to incorporate evidence-based practices into their clinical work will find a pragmatic integration of theory, research, and experience that also includes other respected therapeutic orientations and modalities.

We discuss methods of individual, group, and family therapy with diverse clients from many cultural backgrounds. In addition, we provide specific guidelines for risk assessment and crisis intervention in challenging situations involving sudden loss, violence, suicide, and homicide. Clinicians are often called upon to help intervene with their clients (and in families and communities) after these traumatic events. As news stories in recent years have demonstrated, therapists may face these challenges in small towns and college counseling centers, as well as in major urban areas. Although these topics have been covered elsewhere, this book is unique in that it discusses these issues and relevant interventions in one place with an emphasis on how mental health practice is actually carried out across the range of clinic, agency, hospital, school, community, and private practice settings. This book provides a comprehensive framework for addressing myriad clinical challenges, and the systemic and multisystemic barriers that most therapists will encounter at some point in their careers. It offers models for increasing supervisory, administrative, and organizational support to help clinicians avoid burnout and cope with the challenges of day-to-day practice. Strategies for self-care are discussed that can help therapists to apply to themselves the same compassion and caring that they generously give to their clients.

As we have indicated above, clinical work can be incredibly rewarding, yet extremely taxing. Ongoing supervision and training are essential for all clinicians if they are to remain positive and effective. Unfortunately, experienced and beginning therapists alike often receive little ongoing supervision, while financial considerations and productivity demands have led to fewer opportunities for on-site training. While nothing can take the place of supervision, it is our hope that this book will give isolated and overwhelmed clinicians the hope, encouragement, and antidote to burnout that good supervision and training provide. Ultimately, our goal throughout this book is to empower clinicians with the appropriate tools and interventions to use in the parallel process of empowering their clients.

The Importance of Lifelong Learning

The mental health field is clearly involved in one of the most challenging and important periods in its history as clinicians are expected to apply research findings and use evidence-based practices in their clinical work. For beginning therapists, the numbers of these treatments alone can be staggering. For some senior, experienced clinicians who were trained in theoretical models and treatment modalities prior to this movement, evidence-based practices can also present a challenge. A part of this dilemma rests in the fact that many practitioners in mental health and health professions "continue to implement the practices they learned during training (Isaacs & Fitzgerald, 1999; Pagoto et al., 2007; Turner, 2001)" (Spring, 2007, p. 618) without incorporating advances in the field.

Clinicians with many years of experience in a particular theoretical approach or modality of treatment can often become wedded to one way of working. This may result in clients not receiving the most advanced, best practices available. Orlinsky and Ronnestad (2005) have indicated that the therapists and counselors who are most effective with clients are those who have a commitment to lifelong learning and their personal and professional growth as clinicians.

We operate from a belief that the learning process not only enhances our therapeutic interventions but also helps to keep us engaged in and excited by our work. In Chapter 16, we indicate that ongoing, lifelong learning can often serve as an "antidote to burnout" for front-line clinicians in public agencies, as well as for therapists and counselors in private practice (Boyd-Franklin, 1989, 2003). Openness to change and the willingness to explore new ideas are two of the most important survival skills for therapists. It is our hope to encourage clinicians and agencies to continuously explore new treatment advances, including evidence-based practices, and to consider ways in which they might be incorporated in the service of our clients. This book is intended to provide therapists and counselors with an overview of the treatment approaches that we have found most helpful in our own work, and we strongly encourage clinicians to obtain further training in these treatment modalities.

Challenges of Providing Therapy in the Real World

Today's clinicians confront time pressures, productivity requirements, and expectations that they must do more with less. As managed care has increasingly become the norm, clinicians have to take into account insurance companies' guidelines regarding the types of treatments that can be reimbursed, restrictions on the length of treatment, and varied fee structures for clinical services (Huppert, Fabbro, & Barlow, 2006). Over time, all of these pressures can dampen the enthusiasm that many clinicians bring to their work in their early years. In addition, the debate over evidence-based practices (Goodheart, Kazdin, & Sternberg, 2006; Kazdin, 2008; Norcross, Beutler, & Levant, 2006) and the pressure from federal, state, and local funding sources and managed care companies (Reed & Eisman, 2006) to provide evidence-based services are increasingly pervasive factors for many health and mental health practitioners. Furthermore, many graduate training programs have not prepared clinicians to function optimally in this new service delivery environment.

At the same time, the clients we hope to help may be ambivalent about accepting our services. Therapists are usually well trained in providing treatment to clients who want it, but many clients in the real world are not self-referred and may attach a stigma to therapy. Some clinicians are unprepared for the "resistance" that they may encounter from such clients. Resistance can be especially commonplace among clients who are mandated for treatment by outside agencies, such as the courts, police, child welfare systems, schools, and so on (Boyd-Franklin & Bry, 2000a). Clients unfamiliar with the concept of therapy may have difficulty understanding it as a helpful process. For many ethnic minority clients in poor, urban communities, therapy provided in public agencies may be responded to with understandable suspicion based on past experiences with racism, discrimination, and disrespect encountered in other multisystemic agencies (Boyd-Franklin, 2003). This book offers ways of addressing and working through the ambivalence and mistrust that these clients may bring to therapy (see Chapter 3).

Key Concepts

Evidence-Based Practice in the Real World

For therapists, counselors, and other practitioners, the last decade has been a time of unprecedented change. The evidence-based practice or EBP movement has been one of the most defining characteristics of the mental health field in the 21st century (American Psychological Association [APA] Presidential Task Force on Evidence-Based Practice, 2006; Goodheart et al., 2006; Kazdin, 2008; Norcross et al., 2006). Beginning with the Institute of Medicine (2001), health and mental health organizations have begun to clarify definitions of EBPs for mental health disciplines (APA Presidential Task Force on Evidence-Based Practice, 2006; Gambrill, 2010). The use of EBPs throughout the health and mental health fields has become mandated by funding sources, such as managed care companies (Hayes, Barlow, & Nelson-Gray, 1999; Huppert et al., 2006; Reed & Eisman, 2006) and federal, state, and local government agencies (Carpinello, Rosenberg, Stone, Schwager, & Felton, 2002;

Chambless et al., 1996; Chorpita et al., 2002; Lampropoulos & Spengler, 2002; President's New Freedom Commission on Mental Health, 2003).

Many clinicians who would like to incorporate EBPs feel impeded by real-world factors such as time pressures, productivity requirements, and budget cuts. Other clinicians, who were trained in the field before the advent of EBPs, and have achieved success with clients utilizing other approaches, may be overwhelmed by new expectations and unconvinced that implementing these strategies will benefit their clients.

Goodheart (2006), who was appointed by the president of the American Psychological Association to head the APA Presidential Task Force on Evidence-Based Practice (2006), has pointed out that the debate is centered on what constitutes evidence. We share her point of view regarding the value of evidence-based research interventions, as well as the importance of incorporating other respected findings from diverse theoretical orientations (Goodheart, 2006). With this in mind, we have combined both evidence-based and practice-informed interventions, with clinical expertise and client needs, into our discussions. This book considers the many different points of view regarding EBPs, presents a careful review of some of the main issues in the debate, and makes recommendations for clinicians in responding to these realities (see Chapter 2).

Providing Mental Health Services in a Multicultural World

The number of ethnic minority individuals and families living in the United States continues to grow (McGoldrick, Giordano, & Garcia-Preto, 2005). Although many professional disciplines and schools now address issues related to the treatment of multicultural clients, material is often presented in a superficial manner or relegated to a single course. Such educational efforts cannot adequately prepare therapists to address the needs of a diverse client base. Research has consistently shown that ethnic minority clients often drop out of treatment prematurely, sometimes after only one session (Whaley & Davis, 2007). With this in mind, it is extremely important that therapists emphasize the process of joining and establishing therapeutic rapport in treatment first, before presenting more intrusive assessment and intake forms (Boyd-Franklin, 2003; see Chapters 3 and 4).

Many therapists find themselves working with clients whose ethnic, racial, and socioeconomic backgrounds are different from their own. Each client and family has its own heritage, traditions, values, and survival skills that have helped them to weather adversity. It is important for clinicians to learn how to search for and utilize the strengths and resiliency of their clients. One of the goals of this book is to help clinicians join effectively with clients from different cultural backgrounds and learn to make the most of differences (see Chapter 3). We will also discuss the importance of therapists exploring their own racial and/or ethnic identities, and understanding the ways in which clients may perceive them. The question of raising the issue of race or of cultural difference in the process of therapy and the timing of these interventions will also be explored.

Core Mediational Processes

The concepts of core mediational processes are among the most important contributions of this book. In view of the rapid proliferation of evidence-based practices and other theoretical approaches in the mental health field, there has been a call for the identification of the core underlying mechanisms that are common to many different EBPs (Chorpita, Becker, & Daleiden, 2007; Hayes, Strosahl, & Wilson, 2011; Meichenbaum, 2008). These principles have been described elsewhere as "core processes," "core tasks of psychotherapy" (Meichenbaum, 2008), or "core clinical processes" (Hayes et al., 2011).

The concept of core mediational processes has developed and evolved from our own professional experiences. One of our coauthors, a professor at a major university, also directs a community-based program. She has worked throughout her career to help students incorporate a wide range of therapeutic modalities and interventions in their work with diverse clients. Three of our coauthors are members of a department in which a primary objective is to ensure a greater fit between real-world practice conditions and the dissemination of evidence-based practice strategies. As with all agencies experiencing the currents of systemic change, the process of implementing evidence-based practice models developed at the highest levels of research design has taught these authors many lessons.

During the course of trainings on different evidence-based practice approaches, we often noted that the concepts discussed contained many common elements. This led to our speculation as to whether a core set of processes existed across evidence-based models. Simultaneously, the lessons learned from our implementation efforts inspired us to reconceptualize our approach to service delivery. We began to wonder if an agencywide standard of care comprising a core set of competencies and practice elements was possible. This dialogue and exploration was reinforced by presentations and trainings occurring at the time. For example, Anthony Salerno, then codirector of Evidence-Based Practice Initiatives for the New York State Office of Mental Health, expressed his observation (Salerno, Margolies, & Cleek, 2007, 2008b) that every evidence-based model shares three common denominators: (1) some ele-ment of stage of change assessment and motivational interviewing, (2) some element of psychoeducation, and (3) some element of cognitive-behavioral therapy.

Steven Hayes, author and founder of acceptance and commitment therapy (or ACT; Hayes et al., 2011), has spoken multiple times about moving away from prepackaged best-practice models toward key competencies. In a presentation on the future of social work practice, Lynn Videka, dean of the New York University School of Social Work, emphasized the importance of identifying time-tested best-practice "protocols" that are effective across settings and diagnoses (Videka, 2011). A similar call is reflected in the literature. Hoagwood, Burns, and Weisz (2002), in discussing the need for systematic research and translation of best practices to urban settings, indicate that the mental health community must identify effective mediators of improvement, in other words, change processes that influence outcomes. The authors propose that such mediators would lend themselves more effectively and flexibly to finding "goodness of fit" to organizational and clients' needs rather than some current prepackaged models.

While we are mindful that within each diagnostic category there are nuanced principles and strategies, the core mediational process approach emphasizes extracting common processes from multiple evidence-based models that, when grouped together, will influence change across a broad spectrum of diagnostic categories and presenting problems. This led us to develop a clinical approach, as described in Chapters 4 through 9, that could be broadly disseminated in our agency as well as other practice contexts incorporating a distillation of the common key strategies, interventions, and competencies inherent in evidence-based practices.

The concept of extracting the core components in a number of evidence-based treatments is not a new one. For example, Hayes et al. (2011), in the second edition of their book on acceptance and commitment therapy, discuss the following core clinical processes: (1) present-moment awareness, (2) dimensions of self, (3) defusion, (4) acceptance, (5) connecting with values, and (6) committed action. Present-moment awareness is a mindfulness principle that encourages clients to stay grounded in their present feelings and not be burdened by past pain or worries about the future. Awareness of the different dimensions of the self allows clients to stay open to many varying emotions and experiences. The concept of an observer self can help clients to recognize that they can simply observe their experiences without making judgments about them (Hayes et al., 2011). Clients are encouraged to clarify their core values and connect with the things that are most important to them in life. Finally, while recognizing that they may continue to confront painful experiences, clients commit to pursuing actions that will lead to a meaningful life (Hayes et al., 2011). (See Chapter 8 for further discussion of this approach.) This model can also be helpful to clinicians working with clients with serious mental illnesses.

Meichenbaum has also identified the following core tasks of therapy: (1) developing a collaborative therapeutic relationship that involves empathy, cultural sensitivity and collaboration and assesses client stages of change; (2) educating the client about his or her problem and possible therapeutic solutions; (3) reconceptualizing client problems in a more hopeful fashion; (4) developing client coping skills in interpersonal relationships; (5) encouraging the client to perform "personal experiments" that challenge negative beliefs; (6) ensuring that the client takes credit for changes made; and (7) helping clients identify mental health triggers and coping strategies through relapse prevention (Meichenbaum, 2008, pp. 4–7). Many of these concepts have been incorporated into the core mediational processes discussed within this volume.

In this book, we have identified six key components or core mediational processes that have been especially helpful to clinicians working with clients in today's demanding service delivery systems. These mediational processes reflect a marriage of our core values as clinicians with evidence-based practices and other respected theoretical and clinical literature in the mental health field. The six core mediational processes that we have identified are consistent with those described above (Hayes et al., 2011; Meichenbaum, 2008) and include (1) Joining and Establishing the Therapeutic Relationship (Chapter 4); (2) Psychoeducation and Recovery Principles in Mental Health Services (Chapter 5); (3) Motivational Interviewing (Chapter 6); (4) Cognitive-Behavioral Therapy (Chapter 7); (5) Mindfulness- and Acceptance-Based Principles and Practices (Chapter 8); and (6) Relapse Prevention, Trigger Management, and the Completion of Treatment (Chapter 9). Each of these core mediational processes will be discussed below.

Establishing the Therapeutic Relationship

One of the most consistent research findings in the mental health field has been that the therapeutic relationship is one of the major contributors to treatment outcome, regardless of theoretical orientation, technique, or treatment modality (Horvath & Bedi, 2002; Horvath & Symonds, 1991; Norcross, 2002, 2011a). Thus, this is a central concept stressed throughout this book and we have identified joining and establishing the therapeutic relationship as our first core mediational process.

With the emphasis on evidence-based practice in the field, we have noted a disturbing trend of students and new clinicians becoming so focused on learning and using techniques, that they discount or even ignore the importance of the therapeutic relationship. This tendency, of course, is counter to the underlying message from all schools of therapy that have emphasized the importance of the therapeutic relationship, including cognitive-behavioral therapy (CBT) (J. S. Beck, 2011; Meichenbaum, 2008); mindfulness-based approaches (Hick & Bien, 2010); acceptance and commitment therapy (ACT) (Eifert & Forsyth, 2005; Hayes, Strosahl, & Wilson, 1999, 2011); dialectical behavior therapy (DBT) (Linehan, 1993); motivational interviewing (MI) (W. R. Miller & Rollnick, 2013); psychodynamic therapy (McWilliams, 1999, 2004, 2011; Messer, 2004, 2006); family therapy (Liddle, 2005; Liddle & Rowe, 2010; Liddle, Santisteban, & Levant, 2002; S. Minuchin, 1974; Nichols, 2011; Scapoznik, Hervis, & Schwartz, 2003); and group therapy (Yalom & Leszcz, 2005).

Psychoeducation and Recovery Principles in Mental Health Services

The second core mediational process combines the need for psychoeducation and the incorporation of recovery principles in the delivery of mental health services. Psychoeducation is the process in which the client is provided necessary information about his or her diagnosis, symptoms, and treatment options in order to empower the decisions that he or she makes about treatment. This process can be used to engender a sense of normalization, universality, and destigmatization regarding one's illness (Colom, Vieta, & Scott, 2006; Lefley, 2009; McFarlane, 2002). Additionally, it can help to make the treatment process more transparent, as psychoeducation should include a discussion about the nature of the treatment course and process itself. Psychoeducation can also drive a wedge in a person's overidentification with symptoms, as people tend to misinterpret symptoms as innate truths about themselves. Of course, any psychoeducation effort should be coupled with hope and optimism regarding clients' ability to be self-directed and to achieve a life consistent with their values. In this way, the term recovery, the second part of this mediational process, can help a client to establish a life that is fulfilling both in and apart from his or her mental illness and struggles.

The term *recovery,* originating in the addictions literature (W. White, Boyle, & Loveland, 2005), now has been expanded to include clients who are dealing with mental health issues including serious mental illness

(Ralph & Corrigan, 2005). W. White et al. (2005) have described recovery as a "process of retrieval (regaining what was lost because of one's illness and its treatment) and a process of discovery (moving beyond the illness and its limitations)" (p. 235). Within the mental health field, the idea of recovery has expanded even further, as noted in the Surgeon General's report, with the message "that hope and restoration of a meaningful life are possible, despite serious mental illness" (U.S. Department of Health and Human Services, 1999). Recovery is an integral concept to support individuals to live their lives in the way that is most meaningful to them. Chapter 5 explores the link between psychoeducation and recovery principles in our treatment approach.

Motivational Interviewing

One of the most challenging experiences for new therapists is the realization that clients who are not self-referred may not have made a commitment to change their behaviors prior to treatment. This is particularly problematic because many of the treatment models that therapists have been taught assume a willing client. One of the most powerful models for addressing this issue has been motivational interviewing (W. R. Miller & Rollnick, 1991, 2002, 2013). Motivational interviewing is a collaborative process in which therapists and clients work together to strengthen a "person's own motivation and commitment to change" (W. R. Miller & Rollnick, 2013, p. 12). Given the importance of this approach, we have identified motivational interviewing as the third core mediational process. Chapter 6 discusses the evolution and the changes in this approach over time (W. R. Miller & Rollnick, 1991, 2002, 2013). It also explores the spirit of MI (W. R. Miller & Rollnick, 2013)—its essential orientation to clients—that is composed of four key elements: partnership, acceptance, compassion, and evocation (W. R. Miller & Rollnick, 2013).

Cognitive–Behavioral Therapy

Cognitive-behavioral therapy (CBT) is an evidence-based treatment model that has been adapted and incorporated into evidence-based practices (EBPs) for many different psychological conditions (Barlow, 2008). Given this reality, it is important that clinicians involved in providing therapy in the real world have a solid grasp of this treatment model and be able to incorporate it when appropriate to the needs and presenting problems of their clients. It provides clinicians with a case formulation approach (Persons, 2008) that clarifies the relationship between thoughts (cognitions), emotions, and behaviors (J. S. Beck, 2011). With this in mind, we have identified CBT as the fourth core mediational process. Chapter 7 discusses this model and describes intervention strategies.

Mindfulness- and Acceptance-Based Principles and Practices

Mindfulness- (Bien, 2010; Hick & Bien, 2010; Kabat-Zinn, 1990; M. G. Williams, Teasdale, Segal, & Kabat-Zinn, 2007) and acceptance-based principles (Hayes, Follette, & Linehan, 2004) have been incorporated into a number of evidence-based practices that provide not only excellent treatment interventions but also a philosophical shift in the way in which the treatment of mental illness is viewed by many clients and therapists. These interventions have included acceptance and commitment therapy (ACT) (Hayes, Strosahl, & Wilson, 1999, 2011), dialectical behavior therapy (DBT) (Linehan, 1993), mindfulness-based cognitive therapy (MBCT; Segal, Williams, & Teasdale, 2001), mindfulness-based stress reduction (MBSR; Goldstein, Stahl, Santorelli, & Kabat-Zinn, 2010), and mindfulness-based relapse prevention (MBRP; Bowen, Chawla, & Marlatt, 2011; Marlatt, Bowen, Chawla, & Witkiewitz, 2008).

Mindfulness- and acceptance-based principles and practices are the fifth core mediational process because they represent an approach to empower clients struggling with a wide range of mental health issues. (See Chapter 8 for a discussion of these principles.) Mindfulness, grounded in Eastern philosophy, encourages clients to live in the present. It builds on the observation that human beings often experience difficulty staying grounded in their feelings or experiences, particularly when these are upsetting (Bien, 2010; Hick & Bien, 2010). It addresses the ways in which clinicians can utilize mindfulness in order to stay present in their treatment with each client despite time pressures and productivity demands (Bien, 2010; Hick & Bien, 2010), and incorporates mindful listening (Shafir, 2010) as a key part of the therapeutic relationship and treatment process.

Mindfulness- and acceptance-based principles encourage individuals to accept the fact that they may continue to have some painful emotions in the course of their lives (Hayes et al., 2011). Hayes et al. (2004) have noted that emotional pain in the form of anxiety, depression, grief and loss, etc. is a normal human experience and that it is not the experience of pain that is problematic but our reactions to it and attempts to control it. Rather than engage in self-blame and a judgmental stance, it emphasizes that individuals should not allow upsetting feelings to stop them from pursuing meaningful activities and a productive life.

Relapse Prevention

Relapse prevention is the sixth core mediational process identified in this book. It is extremely important because the process of recovery does not occur in a straight line (Ralph & Corrigan, 2005; W. White et al., 2005) but rather takes many turns and detours along the way (J. S. Beck, 2011). It is up to the clinician to embrace this perspective and cultivate a sense of universality and learning regarding the natural ebb and flow of the change process. Lapses often provide an opportunity to uncover, learn about, and grow from the existing areas of vulnerability in one's recovery path. When clients are able to recognize what they are experiencing and to utilize strategies to recover, a lapse does not have to lead to a full relapse. In fact, we would argue that, most often, recovery is more fully integrated after one undergoes and weathers the inevitable lapses associated with this process, and emerges with resiliency.

Although the terms *relapse prevention* and *trigger management* originated in the addictions field (Marlatt & Gordon, 1985), these concepts are now widely used in the mental health field, particularly in cognitive-behavioral therapy approaches (J. S. Beck, 2011; Ludgate, 2009; Meichenbaum, 2008). In her discussion of relapse prevention, J. S. Beck describes the way in which she helps clients with the essential process of recognizing the plateaus and valleys that they may encounter. When clinicians maintain a consistent stance, helping clients to continuously identify, learn, and internalize ongoing trigger management strategies, it creates a context that fosters lifelong acceptance and change. Chapter 9 discusses this core mediational process in more detail.

Systems Interventions in the Real World

Family Therapy

Many clinicians enter the field with training only in individual treatment approaches. This is unfortunate because it restricts their ability to provide effective care to clients across treatment modalities. Family systems theory provides a key conceptual framework and many important concepts essential for therapists even when treating individual clients. This is particularly true in work with ethnic minority clients and others from more collectivistic cultures, where frequent contact with family and extended family members is expected and continues over a client's lifetime. In such cases, it is critical for therapists to be able to understand the dynamics of the family system as well as the familial and cultural values that affect our clients.

The exposure to family therapy is essential whether clinicians work primarily with children, adolescents, or adults. The ability to provide family therapy is especially valuable when working with children and adolescents. Too often, we have seen cases where three or four children in one family are each assigned to individual treatment with separate therapists, when family therapy is clearly indicated and would provide a more coherent and coordinated treatment approach. In addition, many clinicians may overlook the value of family therapy and psychoeducational approaches with the families of adults, particularly those who are experiencing serious mental illness. Chapter 10 discusses these perspectives.

The Multisystems Model and Interdisciplinary Coordination of Care

Among the greatest challenges clinicians face in the real world of service delivery is the fragmentation of care and the duplication of services (Boyd-Franklin & Bry, 2000a). As a consequence, we have incorporated the multisystems model (Boyd-Franklin, 2003; Boyd-Franklin & Bry, 2000a) and the need for an approach that emphasizes interdisciplinary coordination of care as central concepts in all of our work. Clinicians working with exceptionally stressed inner-city, poor clients and families may find these clients at the mercy of multiple systems (e.g., schools, courts, police, child welfare) that exert a tremendous amount of power in their lives. These clients and families face the daunting task of coordination between agencies that share sparse communication, if any, and may prescribe divergent and possibly mutually exclusive directives. With these multiple players and systems in mind, this book addresses the need for multisystemic interventions and the coordination and streamlining of care (see Chapter 11). Examples are given of ways that clinicians can help such families. In addition, the value of interdisciplinary case conferences that provide the opportunity for service providers from a range of agencies to meet together with the client or family to discuss current issues and formulate an effective treatment plan are discussed.

Group Treatment

The productivity pressures and large caseloads inherent in today's demanding service delivery environments have led to a renewed recognition of the value of group treatment approaches. In treatment settings where there are too few clinicians to serve client needs, groups provide the opportunity to offer excellent treatment to more clients. Many new clinicians have relatively little training in group therapy, as it is often treated as an elective in clinical training programs.

It is important to be sure groups are conceptualized with the real world in mind. For example, we have found that the traditional position that therapy groups forbid contact among group members outside of sessions is often unrealistic. We visualize groups as therapeutic support groups, assume outside contact, and encourage group members to bring these experiences into group discussions. This approach is particularly helpful for isolated clients who may not have family members and friends to support them in their process of change.

Another acknowledgment that clinicians need to make regarding the reality of clinical practice today is that modalities of treatment can and often should be combined in the real world (e.g., individual + concurrent family or group treatment). In Chapter 12, we offer examples of the ways in which these combined treatment modalities can address specific clinical issues. Similarly, therapists working with clients in groups may choose to meet with clients individually in order to address specific treatment issues or in pairs in order to resolve conflicts that may arise in the group process. In this book we reiterate the need to be flexible, in combining modalities in order to address client or family issues.

Risk Assessment, Suicide Prevention, and Crisis Intervention

There are few topics in the mental health field that create more anxiety in clinicians than the process of evaluating risk, particularly with suicidal and homicidal clients (Jobes, 2006; Shea, 2002; Underwood, Fell, & Spinazzola, 2010). This is an extraordinarily challenging aspect of doing therapy in the real world, and graduate programs frequently do not prepare clinicians with the skills to accomplish such a task. With this in mind, Chapter 13 presents an overview of risk assessment and management and discusses implementation in the case of suicide prevention. In this chapter, we also discuss organizational interventions that have been developed to support clinicians in making difficult assessments.

Crises are a normal part of ongoing clinical work, and clinicians in the real world may encounter one of these situations in the course of their careers, but many have received no training in appropriate responses to such events. Chapter 14 explores crisis intervention and postcrisis responses to an act of violence in a mental health clinic, a suicide of a young adolescent in a school, and a homicide in a community.

This chapter presents frameworks that clinicians can adapt to crises in their own work.

Clinician Self-Care

Clinical work can be especially challenging and demanding with clients who have experienced multiple traumas in their lives. Often clinicians and counselors in agencies, clinics, hospitals, and schools have had no training in trauma therapy or counseling. In addition, they may not be prepared for the possibility that they may develop compassion fatigue (as well as vicarious or secondary traumatization; Dass-Brailsford, 2007) as a result of their compassion and empathy for traumatized clients. We draw on the extensive trauma literature on these issues in Chapter 15 to offer guidelines for clinicians in recognizing the effects of vicarious traumatization and to provide the steps they can take to address and prevent it.

We have also drawn upon the literature on vicarious resilience and posttraumatic growth that asserts the positive benefits for clinicians working with traumatized clients. Clinician burnout will also be addressed. Ironically, unlike the other conditions that we have discussed, burnout often results from systemic and organizational issues within our clinics and agencies, which can profoundly affect clinicians over time (Dass-Brailsford, 2007). With these considerations in mind, we have emphasized the importance of self-care for all therapists and counselors throughout their careers. We offer specific suggestions that have been helpful to both new and seasoned clinicians who may experience such challenges in their clinical work.

Supervision, Training, and Organizational Support as Antidotes to Burnout

Over the course of our careers, we have been involved in developing and providing supervision, training, and organizational support to therapists and counselors in clinics and agencies throughout the mental health field. We view these interventions as antidotes to clinician burnout (see Chapter 16). As we mentioned in the first part of this chapter, the process of lifelong learning is a major survival mechanism for therapists and counselors. In our experience, learning innovative ideas and new ways to approach difficult cases, and implementing them in our practices so that more effective treatment can be provided to our clients, can help to invigorate clinicians and enhance their commitment to this work. It is also a useful professional self-care strategy.

Conclusion

In summary, we hope that this book will energize clinicians and encourage them to learn new clinical interventions and to seek diverse forms of training throughout their careers. We also hope supervisors, administrators, and clinic and agency directors will adopt many of the examples of organizational support we have included. Ongoing training and supervision for clinicians is one of the most important investments an agency can make in its staff and is a potent antidote to burnout. Ultimately, through this book, we hope to empower clinicians and provide them with the appropriate tools, anchored in best practices, to more effectively meet the needs of their clients.

CHAPTER 2

Evidence–Based Practice

Introduction

There is an ongoing debate in the mental health field regarding the role of research evidence and its relationship to practice (APA Presidential Task Force on Evidence-Based Practice, 2006; Goodheart et al., 2006; Kazdin, 2008; Norcross et al., 2006). This debate is clearly influenced by contextual and political factors, including managed care insurance companies, public policy, and the movement toward public debate on these issues (Hayes, Barlow, et al., 1999; Huppert et al., 2006; Reed, 2006; Reed & Eisman, 2006). For many clinicians, particularly those who received their degrees over 10 years ago, this may present a confusing puzzle in which they may feel pressured to abandon their own theoretical orientation and treatment interventions that they have practiced throughout their careers (Wofsy, 2006). Even relatively new clinicians, who may have received training in evidence-based practice in graduate school, struggle with the pressures to stay current and informed, on the one hand; while being pressured by productivity requirements and the lack of time on the other hand. In addition, with the adoption of evidence-based practice guidelines in all of the major mental health disciplines and the similar embrace of these guidelines by insurance companies and federal and state policy (Carpinello et al., 2002; Chambless et al., 1996; Chorpita et al., 2002; Lampropoulos & Spengler, 2002; President's New Freedom Commission on Mental Health, 2003), there is a continued expectation that payment for services will be linked to the best evidence-based practice.

With the concerns discussed above, this chapter offers clinicians an opportunity to sort out these issues. It is divided into the following sections: the role of health and mental health care costs and managed care, the history of the evidence-based practice debate, clarification on the definitions of empirically supported or evidence-based treatment, evidence-based practice, and evidence-informed practice (Goodheart et al., 2006; Kazdin, 2008; Norcross et al., 2006). We also explore the challenges of implementing evidence-based practices in the real world.

Health and Mental Health Care Costs, Managed Care, and Evidence-Based Practice

Spiraling health costs and a worldwide concern about the quality of health care systems have influenced the current emphasis on evidence-based practices (EBPs) (Barlow, 1996; Huppert et al., 2006; Institute of Medicine, 2001). These issues have broadened to include mental health care as well. Managed care and the process of third-party payments have transformed the health and mental health care systems in the United States (Hayes, Barlow, et al., 1999; Huppert et al., 2006). As a part of a debate in the mental health field on EBPs (Norcross et al., 2006), Reed (2006) has identified the following as contributing to the discussion of EBPs in the public forum and to the development of EBP as a "public idea":

> In the health care arena, policy makers are indeed faced with a complex problem. Approximately 15% of the U.S. population is uninsured (Cohen & Ni, 2004; U.S. Census Bureau News, 2004). An even higher percentage (24%) has no mental health benefits, and only about half of those have coverage that could be considered reasonable (Maxfield, Achman, & Cook, 2004). We spend more per capita on health care than any other industrialized nation, yet we do not provide demonstrably better care (World Health Organization, 2001). Care is fragmented, with little coordination horizontally across systems or vertically among levels of care (Institute of Medicine, 2001). Health care costs also continue to rise. (p. 15)

In response to these glaring realities, Reed (2006) argues that "Americans have been offered the public idea that the essential problem with the U.S. health care system is uninformed practice, which would be resolved if health care professionals practiced in ways that are consistent with research findings. This is the basic premise of EBP [evidence-based practice]" (p. 15). This has led to a call for evidence-based practices in federal, state, and local funding agencies (Carpinello et al., 2002;

Chambless et al., 1996; Chorpita et al., 2002; Lampropoulos & Spengler, 2002; President's New Freedom Commission on Mental Health, 2003).

In the mental health field, this resulted in a major joint initiative (Reed, 2006) of the National Institute of Mental Health (NIMH) and the Department of Health and Human Services (DHHS) Substance Abuse and Mental Health Services Administration (SAMHSA),

> focusing on promoting and supporting the implementation of evidence-based mental health treatment practices into state mental health systems (e.g., National Institutes of Health, 2004). This initiative focuses on identifying the most effective and feasible methods for implementing EBP in state clinical practice settings and it also provides support to states and localities that are ready and committed to adopting EBP. (p. 16)

As a consequence, scarce mental health funding was targeted to agencies, clinics, and hospitals that were able to demonstrate that they were implementing evidence-based practices and there has been increased pressure on practitioners within these systems to provide evidence-based practice interventions.

The emergence of managed care has had a major impact on the delivery of health and mental health services for almost 40 years. After the passage of the Health Maintenance Organization (HMO) Act by the U.S. Congress in 1973 (Public Law 93-222), managed care continued to expand in the 1970s and 1980s and is still a major force today (DeLeon, VandenBos, & Bulatao, 1991; Reed, 2006; Reed & Eisman, 2006).

Increasingly, managed care, with its goal of reducing the cost and improving the quality of health and mental health care, has embraced evidence-based practice as its guideline in determining which treatments to fund and how many sessions or days to reimburse for outpatient and inpatient treatment, respectively (Huppert et al., 2006). Huppert et al. have emphasized that with increased competition among managed care companies to provide time-limited care at the lowest prices, mental health systems, agencies, and therapists will experience increased pressure to provide evidence-based interventions. Huppert et al. (2006, p. 133) indicated that this process received governmental support when the President's New Freedom Commission on Mental Health (2003, p. 25) recommended that the nation "advance evidence-based practices using dissemination and demonstration projects and create a public–private partnership to guide their implementation; [and] improve and expand the workforce providing evidence-based mental health services and supports."

Evidence–Based Practice:
The Debate in the Mental Health Field

The debate on evidence-based practice has been so pervasive that Messer (2004) has described this as a "culture war" within the field. A part of the argument and the confusion is related to the different terms used within the debate. One area relates to the differences between evidence-based treatment and evidence-based practice. Kazdin (2008) defined evidence-based treatment thus: "Empirically supported or *evidence-based treatment* (EBT) refers to the interventions or techniques (e.g., cognitive therapy for depression, exposure therapy for anxiety) that have produced therapeutic change in controlled trials" (p. 147).

These are defined by the "gold standard" in the field of psychological research, randomized clinical trials (RCTs). Chambless and Hollon (1998) indicated that "efficacy is best demonstrated in randomized clinical trials (RCTs) in which patients are randomly assigned to the treatment of interest or one or more comparison conditions" (p. 7).

Evidence-based practice is not synonymous with empirically supported or evidence-based treatment, and is defined much more broadly (APA Presidential Task Force on Evidence-Based Practice, 2006; Goodheart et al., 2006; Kazdin, 2008; Norcross et al., 2006). In 2001, the Institute of Medicine defined evidence-based practice in medicine as the integration of the best research evidence with clinical experience and patient values. In 2006, the APA Presidential Task Force on Evidence-Based Practice published the following wording regarding evidence-based practice, which expanded upon the Institute of Medicine (2001) definition: "Evidence-based practice in psychology is the integration of the best available research with clinical expertise in the context of patient characteristics, culture and preferences" (p. 273).

Kazdin (2008) offers an even broader interpretation:

> *Evidence-based practice (EBP)* is a broader term and refers to clinical practice that is informed by evidence about interventions, clinical expertise, and patient needs, values, and preferences and their integration in decision making about individual care (e.g., APA Presidential Task Force on Evidence-Based Practice, 2006; Institute of Medicine, 2001; Sackett, Rosenberg, Gray, Haynes, & Richardson, 1996). (p. 147)

Spring (2007) offers the following definition: "Evidence-based practice (EBP) is a process that involves 'the conscientious, explicit use of current best evidence in making decisions about the care of individual patients' (Sackett, Rosenberg, Gray, Haynes, & Richardson, 1996)"

(p. 611). In her view, clinical decision making is the process of integrating the best research evidence with clinical expertise, and patient values (including culture), characteristics, preferences, and circumstances (Spring, 2007).

Broadening the Concept of Evidence-Based Practice

In their book on the topic, Goodheart et al. (2006) offer an even broader definition: "EBP is a larger concept than any one treatment. EBP integrates all scientific evidence and clinical information that is used to guide and improve psychotherapy processes, interventions, therapeutic relationships, and outcomes" (p. 3).

The phrase *and clinical information* opens the door for the inclusion of the accumulated theoretical and clinical knowledge published in the field. Goodheart (2006), who was appointed by the president of APA to chair the APA Presidential Task Force on Evidence-Based Practice, argues that central to the arguments in the field about evidence-based practice are differences in "how evidence is defined and how the endeavor of psychotherapy is viewed" (p. 39). She proposes the following streams of evidence that facilitate "scientifically informed practice and are needed for clinical decision making": empirical research, a diverse theoretical and clinical literature, effectiveness data that are based on "real world outcomes in diverse communities" (p. 45), clinical interviews and observations, and the response of the patient to the treatment.

In her discussion of psychotherapy, Goodheart (2006) states:

> Psychotherapy is *first and foremost a human endeavor*. It is messy. It is not solely a scientific endeavor, nor can it be reduced meaningfully to a technical mechanistic enterprise (Goodheart, 2004). The evidence-based movement can disempower practitioners relative to researchers to the extent that clinical skill is equated solely with applied science and to the extent that science is restricted to randomized clinical trials of treatment practices (Tannenbaum, 1999). (p. 41)

Throughout this book, we have adopted a broader definition of evidence. With Goodheart (2006), we value the role of research evidence in informing clinical work. In keeping with the long tradition of psychotherapy, however, we also value the fact that therapists who practice in the real world often draw on a wide range of accumulated theoretical and clinical knowledge, including books and articles from diverse theoretical orientations to inform their work:

> *Psychotherapy draws on many theories.* These theories include behavioral, cognitive-behavioral, psychodynamic, family systems,

humanistic, feminist, integrative, and cultural competence orientations, among others.

In diverse practices and clinical settings, underlying theories may
differ somewhat, but most experienced clinicians are integrationists
(Lambert, Bergin, & Garfield, 2004). . . . Good clinicians borrow
from each other and borrow what works. Some psychotherapy-related
theories contain constructs that are easy to isolate and measure; others do not. There are very few differences among bona fide therapies
that have been widely practiced over time and that have a coherent
theoretical structure and research underpinning (Wampold, 2001).
Good clinicians also become aware of new and emerging approaches,
such as cultural competence guidelines that evolve as society and
practice changes. (Goodheart, 2006, p. 42)

Access to Evidence–Based Practice Research Databases

One of the great assets of the Internet age is the ability to access resources
and information at the touch of a button. While this access can lead to
increased knowledge—facilitating better care and enhanced implementation supports for new, cutting-edge treatments—it is a resource that
must be used with discernment. Indeed, a Google search on the topic of
evidence-based practice generated 18,200,000 hits. Several resources,
however, are easily accessible and support best-practice work across a
number of diagnoses. Box 2.1 lists some of the resources that we have
found helpful in our work with youth, families, and adults.

Clinical Expertise

All of the major definitions of evidence-based practice emphasize and
value the role of clinical expertise. This is an important concept because
the experience and knowledge of a therapist is one of the most important
factors in clinical decision making (Goodheart, 2006; Spring, 2007).
Goodheart emphasizes the role of clinical expertise in psychotherapy:
"Psychotherapy requires clinical expertise because it is a complex interpersonal process that takes place in a context of uncertainty and ambiguity and under the press of clients' urgent needs" (p. 49).

Given the pressures of real-world clinical practice, therapists call
on their experience to make the difficult decisions that are necessary
to maintain the therapeutic relationship, honor the client's perspective,
and move the treatment toward a good outcome (Goodheart, 2006). So
where does this leave the new inexperienced clinician? In many cases,
clinical expertise is obtained through a combination of reading the
broad theoretical and clinical literature, training in specific psychological treatments, research evidence, good supervision (see Chapter

BOX 2.1. Evidence-Based Treatment Resources

General Resources

- **Association for Behavioral and Cognitive Therapies** *(www.ABCT.org)*.
- **American Psychiatric Association** ("Practice Guidelines" page at *www.psych.org*).
- **National Association of Social Workers** ("Practice and Professional Development" page at *www.socialworkers.org*).
- **National Guideline Clearinghouse** *(http://guidelines.gov)*.
- **SAMHSA National Registry of Evidence-Based Programs and Practices** *(www.nrepp.samhsa.gov)*. Contains EBP manuals, research, and contact information for the model developers and trainers.

Working with Youth

- **Society of Clinical Child and Adolescent Psychology** ("Evidence-Based Treatment for Children and Adolescents" page at *http://effectivechildtherapy.com/sccap*).
- **American Academy of Child and Adolescent Psychiatry** ("Practice Parameters" page at *www.aacap.org*).

Working with Serious Mental Illness

- **American Psychological Association** ("Training Grid: Best Practices for Recovery and Improved Outcomes for People with Serious Mental Illness/Serious Emotional Disturbance" page at *www.apa.org/practice/resources/grid/index.aspx*).

Journals and Publication Search Engines

- ***Psychiatric Services: A Journal of the American Psychiatric Association*** *(http://psychservices.psychiatryonline.org)*. All articles are publicly available for 1 year postpublication date.
- **PubMed: U.S. National Library of Medicine and the National Institutes of Health** *(http://pubmed.gov)*. Contains article abstracts and PDFs.

16), and the response of the clients that they encounter in real-world settings.

Thus, Goodheart (2006) and other practitioners in the field who respect research evidence have also begun to question the hierarchy of many definitions of evidence-based practice that privilege research evidence as the main form of evidence:

The purpose of practice and science necessarily differ. Practitioners learn over time to use evidence without subscribing to specific hierarchies of which type of evidence is most important because usefulness varies widely depending on context. The discussion of evidence focuses on practitioners' need to seek information from a broad range of research; from the literature of reasoned theories and consensus and diverse forms of knowledge; from the fruits of clinical observation and inquiry; and from clients' contributions, responses, and progress. (p. 56)

In our definition of *clinical expertise* we include not only the expertise of the individual clinician but also the broader theoretical and clinical literature available in the field in addition to research regarding evidence-based treatments, as well as the ability to access the clinical expertise of senior clinicians through the processes of supervision and consultation. These components taken together add to the clinical expertise of the individual clinician and impact the process of clinical decision making. With this in mind, as indicated above, we have incorporated throughout this book research evidence as well as the important theoretical and clinical knowledge in areas such as multicultural competence, family therapy, group therapy, risk assessment, and crisis intervention that therapists can access in their goal of addressing the needs of their clients.

Patient Values, Needs, Cultures, and Circumstances

As stated above, the APA Presidential Task Force on Evidence-Based Practice (2006) report included the "context of patient characteristics, culture, and preferences" (p. 273). In the process of their deliberations, the task force clarified the differences between empirically supported treatments (ESTs) and evidence-based practice (EBP). One key area they identified was in the prioritization of the needs of the patient in the process:

ESTs [empirically supported treatments] start with a treatment and ask whether it works for a certain disorder or problem under specified circumstances. EBPP [evidence-based practice in psychology] starts with the patient and asks what research evidence (including relevant results from RCTs) will assist the psychologist in achieving the best outcome. (APA Presidential Task Force on Evidence-Based Practice, 2006, p. 273)

They also embraced a definition that elaborated the patient's needs more fully:

Normative data on "what works for whom" (Nathan & Gorman, 2002; Roth & Fonagy, 2004) provide essential guides to effective practice. Nevertheless, psychological services are most likely to be effective when they are responsive to the patient's specific problems, strengths, personality, sociocultural context, and preferences (Norcross, 2002). . . .

EBPP involves consideration of the patient's values, religious beliefs, worldviews, goals, and preferences for treatment with the psychologist's experience and understanding of available research. (APA Presidential Task Force on Evidence-Based Practice, 2006, p. 278)

There have also been extensive debates over the role of patient characteristics in evidence-based practice. Personality characteristics as well as comorbidity and dual or multiple diagnoses in each client have led some critics of evidence-supported treatments to argue that some RCTs have focused on a narrow definition of a particular diagnosis (Goodheart et al., 2006; Kazdin, 2008; Norcross et al., 2006). Some critics have raised the concern that clients in the real world are often more complex in their clinical presentations and diagnoses than clients who have been rigorously screened for most RCTs (Norcross et al., 2006). The APA Presidential Task Force on Evidence-Based Practice (2006) also acknowledged this reality. They stated that

most patients present with multiple symptoms or syndromes rather than a single discreet disorder (e.g., Kessler, Stang, Witchen, Stein, & Walters, 1999; Newman, Moffitt, Caspi, & Silva, 1998). The presence of concurrent conditions may moderate treatment response, and interventions intended to treat one symptom often affect others. (p. 279)

Diverse Populations: Challenges for Evidence-Based Practice in the Real World

One important challenge faced by those attempting to implement EBP in the real world is that relatively few evidence-based practices have been adequately evaluated across cultural, racial, ethnic, and socioeconomic groups (Spring, 2007). For many clinicians in the real world of practice, diversity is the norm in their practices particularly in public agencies, clinics, and hospitals in urban areas. The APA Presidential Task Force on Evidence-Based Practice (2006) acknowledged the need for the inclusion of gender, gender identity, culture, ethnicity, race, age, family context, religious beliefs, and sexual orientation. In addition, Olkin and Taliaferro (2006) have argued that evidence-based practices have ignored people with disabilities.

As a part of their book *Evidence-Based Practices in Mental Health*, Norcross et al. (2006) asked a number of experts to address the question of how well evidence-based practices address the different dimensions of diversity. In addition to the response of Olkin and Taliaferro (2006) regarding the lack of inclusion of persons with disabilities in evidence-based research, Sue and Zane (2006) argued that ethnic-minority populations have been neglected by evidence-based practices. Similar conclusions were drawn with respect to gender (Levant & Silverstein, 2006) and lesbian, gay, bisexual, and transgendered clients (Brown, 2006).

Several authors have explored the interface between the needs of ethnic minority populations and evidence-based practices in mental health services (Bernal & Scharron-del-Rio, 2001; Miranda et al., 2005; Sue & Zane, 2006; Whaley & Davis, 2007). All of these publications have drawn attention to the underrepresentation of ethnic and racial minority groups in research on evidence-based treatments (Whaley & Davis, 2007). Atkinson, Bui, and Mori (2001) have argued that empirically supported treatment and multicultural counseling have "fairly distinct and somewhat antithetical goals" (p. 570). However, Whaley and Davis (2007) have asserted that these two perspectives are more complementary than many researchers and clinicians have realized but that this convergence has not been recognized because of the "lack of research devoted to the development of culturally competent evidence-based practices" (p. 563).

As we demonstrate in Chapter 3, this oversight is particularly problematic because of the increasing numbers of ethnic minority clients represented in the sociodemographic shifts in the population of the United States (Whaley & Davis, 2007). There is agreement in many sources that the mental health system must begin to address these changes and meet the needs of multiculturally and socioeconomically diverse populations (American Psychological Association, 1993, 2003; APA Presidential Task Force on Evidence-Based Practice, 2006; Bernal & Scharron-del-Rio, 2001; Comas-Diaz, 2006; Miranda et al., 2005; Sue, 1998; Sue & Torino, 2005; Sue & Zane, 2006; Whaley & Davis, 2007).

These concerns have led to questions regarding the relative efficacy of traditional empirically supported treatments and culturally adapted therapy. Miranda et al. (2005) and Whaley and Davis (2007) have carefully reviewed the research on interventions with ethnic minority populations. Whaley and Davis in their review concluded:

> [Miranda et al. (2005)] found that both traditional empirically supported treatments and adapted interventions are effective with ethnic/

racial minority populations. However, they pointed out that standard and culturally adapted psychosocial interventions have not been compared in an RCT (Miranda et al., 2005). (p. 571)

Although there has been some progress, Sue and Zane (2006) have indicated that the majority of research has been done with White populations, which has limited its applicability to many ethnic minority populations and other marginalized groups (Berger, 2010). For example, Berger (2010) described the process of performing literature searches to identify the best evidence-based practices in working with marginalized populations. Repeatedly she encountered the lack of research with these groups. She has identified three factors that contribute to this scarcity of knowledge:

> Three factors contribute to the scarcity of knowledge about marginalized populations: sample selective bias, difficulty in accessing "hidden populations (e.g., homeless people, undocumented immigrants), and, the absence of culture-sensitive measurement instruments. First it is not uncommon for studies to maintain the "purity" of the sample by excluding people with multiple and severe problems or co-morbidities. This is especially true in controlled trials, which have been placed at the top of the hierarchy of evidence and tend to have homogeneous participant selection criteria (Sue & Zane, 2006).
> Second, even when researchers target a diverse sample, marginalized, disenfranchised, minority, poor and severely troubled populations are more difficult to access and recruit for participation in research because of fear (e.g., in the case of undocumented immigrants), lack of trust in establishments, shame as well as motivation to participate (Emani & Monir, 2007; Faugier & Sargeant, 1997; Miles, 2008). Finally, even when researchers succeed in identifying and accessing such population groups, studying them is more challenging because of language barriers, literacy issues, and the absence of culturally appropriate, sensitive, valid and reliable measures which are appropriate for use in different populations and of norms for diverse population groups (Aisenberg, 2008; Sue & Zane, 2006; T. Weiss & Berger, 2006). (p. 183)

Thus, as the debate over these issues continues, the development and testing of culturally adapted treatments as well as the comparison of these approaches to traditional empirically supported treatments is still in its early stages. Since many traditional evidence-based or empirically supported treatments have never been tested with ethnic minority and other diverse groups, clinicians in the real world of practice are often in a dilemma that requires them to rely more heavily on their own clinical expertise as well as the literature on the treatment of multicultural and other diverse populations, and feedback from their clients on their responses to these treatment approaches.

Evidence-Informed Practice

Another perspective in the field has argued that the realities of mental health and health delivery systems are such that many practitioners may in fact be practicing _evidence-informed practice_. _Evidence-informed practice_ goes beyond the definition of evidence-based practice and is considered by some to be a "more pluralistic," "less doctrinaire," and a more "practitioner friendly" approach (Epstein, 2011, p. 2). Rycroft-Malone (2008) argues that the field recognizes the:

> appropriateness of randomized controlled trial [RCT] for evidence of effectiveness, but that other forms of evidence also inform clinical decision making and the delivery of health care. This more inclusive view of evidence has prompted the term evidence-"informed" instead of evidence-"based" practice (Davies et al., 2000). (p. 405)

At one end of those who advocate for "evidence informed practice" are those who support the inclusion of other forms of research such as qualitative studies, single-case study designs, and pragmatic case studies, in addition to randomized clinical trials (RCTs) (Fishman, 2009; Messer, 2004, 2006). At the other end are Nevo and Slonim-Nevo (2011) who provide a different conceptualization of evidence-informed practice:

> Evidence-informed practice (EIP) should be understood as excluding non-scientific prejudices and superstitions, but also as leaving ample room for clinical experience as well as the constructive and imaginative judgments of practitioners and clients who are in constant interaction and dialogue with one another . . . In particular we argue that research findings should not override, or take precedence over, clinical experience and clients' wishes, values and knowledge. Rather empirical evidence is better regarded as one component in the mutual and constantly changing journey of client and practitioner. (p. 3)

Many of the proponents of evidence-informed practice (Epstein, 2011; Nevo & Slonim-Nevo, 2011; Rycroft-Malone, 2008) have actually taken positions similar to that of Goodheart (2006) discussed above. In our view, mental health practitioners certainly should examine the research evidence and search for best-practice interventions that have been rigorously tested in the field. However, there is a gap in research evidence that often exists, particularly for poor ethnic minority clients living in urban areas, who make up the caseloads of many front-line clinicians, and often are not represented in evidence-based treatment studies, particularly RCTs. In these cases, we recommend a broader view of evidence-based practice described by Goodheart or the evidence-informed practice model (Epstein, 2011; Nevo & Slonim-Nevo, 2011; Rycroft-Malone, 2008) described above.

Our discussion in the second part of this book of core mediational processes illustrates this point. Many of these processes are based on research evidence and evidence-based interventions. At the same time, we have incorporated the clinical expertise of sound theories and respected clinical interventions in the field. We have also drawn on our own experiences as clinicians, supervisors, and administrators as well as the values, needs, preferences, and feedback from our clients.

Evidence-Based Relationships

Another aspect of this entire debate has been the research on *evidence-based relationships* (EBRs; Norcross, 2002, 2011) or *evidence-supported relationships* (ESRs; Messer, 2004, 2006). As we have noted in Chapter 4, the therapeutic relationship is central to the process of therapy and "accounts for 30% of the variance in outcome in psychotherapy, second only to patient factors, which account for 40% of the variance (Assay & Lambert, 1999; Lambert, 1992; Lambert & Barley, 2002)" (Carter, 2006, p. 69). As we have indicated throughout this book, research has repeatedly and consistently demonstrated that the therapeutic relationship is one of the most important variables in treatment outcome regardless of the theoretical orientation of the clinician, the specific therapeutic techniques, or the treatment modality (e.g., psychodynamic, humanistic, cognitive behavioral, family systems, group dynamics; Duncan, Miller, Wampold, & Hubble, 2009; Norcross, 2002, 2011a). Norcross (2002, 2011a) and his contributors established this through extensive meta-analyses of numerous research studies across theoretical orientations.

Research has demonstrated that no particular type of therapy has been shown to consistently produce better outcomes than others (Wampold, 2001). Messer (2004, 2006), in response to these studies, presents complex cases that call upon his own psychodynamic orientation, and a "knowledge of ESTs [empirically supported treatments], ESRs, therapist variables, client factors, and their interaction; the recognition of intrapsychic and interpersonal themes; a degree of psychotherapy integration; and an appreciation of unique patient needs (Messer, 2004)" (Messer, 2006, p. 40). These concerns have also led clinicians such as Carter (2006) in Goodheart et al.'s (2006) book on EBPs to argue for "theoretical integration and technical eclecticism" (p. 73). She argues that these two factors taken together provide a useful framework if it "provides procedures for integrating diverse perspectives into a system that is applicable for the particular clinician–patient pair, to the particular patient problems, and in the particular context (Feixas & Botella, 2004)" (Carter, 2006, p. 73).

Challenges in the Implementation of Evidence-Based Practice in the Real World

There are many challenges in the implementation of evidence-based practice, and there are even more in developing studies to test the effectiveness of these evidence-based treatments in clinical settings (Kazdin, 2006, 2008; Weisz & Addis, 2006). A part of the dilemma is that most evidence-based treatments have been studied in efficacy studies that are quite different from effectiveness studies (Kazdin, 2006). Efficacy studies "are conducted in controlled settings and under conditions that depart from clinical practice" (p. 153).

These conditions include, for example, careful inclusion and exclusion criteria that often exclude clients with comorbid conditions, which are more typical of the real world of clinical practice (Kazdin, 2008). Effectiveness studies on the other hand, are "conducted in clinical settings with a diverse set of patient, therapist, and treatment administration characteristics" (Kazdin, 2006, p. 153). As a result of the highly controlled nature of many evidence-based treatments, concerns have been raised about the "generalizablity of the findings to clinical practice" (p. 153) in real-world settings. As indicated above, for all of these reasons, effectiveness studies testing real-world implementation have definitely lagged behind the development of evidence-based treatments (Goodheart et al., 2006; Kazdin, 2006, 2008; Norcross et al., 2006).

In addition, both the implementation of these evidence-based practices in the real world and the testing through effectiveness studies require the partnership of groups of people with different interests, goals, objectives, incentive systems, work pressures, and the demands of daily work (Weisz & Addis, 2006). These might include clinical practitioners, researchers, trainers, organizational leaders, and administrative staff (Berger, 2010; Kazdin, 2006, 2008; Steinfeld, Coffman, & Keyes, 2009; Weisz & Addis, 2006). Weisz and Addis, for example, compared and discussed the differences between the two worlds of clinical practice and clinical research.

From a clinical practitioner's point of view, the emphasis is on providing effective services to clients. Mental health practitioners and the agencies in which they work experience pressures related to the number of clients seen, total hours of clinical care provided, productivity requirements, and reimbursement by managed care insurance companies (Weisz & Addis, 2006). These pressures are quite different from those experienced by clinical researchers many of whom are in academic settings. As Weisz and Addis have stated:

> [For researchers] in clinical trials, a premium is placed on findings showing that a particular treatment both is delivered exactly as designed and produces better outcomes than those found in control or comparison groups. . . . Promotion and tenure decisions may depend on both research quality and success in generating grant support. Such pressures may lead to clinical trial procedures that emphasize experimental control and the likelihood of good results, sometimes at the expense of clinical representativeness and relevance to everyday clinical care (see Weisz, 2004). (p. 181)

Despite these obvious differences, numerous experts have called for a partnership between clinicians and clinical researchers and have demonstrated ways in which these relationships can be developed (Kazdin, 2006, 2008; Weisz & Addis, 2007).

Despite the relatively large number of evidence-based practices now available, therapists in the real world have continued to report relatively low use of EBPs (Connor-Smith & Weisz, 2003; Drake et al., 2001; Gotham, 2004, 2006; Steinfeld et al., 2009). There are a number of different possible explanations for this gap. On the one hand, the burden for staying current in terms of the dissemination of these evidence-based practices has often been placed on the individual practitioner (Goodheart et al., 2006). Representatives from a number of different health and mental health disciplines have questioned the practicality of this approach given the time and productivity demands as well as the often questionable access to Internet databases for many individual practitioners (Berger, 2010; Epstein, 2011; Rycroft-Malone, 2008).

Another approach has been the implementation of evidence-based practices within agencies, clinics, and hospitals locally and in wide-scale dissemination efforts (Carpinello et al., 2002; Hoagwood, Burns, Kiser, Ringeisen, & Schoenwald, 2001; Jensen, Hoagwood, & Trickett, 1999; Salerno et al., 2011; Steinfeld et al., 2009; Weisz & Addis, 2006). Steinfeld et al., for example, have described the process necessary to implement cognitive-behavior therapy for anxiety and depression in a large mental health system. They emphasize the importance of high-level organizational support for the training program throughout the agency. Another interesting aspect of their implementation project was the recognition of individual differences among practitioners in their response to the training in the CBT model. The responses of clinicians in their report are typical of the range of responses among mental health providers:

> Whereas many staff expressed strong interest in further training, some indicated serious reservations regarding an EBP training program. The majority of staff members were senior in their careers; had less exposure in their graduate education to EBPs; and were concerned about time, cost implications, and the impact of training on their workload. They expressed concerns about how an EBP could be adapted to their practice style, which often involved seeing patients for relatively brief periods of time (4–6 sessions). They were concerned that CBT was too mechanistic and not sensitive to relationship components of psychotherapy. (Steinfeld et al., 2009, p. 411)

These concerns are not new and have been expressed by many clinicians and clinical scholars throughout the field (Goodheart, 2006; Messer, 2004, 2006). What was striking in Steinfeld et al.'s (2009) report, however, was that these points of view were respected and valued in the implementation process. For example, they began with a group of clinicians who initially expressed interest in learning CBT. This group was provided with a combination of large trainings and ongoing group supervision and consultation. A year later, after the initial trainings, a concerted effort was made to engage clinicians who had initially been reluctant to seek the training. By this time, there was a group of clinicians who had experienced some success with the new model and were able to share their experiences. In our experience, this type of gradual implementation is helpful to clinical staff. See Chapter 16 for a more complete discussion of our own experiences with implementation of evidence-based practice within a large mental health agency and the importance of organizational support of training.

What Can Practitioners Do?

One of the challenges for clinicians from all of the mental health disciplines has been the need to push beyond our personal and professional "comfort zones" and explore and become exposed to new developments and the evidence-based practices in the field. This does not mean that one needs to abandon one's core theoretical orientation and training. As Messer (2004, 2006), Goodheart (2006), and Carter (2006) have indicated, evidence-based research can be one part of the considerations that can influence clinical decision making with a particular client. It is indeed unfortunate that the "culture war" (Messer, 2004) may prevent clinicians from exploring new approaches and new ways of conceptualizing best practices in the care of our clients. This book offers clinicians a way of integrating evidence-based research as one facet of evidence-based practice and evidence-informed practice that might also include the incorporation of respected theoretical approaches and clinical interventions, clinical expertise, and the needs, values, cultures, and preferences of the clients who we treat.

At the other end of the spectrum are practitioners who would like to encourage their agencies to provide training in EBPs and research on their effectiveness. Kazdin (2006, 2008) and Weisz and Addis (2006) have argued for partnerships between clinical practitioners and clinical researchers and have given examples of the ways in which these partnerships might work. Berger (2010) has offered a number of suggestions for practitioners interested in increasing their own knowledge base in terms of EBPs and in participating in effectiveness research. Clearly, all health and mental health practitioners should take full advantage of continuing education trainings offered in the field. Berger has also encouraged clinicians to advocate within their agencies for training in EBPs in new areas as well as "consultation with specialists who have expertise in research in fields of their interest" (p. 184). She also encourages clinicians to help to facilitate partnerships between their agencies and academic researchers who have developed EBPs. This can be a win–win situation for all involved (Berger, 2010; Kazdin, 2006, 2008; Weisz & Addis, 2006).

Conclusion

The incorporation of evidence-based practice can be challenging for agencies as well as both new and experienced clinicians. As the healthy debate regarding evidence-based practice, evidence-informed treatment, and best-practice implementation continues, value must be placed on clinical experience, relevant research, respected clinical publications from various orientations, the complexity and diversity of clinical populations, and the therapeutic relationship. Access to information regarding best practices should be made available so clinicians, researchers, and clients alike may pursue continuous learning. Furthermore, clinicians are encouraged to go outside of their comfort zone and integrate best-practice literature into their clinical decision making. Future chapters in this book highlight core mediational processes derived from diverse evidence-based practices, as an alternative to the adoption of a "one-size-fits-all" treatment model.

CHAPTER 3

Incorporating Multicultural, Racial, and Socioeconomic Diversity

Introduction

Many training programs in the mental health field are now incorporating multicultural competency as a central component. The nature of today's extraordinarily diverse population in terms of socioeconomic, racial, and cultural backgrounds, as well as sexual orientation and other factors, dictates that such training is a necessity. Unfortunately, this training in some cases is relatively superficial or is limited to one course and is often not accompanied by careful supervision of a wide range of clients from different backgrounds. In addition, the high level of immigration from many different parts of the world brings an increased complexity to many cases. Even experienced clinicians may find themselves treating clients and families from a particular country of origin for the first time, having had no prior opportunity to acquaint themselves with this country's cultural norms and values. With these challenges in mind, we consider incorporating multicultural, racial, and socioeconomic diversity and strengths as a central part of the therapeutic process.

This chapter first explores the relevance of familial, cultural, or religious values for *all* clients and the importance of joining and establishing a therapeutic relationship with clients from ethnic minority backgrounds, who may be new to the therapeutic process. Throughout this chapter the necessity of avoiding stereotypes and assuming an "asking stance" (Cave, as cited in Salerno et al., 2007, 2008b) is emphasized. We raise clinically relevant points about a number of different ethnic and racial groups, both to illustrate their diverse needs and to exemplify how to conceptualize clinical interventions. Although a thorough exploration of all diverse groups is beyond the scope of this chapter, clients from many different cultural and racial backgrounds and socioeconomic levels will be discussed as a means of acquainting both new and seasoned therapists with the heterogeneity of clients who they might encounter in the real world. Clients presented within this chapter include poor clients, undocumented immigrants, African American, Latino, Asian, and Asian Indian clients and families. (See McGoldrick et al. [2005] for a more comprehensive review of the values, culture, and treatment of a wide range of ethnic and racial groups.) Finally, the importance of the therapist's use of self in the treatment of diverse clients is explored throughout.

The Relevance of Familial, Cultural, or Religious Values for All Clients

It is important to honor and respect the life journey of each client or family. It is essential to clarify that the importance of exploring the familial, cultural, religious or other values, and traditions of *all* of our clients pertains to those from the majority culture, that is, White clients, as well as those from ethnic minority groups. As a part of our core mediational process of joining and establishing therapeutic rapport (see Chapter 4), we ask about the values that are important to all of our clients. For example, during the first session, we will usually ask questions similar to the following:

> People often tell us that they have a long tradition of values in their own lives and sometimes from their families or their cultures that have shaped who they are. What are some of your values and those in your family? What are some of the ways that people in your life have dealt with the tough times? (Wofsy & Mundy, 2011b)

It is also often helpful for a therapist to ask directly, "What strengths have helped you and your family to survive in the face of adversity?" Some clients will respond directly with their own beliefs about the role and value of family; others may talk about spiritual or religious values that have sustained them. As clients begin to answer, therapists often see another side of their clients—one that is based on their strengths and hopes. This series of questions also presents an excellent example of what we have described throughout this chapter as the asking stance of the therapist (Cave, as cited in Salerno et al., 2007, 2008b). The therapist is not the expert; the clients are experts on their own lives.

The Importance of Joining and Establishing a Therapeutic Relationship in a Multicultural World

As we discuss in Chapter 4, joining and establishing a therapeutic alliance and positive therapeutic relationship are essential in our work with all clients. These strategies are even more important when working with some ethnic minority and/or poor clients who may be new to the process of therapy. For many ethnic minority clients (African American, Caribbean, other clients of African descent, Latino, and Asian), therapy may be stigmatized within their cultures (Boyd-Franklin, 2003; McGoldrick et al., 2005). In addition, some African American clients may have a "healthy cultural suspicion" of therapy (Boyd-Franklin, 2003). Too often, therapists rely on an initial impression of these clients and label them as "resistant," which may result in a mutual withdrawal from the treatment process. It is extremely important for therapists not to take this initial resistance personally and to learn how to join effectively.

The key point for therapists to recognize is that "resistance" may be an instinctive reaction to experiences clients have had with racism, discrimination, sexism, ethnic stereotypes, poverty, and homophobia. This is especially true for many ethnic minority clients, particularly those who are poor, who have had significant interactions with multisystems including schools; child welfare and child protective services; the welfare department; housing; the police, courts, and the justice system; and medical, health, and mental health systems. It is all too common for these clients to come away from such experiences feeling disrespected and possibly even humiliated. Another factor contributing to perceived resistance is a strong cultural objection to exposing their lives to strangers. Some African American clients, for example, have been raised to keep family business in the family and to not "air their dirty laundry in public" (Boyd-Franklin, 2003, p. 23).

Avoiding Stereotypes: Multicultural Perspective and the Asking Stance

It is important to remember in the discussion of cultural issues in the treatment of African American, Latino, and Asian clients that there is enormous diversity in each ethnic and racial group. Although an in-depth exploration is beyond the scope of this chapter, it will refer clinicians to important work in the multicultural literature and focus on highlighting areas where challenges to best practice may occur for clinicians in working with clients from different racial, ethnic, cultural, religious, sexual orientation, and socioeconomic groups.

Boyd-Franklin (2003), in her discussion of the importance of cultural competency in the treatment of African American clients and families, cautions clinicians about the need to avoid stereotypes in working with clients from different ethnic and racial groups. This approach may also be extended to clients with different socioeconomic realities as well as all ethnic and racial groups. She argues that although the lens of cultural strengths can be a helpful one, it can become a stereotype if it is applied automatically without careful consideration of individual differences. She uses a camera lens analogy to clarify this point: knowledge of a particular cultural or racial group is like the camera lens—it is essential to take the picture, but it must be adjusted for each new client we treat.

In addition to studying and learning about different cultural groups, clinicians are reminded to also adopt an asking stance (Cave, as cited in Salerno et al., 2007, 2008b), as discussed above, in which therapists recognize their clients' expertise in their own family and cultural background and respectfully inquire about their clients' experiences. This chapter explores a number of issues related to culture, race, and socioeconomic background that therapists should be aware of in their clinical work with poor clients, as well as African American, Latino, and Asian clients and families.

Working with Poor Clients and Families

Many clinicians, particularly beginning therapists or counselors working in nonprofit agencies or clinics in urban areas or in poor rural areas, often find themselves shocked when they realize the extent to which, and the ways in which, poverty impacts the lives of their clients. Even experienced clinicians can be frustrated and overwhelmed when confronted by the ongoing realities of homelessness, a lack of food, a lack of money, substandard housing, unemployment, poor schools, high dropout rates, crime, dangerous neighborhoods, gang violence, substance abuse and drug dealing, racial and ethnic profiling by police, poor health care, and a lack of health insurance (Boyd-Franklin & Bry, 2000a). In fact, in Chapter 15, we argue that not only can this situation be traumatizing for our clients but it can result in vicarious or secondary traumatization for clinicians.

Burns and Hoagwood (2002) highlight the wide gap between university-based research settings where best-practice models are often developed and poor, urban areas where such practices are needed. The authors propose a six-step research and implementation model that seeks to conduct best-practice studies to identify the challenges unique to these areas and establish well-tested methods when working with this population.

A common error in the mental health field has been the equating of the terms *poor* with *ethnic minority*. It is important for clinicians to remember that there are many White clients and families that may also live in poverty (Boyd-Franklin & Bry, 2000a). The White poor can sometimes be invisible to schools and mental health agencies because the color of their skin may obscure their true level of need. By the same token, it is also important for clinicians to remember that many ethnic minority clients may be middle or upper class (Boyd-Franklin, 2003).

Boyd-Franklin and Bry (2000a) also caution therapists to be aware of the large number of clients who may be considered "working poor" (p. 12). These clients and their families often work extremely long hours at multiple low-wage jobs. Such hard work does not result in any measure of financial security as the jobs often lack benefits, such as health insurance, and the most basic worker protections. Employees in this situation are aware that they can be fired at will with no recourse and thus may not be available to attend school meetings or to take their children to therapy. Without knowing of these families' situations, some counselors may harshly judge these parents or clients.

Challenges for Poor, Undocumented Immigrant Clients and Families

Some clients from a poor, immigrant background may be undocumented or have family members who are. Coming to the attention of a school, hospital, clinic, the police, or a court can be threatening to them because of their concern that such contact may result in the deportation of family or household members. Intake or assessment forms that contain many personal questions may invoke fear and may result in clients dropping out of therapy after the first session. Thus, clinicians are encouraged to join and establish therapeutic rapport before personal information is requested from clients.

Therapy with Poor Clients

Harry Aponte (1994a) in his book, *Bread and Spirit: Therapy with the New Poor*, makes the following observations[1]:

---

[1]Excerpts from Aponte (1994a) are reprinted with permission from W. W. Norton & Company, Inc. Copyright 1994 by Harry J. Aponte.

The poor need to feel control over their own lives. They must experience therapy as a place where they discover their inner potential to determine their lives' direction. Therapy makes this possible when the poor are not treated as helpless victims of the unconscious, of family systems, or of society. Therapy helps them believe in their ability to direct their own emotions, attitudes, and actions in the face of horrendous problems. From within themselves, they can achieve the freedom to exercise fully their ability to make attitudinal and spiritual choices, even if they are not able to change their economics. Outside themselves, they can make choices and changes about family, friends, and officials. They do not have to stay put. With some backing, they can expect more not only of themselves, but also of the world around them. (pp. 9–10)

Aponte (1994a) also cautions therapists to recognize that a part of their task must rest with respecting the values, culture, and spirit of their clients. He cautions us about thinking solely of the services that we provide to a community without the emphasis on our partnership with individuals, families, and communities. As indicated throughout this book, our goal is empowerment, not merely helping or advocacy. Aponte (1994a) reminds us that it is not our job as providers to impose our own values on our clients:

It means working in partnership with the community that exists; the mandate for service providers is to serve, not colonize. People and families come into being, develop, and are sustained by their personal traditions, structures, and beliefs—not by services.

Service providers who try to substitute their personal political and social views for a community's views about moral behavior and family relationships stifle the souls of communities. . . .

In the poor, professionals face a diversity of racial, ethnic, cultural, and religious values that may well contradict their own core beliefs about family structure, sexual mores, and social hierarchy. (pp. 11–12)

Recognizing the strengths and resilience of poor clients is also essential in our work. As Aponte (1994a) reminds us:

People can be poor economically and still be emotionally, familially, and socially healthy—at least as healthy as anyone else. With their communities and cultures intact, the poor can maintain their identity, self-esteem and sense of belonging. They have their trust in family and friends, as well as in their social network—public institutions and economic infrastructure. Instead of withdrawing in despair or becoming predatory in anger, they take care of themselves, their families, and their neighbors. The intactness, order, and connectedness of the social ecosystem are reflected in personal living.

People with intact communities and cultures also know power in a healthy, natural and benign form that allows them to assume a society that will respond to their voices. They feel they belong to a society that gives to them and to which they want to give. They can endure material deprivation because the spirit is nourished with self-esteem, caring personal relationships, and trust in the community. There is a sense of meaning and purpose at home and in the community. (pp. 13–14)

These phenomena will be discussed further below as we explore protective cultural factors and strengths for our clients and their families in the face of stressors such as poverty, racism, and societal injustice, including the role of churches and other faith-based organizations in some cultures and communities, and that of a connected, strong kinship network of extended family members and close friends.

Therapists' Use of Self in Multicultural Treatment

One of the most important determinants of a successful outcome is the ability to help to create a trusting therapeutic relationship with a client. While recognizing that clinicians are trained in particular therapeutic modalities, we have found that the process of the therapist's use of self (Aponte, 1994a; Boyd-Franklin, 2003), that is, the therapist's use of him- or herself in the treatment, can make the difference as to whether the client remains in therapy or drops out. As we explore further in Chapter 4, conveying such qualities as warmth, empathy, openness, and respect toward clients through the "person of the therapist" (Aponte, 1994a, p. 153) can be particularly important when working with poor clients and/or clients from ethnic minority groups who may be new to therapy and who may have to overcome a preexisting cultural stigma associated with seeking treatment.

In order for therapists to be open, responsive and authentic with clients who are from all socioeconomic, ethnic, racial, and sexual orientation groups, the therapists must first do some work discussing, clarifying, and exploring their own cultural, racial, ethnic, religious, gender, and sexual orientation backgrounds. This can lead to a process of values clarification (Aponte, 1994a; Boyd-Franklin, 2003), which can help therapists to understand their own issues and beliefs and empower them to work with clients whose worldviews, values, and experiences might be quite different from theirs.

Training the Person of the Therapist
for Cross-Cultural Work

Aponte (1994a), Boyd-Franklin (2003), McGoldrick et al. (2005), and Pinderhughes (1989) have all explored the process of training therapists to work with clients from cultural, racial, and socioeconomic backgrounds different from their own. All have argued that reading alone is not sufficient to produce cultural competency in cross-racial or cross-cultural clinical work. Pinderhughes addresses the need for therapists to look at themselves directly, "It is not possible to assist clients to examine issues concerning cultural identity and self-esteem if helpers have not done this work for themselves" (p. 19). ✷

Pinderhughes's (1989) model describes therapists' training in this area as "exploring within a group format the participants' own feelings, perceptions, and experiences vis-à-vis ethnicity, race, and power" (p. 211). This model emphasizes the value of sharing in a culturally and racially diverse group and explores values on "both personal and societal levels" (p. 212). Once this initial discussion of their own values and experiences has occurred, clinicians are more prepared to discuss their clinical work with clients from different cultural, racial, and socioeconomic backgrounds.

In his discussion of this issue, Aponte (1994a) states:

> The extent to which therapists understand and have resolved their own stories will determine how sensitive they are to their clients' stories. Their ability to deal with the pain associated with their own ethnicity, race, and economic struggles dictates their ability to work with the personal meanings and emotions associated with similar issues in their clients' lives. (p. 155)

Values Clarification

Each counselor or therapist brings his or her own personal values to the treatment process. New therapists are often not only surprised to discover how much their own cultural or racial or socioeconomic background has shaped their values but how much their religious, spiritual, or moral beliefs may influence their responses to clients' situations and the clients themselves. Boyd-Franklin (2003) states that "Values clarification is an ongoing, lifelong activity. It is not a task done once in training and then completed, but a process of continuously exploring one's own reactions, countertransferences, and beliefs as one works with [clients and] families" (p. 191). Aponte (1994a) in his discussion of the role of values in therapy makes the following observation:

Values frame the entire process of therapy. Values are the social standards by which therapists define reality, identify problems, formalize
evaluations, select interventions, and determine therapeutic goals. All
transactions between therapists and clients involve negotiations about
the respective value systems that each party brings into the therapeutic process. (p. 170)

The Negotiation of Values in Therapy

One of the foundations of multicultural approaches to treatment, particularly cross-cultural or cross-racial therapy, involves the negotiation of
values (Aponte, 1994a; Boyd-Franklin, 2003). Aponte states that when
a therapist and a client engage in therapy, "they embark upon a personal
relationship framed by professional parameters" (p. 169). He argues that
values are central to therapeutic relationships:

> My contention here is that value biases are pervasive in all aspects of
> therapy. The question is not one of whether the therapist's values will
> come face to face with [the client or] the family's values in the crucible
> of therapy, but how. How can therapists work with their professional
> and personal values to benefit the [clients and] families they treat?
> Negotiating values that form the basis of problem definition, assess-
> ment, therapeutic interventions, and goal-setting becomes central to
> the therapeutic process. (p. 175)

Rather than restate the extensive literature on multicultural issues
in therapy (Aponte, 1994a; Boyd-Franklin, 2003; Boyd-Franklin & Bry,
2000a; McGoldrick et al., 2005), the remainder of this chapter addresses
the challenge of the negotiation of values in the treatment of clients from
different racial, ethnic, and socioeconomic backgrounds. Case examples
illustrate the real-world experiences of therapists from similar and different backgrounds who have struggled with the process of negotiating values in therapy with clients and families, as these challenges often
inhibit effective utilization of best-practice methods.

Challenges and "Mistakes" as Opportunities
for Deepening the Therapeutic Relationship
in Multicultural Treatment

When beginning clinicians learn for the first time about the process of
working with clients from diverse backgrounds, they often are fearful
that they might unintentionally "make a mistake and offend someone."
This fear, frequently a result of a sincere desire to communicate respect
and positive regard for their clients, can make clinicians overly cautious

in the therapeutic process and inhibit their ability to be genuine and to use themselves in an authentic way with their clients. White therapists may be particularly vulnerable to such fear when beginning to work with ethnic minority clients.

One of the concepts that can be helpful in this situation is the notion of "learning from our mistakes"—understanding that challenging moments in therapy can often lead to a process of deepening the therapeutic relationship. Our clients can sense when we are sincere and sometimes just saying, "You seemed upset when I said that; can we talk about it?" can open the door for a more "real" relationship. For example, Boyd-Franklin (2003), in her book on therapy with African American clients and families, discusses the "concept of vibes." These vibes are intuitions on the part of Black clients that help them to sense whether respect is sincere and can also be a way to protect themselves and their families from negative experiences. If a clinician of whatever background is open, warm, and caring, clients will sense this and respond.

Working with African American Clients and Families

As discussed above, among the challenges faced by clinicians working with African American clients, particularly in cross-racial treatment, are that many clients may be new to therapy, may not have been self-referred, and may have a cultural stigma about therapy. Boyd-Franklin (2003) has noted the healthy cultural suspicion that some African American clients may bring to therapy. Therapists who are not prepared for this reality may take this personally and not recognize that it may have nothing to do with them, but may be related to their clients' experiences with racism, disrespect, and discrimination. In addition, in response to intrusion into their families by outside agencies, some African American families have raised their children to be careful in discussing family business outside of the family. This may lead therapists to feel that some African American clients may seem secretive and reluctant to trust initially. Too often, an African American client may be dismissed as resistant to treatment. Boyd-Franklin (2003) encourages therapists to join past this initial response and establish therapeutic rapport with these clients. She gives many examples of this process and appropriate therapeutic responses.

The assumption that all clients enter the treatment room wanting therapy is problematic with clients who have suspicions of the treatment process. Boyd-Franklin and Bry (2000a) caution supervisors to help new therapists to recognize that these initial reactions are merely the beginning of an elaborate dance between African American clients and therapists. This does not necessarily lead to an end to therapy, particularly if clinicians can be helped to address these issues in a culturally competent manner. With this in mind, Boyd-Franklin (2003) emphasizes taking the time necessary to establish a therapeutic alliance with members of this racial group as an important component of culturally competent practice. Therapists are reminded that joining and establishing therapeutic rapport with these clients and families is essential before asking questions from intake forms or assessment questionnaires (see Chapter 4).

This need for clinicians to spend some time in the initial session joining and connecting may be considered contrary to some evidence-based treatment approaches that begin with a comprehensive assessment. Clinicians in many settings also struggle with intake forms that require a great deal of data collection before a therapeutic relationship has been established. Unfortunately, asking these personal questions may be perceived as intrusive by some clients and this may contribute to the high dropout rate of African American clients after the initial session (Boyd-Franklin, 2003). Agencies should also consider cultural competency training for all staff members, such as phone-intake workers, receptionists, and administrative personnel, so that African American clients do not perceive experiences of disrespect.

Strengths of African American Clients and Families

Extended Family Networks

Families, which may include extended relatives including mothers, fathers, brothers, sisters, grandmothers, grandfathers, aunts, uncles, and cousins (Boyd-Franklin, 2003), are an extremely important strength in the lives of many African Americans as well as other ethnic minority clients discussed in this chapter. It is also common for African American families to "adopt" non-blood-related persons with whom they are close, such as neighbors, community members, church family, godmothers, godfathers, play mothers and fathers, play sisters, brothers, and cousins (Boyd-Franklin, 2003). Extended family members and close family friends may be involved in the lives of African American clients.

One theme, consistent across many of the ethnic minority groups discussed in this chapter, is the expectation of interdependence among extended family members. This can be challenging for therapists who have been trained in Euro-western therapy models that emphasize independence, autonomy, separation/individuation from family in adulthood, and the importance of pursuing what is in the individual's best interest. While African Americans may be raised to be independent thinkers, they often, paradoxically, function interdependently within their families. This can be confusing for some therapists, particularly when working with African American women who present as strong and independent in their interactions with the outside world, but who carry tremendous burdens within their families.

Spirituality and Religion in the Treatment of African American Clients

Research has shown that spirituality and religion are vital components of the cultural beliefs of many African Americans (Lincoln & Mamiya, 1990; Taylor, Chatters, Bullard, Wallace, & Jackson, 2009; Taylor, Chatters, & Levin, 2004). In a national Gallup poll (2006), Gallup and Newport found that 85% of African Americans surveyed reported that religion was very important in their lives. Despite the central role of spirituality and religion in the lives of many Black people, Boyd-Franklin (2010) has indicated that this topic has received relatively little attention in the training of mental health professionals. As a consequence, even when counselors are aware that this is an important issue they may not have sufficient exposure to the process in order to explore it with African Americans in treatment.

A further complication is the tremendous diversity of religious and spiritual beliefs and practices within the African American community. The majority of African Americans identify as Christian, with 78% as Protestant, 5% as Catholic, and 1% as Jehovah's Witnesses; 1% identify as Muslim (Pew Forum on Religion and Public Life, 2009). Those who do not practice any formal religion might maintain strong spiritual beliefs in God, and there are African Americans who have no religious or spiritual beliefs. Additionally, individuals and families may choose to leave out their spirituality and belief systems when values are explored.

Some therapists may be surprised to discover that certain African Americans, particularly religious individuals, may consider therapy "antispiritual" (Boyd-Franklin, 2003, 2010; Boyd-Franklin & Lockwood, 2009; Constantine, Lewis, Conner, & Sanchez, 2000; Richardson & June, 1997). Although the mental health field has made progress in recent years in acknowledging the role of spirituality and religion in the lives of many individuals from different cultural and religious groups, some individuals are familiar with the animosity with which their beliefs were treated: "Many African Americans still remember unfortunate periods in the history of psychology in which religious beliefs or spirituality were pathologized and demeaned as 'religiosity' or were ignored as irrelevant to psychology" (Walsh, 2009). As a consequence, even those who are otherwise willing to refer someone for counseling may feel comfortable only when assured that the therapist will not challenge the person's religious beliefs. It is not unusual, therefore, to receive a request for referral to a "Black Christian therapist" (Boyd-Franklin, 2010, p. 986). With this in mind, Boyd-Franklin (pp. 986–989) presents the following case in which a White therapist encounters this issue with an African American client.[2] The therapist's nondefensive posture and effective use of self is an excellent example of culturally competent treatment.

Barbara, a 35-year-old African American woman, was referred by a friend to a local mental health agency because she was experiencing distress related to her couple relationship. She was assigned to Mary, a White therapist. In the first session, Barbara looked surprised as her therapist greeted her. She responded that she had requested a "Black Christian therapist." Mary was concerned because she was White and not particularly religious.

She resisted the urge to become defensive and said to Barbara, "It seems that having someone of your own race and faith is very important to you; can you tell me more about this." Barbara explained that she had grown up in a Black church with a strong belief in God, and that it was important to her that her therapist understand how her religious beliefs shaped her decisions. The therapist validated the importance of Barbara's religious beliefs in her life. She explained to Barbara that the agency did not have any Black therapists on staff. She invited Barbara to give the therapy a try for a few sessions to see how she felt. If she was not comfortable, Mary would try to help her find a Black Christian therapist outside of the agency.

In this session, the therapist asked Barbara to tell her more about her church background. Barbara's minister had been a father figure to her. She spoke of the importance of her faith in her life and how much being a Sunday school teacher meant to her. The therapist validated the significance of her spiritual beliefs and the role of her minister and her church family in her life as well as exploring Barbara's concerns. By the end of the session, Barbara was more relaxed and she agreed to "give therapy a try."

In the second session, Barbara hesitantly explained that for the past year, she had been dating a young African American man, Bill, who had been introduced to her by a friend. Although Bill had been raised as a Christian, he was no longer religious. They had begun to discuss the possibility of a future together involving marriage and children. Barbara desperately wanted to be married to Bill and to have children, and she reported that she loved him, but she foresaw problems for the relationship if Bill continued to fail to embrace the religious beliefs that were so important to Barbara.

---

[2]Copyright 2010 by the Division of Counseling Psychology of the American Psychological Association. Adapted with permission from Sage Publications, Inc.

When the therapist asked if Barbara and her boyfriend had ever considered seeking counseling to address these issues, Barbara reported that she had asked him whether he would meet with her minister so that they might undergo pastoral counseling together. Bill refused, fearing that he would be "outnumbered" by Barbara and her minister. Barbara and her therapist had begun to establish more of a therapeutic rapport. They continued to discuss Barbara's relationship in more detail. After two months, the therapist asked Barbara whether her boyfriend would consider coming in for a session to help the therapist understand his point of view.

Her boyfriend initially refused but Barbara persisted and he finally joined a session. He told the therapist clearly that he did not feel that he and Barbara needed counseling as he did not have any faith in counseling. He expressed his belief that their love was sufficient to overcome any obstacles they would face as a couple. They loved each other and that was enough. The therapist accepted Bill's statement nondefensively and asked him to tell her more about his view. He explained that his mother was a religious Baptist, like Barbara, and she had forced him to attend church as a child. He swore that when he grew up he would never allow anyone to pressure him into church attendance.

The therapist turned to Barbara and asked her if she was aware of Bill's early experience. This was the first she heard of it and had only been aware that he had been raised Christian. The therapist asked Bill to tell Barbara more about his feelings and he shared that his mother's minister had preached a great deal about "hell and damnation," an approach to religion Bill found off-putting. Barbara was surprised by this revelation, which led to a productive discussion of the differences between Barbara's church and Bill's early experiences. Bill reported that he still had strong spiritual beliefs that were a part of his life but that he avoided church affiliation. The therapist encouraged Bill to share his spiritual beliefs with Barbara in the session and she pointed out their common spiritual values.

At the end of the session, Bill and Barbara were surprised at the amount of material that they had discussed. The therapist had encouraged them to talk to each other and not just to her and, for the first time, Barbara had begun to understand Bill's hesitation about church involvement. Barbara and Bill agreed to come together for more sessions. In future sessions, Barbara was able to share with Bill the joy that she experienced in her church. In examining his family-of-origin issues, Bill realized that he had been equating Barbara's requests for him to attend church with his mother's demands as a child. The conflation resulted in a classic "pursuer–distancer" relationship. With the therapist's help, Barbara was able to stop pursuing his church involvement. The therapist asked Bill if he would consider visiting her church one Sunday on his own just to "check it out." She suggested that Barbara not push for this and that Bill would only go when he was ready and was not obligated to attend the same service as Barbara attended.

In a future session, Bill reported that he had attended a service at her church by himself and had been surprised by how much he had enjoyed the music and the "message" of the sermon. He began occasionally attending with Barbara, but pointed out that he would make that decision and did not want her "bugging" him. It was clear that he now appreciated the importance of Barbara's church home in her life. He also repeated his message that although he had a sense of spirituality in his life, he was not ready to join her church at this time. Because she now understood his resistance more clearly and had a greater understanding of his spiritual beliefs, Barbara was able to accept his position. She reported that she would continue to pray for him. The therapist emphasized throughout the treatment their love for each other and the need not to allow old family patterns, including their earlier religious experiences, to interfere with their lives now.

This case illustrates a number of aspects of cultural and religious sensitivity on the part of a White therapist working with African American clients. Although the therapist was initially surprised when Barbara stated her preference for a Black Christian therapist, she did not respond defensively. Mary explored Barbara's religious beliefs and communicated her understanding of why Barbara had made the request— an acknowledgment that can be important to African American clients. After explaining that there were no Black Christian therapists on staff, Mary encouraged Barbara to give therapy a try with the provision that Mary would help Barbara find a referral if she was still not comfortable after a few sessions. Mary also showed a great deal of cultural and religious sensitivity in engaging Bill, a Black man with a great deal of hesitancy and suspicion about the counseling process. As indicated above, Bill is also an example of a Black person who was raised in a church, considered himself spiritual but not religious, and who avoided religious affiliation as an adult.[3]

Raising the Issue of Race in Cross-Racial Treatment

As the example above indicates, another area that can present challenges for many White therapists and those from other ethnic and racial groups has been the question of whether and when to raise the issue of race or racial difference in cross-racial therapy. In some cases, such as the example of Barbara above, some African American clients may raise this

---

[3] All identifying details have been changed in this and all other case examples in this book in order to protect the confidentiality of the clients involved. In some cases, details from more than one case have been included in order to further disguise the clients' identities.

issue directly by requesting a Black therapist. Mary did not personalize Barbara's statement despite her unspoken concerns about her status as a White woman who was not particularly religious. The therapist's response—asking Barbara to tell her more about why having a "Black Christian therapist," that is, someone of her own race and the issue of faith, was so important to her—was direct and nondefensive. Whether race or religion is raised by the client or family, the therapist responding directly, as the therapist did in the case above, can be an equally helpful strategy.

In cases where clients do not introduce the issue of race in cross-racial treatment, some therapists are more reluctant to bring it up. Boyd-Franklin (2003) has indicated that, in fact, raising the issue can be helpful in the cross-racial treatment process. Timing is everything and the therapist may want to begin by joining and building a therapeutic alliance for a few sessions before the issue is raised. The asking stance (Cave, as cited in Salerno et al., 2007, 2008b) is direct, respectful, and conveys an active willingness to hear the client's or the family's response(s).

If a therapist from a different cultural or racial group raises the question "How do you feel about working with a White [Latino, Asian, or other ethnic or racial group] therapist?" clients and families can respond in different and sometimes unexpected ways. Some will quickly indicate that this is not a problem for them. For others, the mere fact that the therapist has asked the question conveys the message that "anything can be discussed here, clearing the air and removing a possible obstacle to the development of trust" (Boyd-Franklin, 2003, p. 184). In addition, the question about the client's feelings about the race or culture of the therapist may lead to meaningful discussions between clients or families and clinicians in cross-racial or cross-cultural treatment.

Boyd-Franklin (2003) has indicated that in some cases the question might lead to the expression of anger or disappointment by the client, particularly one who was requesting or hoping for a Black therapist. The case below captures both the initial anger of the client, the therapist's nondefensive response and, ultimately, a meaningful discussion about the issue of race.

———

Kareem, a 51-year-old divorced African American man, entered treatment because of his depression. He was living at a homeless shelter and had been unemployed, with no health insurance, for 3 years. Initially, he presented as sad and angry about the loss of his job at a bank where he had worked for 10 years. He was assigned to Chris, a 30-year-old White male social worker, who was affiliated with the program providing mental health services at the shelter. In the first session, Kareem told the therapist that he had been a faithful worker at his job for many years and he was angry that he was the "last hired, first fired, like many Black men."

Chris could feel Kareem's anger and was not sure how to respond. He decided to reflect it and stated, "It sounds like you were furious and felt betrayed." Kareem responded with anger, "You're damn right! I am furious! I gave that job the best years of my life and it counted for nothing! I am a Black man with a college degree and I am living in a homeless shelter! You're damn right; I am furious!"

Chris responded, "You have a right to be furious." He asked Kareem to relate his experience. Angrily, Kareem explained that the "bottom had fallen out of the banking business and his employer started cutting people." He was one of the first to be laid off. With a great deal of bitterness, he told Chris that they didn't even give him the courtesy of notice. He barely had time to get a few personal items from his office before Security escorted him out of the building. When Chris asked how that felt for him, Kareem replied, "humiliating."

Kareem was able to exist, however barely, for the first 2 years while he received unemployment benefits. Once they expired, he could no longer afford to keep his apartment. He moved in with a former girlfriend for a while but she had "thrown [him] out." Despite all these difficulties, he made great efforts to find work. He had sent out "tons of resumes," gone to many job fairs and, as a result, had some interviews, but received no job offers. Chris reflected the sense of anger and hopelessness that Kareem seemed to be feeling when Kareem asked, "Who's going to hire a 51-year-old Black man?" The session ended with Kareem, who had initially been bending over looking angry and dejected, standing up and walking out with some sense of dignity.

In the next session, Chris asked how things had been going for him at the shelter. Kareem reported that two men had jumped him and beat him up for the few cigarettes he had in an old pack. Chris stated to Kareem, "You seem to me to be a proud man with a good education and this whole experience has been hard for you." Kareem replied, "How would you know, you have a job?" Chris acknowledged the difference in their employment situations and replied, "I wondered what it has been like for you to talk with a White man with a job about all of the challenges you have faced." Kareem replied angrily, "How the hell do you think it feels? You are a young White boy with a good job and I am a homeless Black man with nothing!" Chris again reflected, "Yeah and you are furious about all of this." Kareem replied, "You are damn right!"

Chris was not sure how to proceed in light of Kareem's anger. Finally Chris followed his "gut hunch" and took a chance. He looked Kareem directly in the eye and said, "This whole thing is terrible. You are a Black man with a college degree and you have been treated like garbage. I can understand why you would be angry about everything and now you have to talk to a young White man. It must be awful for you. . . . "

Kareem again replied, "Yeah, you're damn right," but with lessened rage. He then added: "It's hard out here today for a Black man. Nobody cares about you. They throw you away like you're nothing." Chris replied, "Yeah, I hear you. Can you tell me more about what you have been through?" Kareem began telling Chris the saga of his time "living on the streets." Chris replied, "You know, you have been through a lot and you have a right to be furious, but when I look at you, I see a strong Black man. You are a survivor. You have to not let these experiences stop you." Kareem replied, "You're damn right!"

The therapeutic alliance, although still fragile, had started to form.

This case captures many aspects of the challenges clinicians often face in the process of raising the issue of race in therapy. The anger and rage that Kareem expressed had been building for some time—a common reaction among African Americans to the history of racism and discrimination in this country (Boyd-Franklin, 2003; Cose, 1993; Franklin, 2004), and particularly true for Black men who are often treated as if they are "invisible" (Franklin, 2004). Although he had worked hard all of his life, Kareem had experienced the "last hired, first fired" policy, a situation faced by many African Americans.

When Chris sensed Kareem's anger, he was frightened and unsure where to go with it. Chris decided to reflect that anger and stay present in the session with Kareem. When Kareem challenged Chris's ability to understand him because he had a job, Chris intuited that Kareem might have left unsaid, but was feeling, the additional difference that Chris was "a young White man with a job." Although the timing of this question when Kareem was so angry might not have been ideal, Chris's willingness to be genuine and to follow his intuition ultimately facilitated the joining process and the beginning of the therapeutic alliance.

Finally, Chris followed his "gut hunch" and spoke directly about how unfair all of this had been. He addressed Kareem's strengths by referencing his education, his pride, and the fact that he was "a survivor." In our experience, this survivor reframe has often been a helpful one with African American clients who are angry about experiences of racism and discrimination (Boyd-Franklin, 2003).

This was not an easy session. We could spend a great deal of time analyzing the process and debating if "mistakes" had been made, but Chris conveyed true empathy and compassion to Kareem and, even more important, he recognized Kareem's pride and conveyed that he could also handle his anger. This young White therapist's willingness to raise the issue of race and follow his "gut hunch" created an opportunity for the beginnings of a therapeutic relationship between these two men.

Working with Latino Clients and Families

Issues of diversity are never more present than in our work with Latino clients. There is often controversy over the terms used to describe these groups in the United States. Garcia-Preto (2005) makes the following distinctions between the terms *Hispanic* and *Latino*:

 Hispanic refers to the influence of the Spanish culture and language on a group of people who suffered years of colonization. The term doesn't take into account indigenous cultures, therefore prioritizing the dominant European cultures (Quinones-Rosado, 2000).

In contrast, *Latino/Latina* does not refer to Spain, but rather to Spain's former colonies in Latin America, indicating people who come from South America, Central America, and Mexico, including territories in the United States that were taken from Mexico and some of the Caribbean islands. (p. 155)

The following persons are identified as Latino in the United States: "Cubans, Chicanos, Mexicans, Puerto Ricans, Argentineans, Colombians, Dominicans, Brazilians, Guatemalans, Costa Ricans, Nicaraguans, and Salvadorans" among others (Garcia-Preto, 2005, p. 154). In addition, persons from other Central and South American countries such as Honduras, Panama, Belize, Ecuador, Chile, Venezuela, Paraguay, Bolivia, Peru, and Uruguay may also be considered Latinos in the United States. She also indicates that Brazilians, despite their country's original colonization by Portugal and the fact that they speak Portuguese, are often classified as Latinos when they enter the United States. Garcia-Preto indicates that many Latinos do not identify with this term, but with their countries of origin. When clinicians ask clients about their cultural background, clients are unlikely to respond, "Latina(o)", but, rather, "Puerto Rican," "Cuban," "Mexican," and so on. McGoldrick et al. (2005) explore the similarities and differences between these different groups and the therapeutic implications for treatment.

Separation of Families through Immigration

Familismo or love and connection to family and extended family members is an extremely important value in Latino families (Garcia-Preto, 2005). In their countries of origin, many Latino clients have lived in close proximity to their family members and have relied on them for support (Falicov, 1998). Immigration policies in the United States often dictate prolonged and painful separation of individuals from their families (Boyd-Franklin & Bry, 2000a; Falicov, 1998; Garcia-Preto, 2005,

McGoldrick et al., 2005). It is important for clinicians to understand the relationship between the immigration process, specifically as it pertains to obtaining a "green card," and prolonged absences from family members. Boyd-Franklin and Bry (2000a) state:

> One common scenario for Latino immigrant families has been the experience of parents (often mothers) who leave children behind in their country of origin. Frequently, parents come (together or separately) to the United States on a travel visa or enter this country illegally. They must then find employment and someone who will sponsor them, usually an employer, for a "green card." The green card is a permit that allows an individual from another country to live and work in the United States. After obtaining a green card, a person can "sponsor" or bring other family members to the United States. Unfortunately, this process can take 6–7 years (or more). In addition, it may take another 6–7 years for the parent(s) to save enough money to bring over each of their children. Children left behind at a young age may well be teenagers by the time they are reunited with their parents. (p. 30)

Within the United States, women may come in advance of their spouse or partner as it is often easier for them to obtain employment. Because the mother–child bond is a close one in most Latino cultures, particularly the mother–son relationship (Garcia-Preto, 2005), the enforced separation between a Latina and her loved ones, particularly her children, may create extreme emotional distress. The following case illustrates the challenges that many Latinas may face in separating from their children and loved ones as a result of immigration.

Marta, a 30-year-old Latina from El Salvador, was hospitalized for suicidal ideation. She was placed on antidepressant medication and was referred to a local mental health clinic for outpatient treatment. Emily, a White clinician, was assigned to work with Marta. In her first session, Emily joined with Marta and began establishing a therapeutic relationship. Marta had been in the United States for 5 years and was bilingual, although she often struggled to find the right word to express herself in English, particularly when she was trying to describe her feelings and emotions. Emily spoke no Spanish but they were able to struggle together with the language challenges.

In the first session, Marta appeared depressed. When asked, she stated that she was not feeling suicidal at that time. She reported that she was sad because her baby had died. With gentle questioning from the therapist, Marta revealed that she had been separated from her son for the 5 years she had been in the United States, hoping to find work so that her son might have a better life. Her parents had cared for him in El Salvador. He had become sick and had died suddenly about 2 months before her hospitalization. She could not leave the country even to go to his funeral. She burst into tears and sat sobbing in the session.

Not sure what to do, Emily handed her a tissue and touched her hand. She said, "That must have been terrible for you." She sat quietly and allowed Marta to cry out her sadness and intense feelings of loss. During that week, Emily met with her supervisor because she was having trouble understanding why Marta had not flown immediately to see her child when he became ill. Emily understood Marta's impoverishment, but could not comprehend this being such an obstacle—couldn't Marta have borrowed the money? Didn't she have any savings? The supervisor was concerned about Emily's lack of empathy toward Marta and encouraged Emily to ask her about her son. The supervisor, also recognizing that Emily's upper-middle-class background had protected her from the realities of the level of poverty that Marta experienced, encouraged her to ask more about Marta's life in the United States. Her supervisor also explained the implications of Marta's immigration status: Without a green card, Marta was not legally permitted to live or work in the United States and she would not be allowed back into the country if she left. Her supervisor also suspected that Marta had struggled to enter this country and she encouraged Emily to ask about this.

In the next session, Emily asked Marta about the birth of her baby. Marta revealed that she had become pregnant by a young man from another village who refused to marry her. She was not only scared, but experienced a great deal of shame in her family and in her village. When Emily asked her to describe her son, Marta smiled for the first time in the session. She said, "Oh, he was a beautiful boy." She pulled a tattered picture of an adorable, smiling 6-month-old baby from her wallet, a picture that had been taken just before Marta left for the United States. The therapist agreed with her that her son was a beautiful boy. Marta's mother had agreed to care for her son until Marta was in a position to bring him to the United States. Marta said that she had no idea it would take so long and be so hard. Emily stated, "You must have loved him a great deal." Marta began sobbing. She kept repeating, "If I had known he was that sick and would die so quickly, I would have given up and gone home."

Marta explained that her father had become ill and could not work his small piece of land in El Salvador. She decided to try to escape her family's poverty by going to the United States, getting a job, sending money back to her mother and father, and eventually bringing her child over. The therapist reflected Marta's strength and devotion as a mother to want to provide a better life for her son and her family. Marta's response to this validation was dramatic. She seemed to relax and, although she continued to cry, her tears were gentle tears and not the heart-wrenching sobs she had cried earlier.

With this session, Emily's view of Marta had shifted and she felt genuine empathy and sadness for her. Marta felt understood for the first time and began to share more of her feelings and experience with her therapist.

In the next session, Marta shared with her therapist her horrifying experience entering the United States. She had started her journey in Mexico where she worked for a number of months until she raised enough money to pay a "coyote" to transport her to the United States. She sobbed as she described being hidden in the sweltering trunk of a car with two other people and no water. When they were released in the United States, they were forced to run for cover in a desert area. Marta twisted her ankle but was helped by a fellow passenger to get to the town nearby where his daughter lived in a small one-bedroom apartment that she shared with her husband and child. This woman was about Marta's age and she took both her father and Marta in to live with her family. She helped Marta to find work in a small factory in the area. Marta was paid little and almost half of that went to the woman who took her in for her "room"—a portion of the floor to sleep on. Each month, Marta sent the rest of her salary home to her family to help care for them and her son.

Emily was stunned and touched by Marta's story and the hardships she had endured. She reflected to Marta how much courage and determination she had shown in surviving so many horrible experiences. This was the beginning of a true therapeutic relationship that allowed Emily and Marta to work together to address Marta's sadness, profound grief and loss, and her feelings of guilt at not having been able to save her child.

This case reveals many of the challenges faced by many undocumented Latinas and Latinos in this country as they try to achieve legal immigrant status. It also captures the trapped and hopeless feelings that many immigrants experience when they cannot return to their families in times of illness, death, and loss for fear that they will not be able to reenter the United States. Initially, it was a struggle for Emily to understand Marta's reality, which was so different from her own. With her supervisor's help, she was able to join and to begin to establish a therapeutic relationship by asking about and acknowledging Marta's love for her child, at which point Marta was able to feel Emily's empathy and compassion for her. Emily's validation of Marta's resilience, strength, and courage in her struggle to provide for her family further strengthened their therapeutic relationship. They were then able to begin the process of healing the sadness, grief, and loss that Marta was experiencing.

Language Concerns

With the exception of Brazilian clients, who may speak Portuguese, many Latino clients may be monolingual (Spanish) or bilingual (Spanish–English) speakers. Clients who speak only Spanish or little English often

cannot receive effective treatment in facilities, such as mental health centers, social service agencies, hospitals, medical facilities, courts, banks,
post offices, and schools, if there are no staff members who are fluent
in Spanish. In other situations, children or adolescents may be used as
translators when they are more fluent in English than their parents. This
unfortunate practice should be avoided because it often reverses the generational boundaries, puts the child prematurely in a parentified role,
and may ultimately lead to disrespect of the parent by the child or adolescent (Garcia-Preto, 2005).

The following case illustrates this dilemma and reinforces the need
for recruiting clinicians who are fluent in Spanish and other languages
to training programs in the mental health field.

Ms. Achara, a 45-year-old Dominican woman, was frequently called to the
school to respond to complaints about her 13-year-old son Jorge's behavior.
She was almost exclusively Spanish speaking, although she could speak a
few words of English. During the school year, she had repeated experiences
of meetings in which she listened to teachers' complaints about her son and
nodded politely. At some point in the discussion, she would indicate that she
did not know what to do to help him. This would usually lead to a flood
of suggestions that she did not understand. Occasionally, a school official
would ask Jorge to translate for his mother, but given that the official could
not understand Spanish, there could be no corroboration that Jorge was
giving his mother an accurate translation. Finally, Ms. Achara began avoiding the school and would not take or respond to calls from his guidance
counselor.

In November of that school year, a Spanish-speaking counselor intern
was assigned to work with Jorge. In his discussions with him, the intern
learned why the parent meetings at the school had been so ineffective. He
obtained the mother's cell phone number from Jorge and left a message in
Spanish for her, letting her know that he was working with her son. Ms.
Achara was so relieved to hear from someone who spoke her language that
she returned the intern's call that afternoon. She explained that she worked
in a factory and was no longer able to get off during the day to attend school
meetings. He offered to arrange to meet with her and her son in the evening
at his university's training clinic.

She arrived a half hour late for the meeting and explained that she had
to wait until her husband, Jorge's stepfather, returned from work because he
had the only car in the family. The intern first met with Jorge and his mother
together, joined with each of them, and asked a little about where they were
from. They discussed their Dominican cultural background and eagerly
reported that they planned to "go home" to the Dominican Republic soon
for Christmas. The counselor asked about her relatives back home and she

talked about her large extended family including her three older children. He asked who was here to support her and her son and she reported that it was just her husband and some friends.

The mother then explained her relief that the counselor spoke Spanish. She expressed her frustration at not being able to understand the teachers and counselors at the school and she spoke of her worries about her son. Ms. Achara explained that he had always been active and that it was hard to get him to sit still and listen at home and in school. The counselor asked her to talk with Jorge about her concerns. Jorge was honest and admitted that it was frustrating for him also. At the end of the session, the intern had joined well and established therapeutic rapport with both Ms. Achara and Jorge. They both agreed to meet weekly to address the issues that Jorge was facing at school. The therapist also introduced the possibility that Jorge's stepfather might join the sessions. Although both mother and son expressed doubt at this suggestion, the seed had been planted for the future.

This case illustrates one of the greatest frustrations shared by clients and families of many different ethnic and cultural backgrounds when they immigrate to the United States speaking only their native language and little English. In some cases, interpreters are available, but in many hospitals, clinics, agencies, and schools the availability of interpreters is haphazard at best. Often, anyone who speaks the same language is asked to serve as translator, regardless of training or understanding of the treatment process. This is a common occurrence when family members (often parents and grandparents) attend school meetings or therapy sessions. In this case, the mother knew only a few words and phrases in English and was unable to understand her son's teachers and counselors. Another complication is that poor and working poor families often do not have jobs that allow them the flexibility to take time off from work during the day in order to attend important meetings regarding their children. The use of children or adolescents as interpreters for their parents in these situations is also highly problematic (McGoldrick et al., 2005). As discussed above, it reverses the generational boundaries and places parents in an awkward and difficult position. In some circumstances, it exposes children to the private issues of their parents in inappropriate ways.

There has been some response to a necessity for interpreters in hospital settings. Some major hospitals now employ interpreters who can participate in medical consultations, as well as mental health and social service meetings. Yet difficulties remain in terms of preparation and training. There are no professional standards for interpreters. In addition, some clients have confidentiality concerns when translators live in the same community. A further complication is that, as with Jorge's mother in the case above, some Latina(o)s are deferential to authority figures, such as school officials and medical personnel, and may be reluctant to mention their concerns directly. In Jorge's mother's case, she simply stopped coming to meetings.

As indicated above, this case also speaks to the importance of recruiting and training clinicians from Latino, Asian, and other ethnic groups who are fluent in the languages of their clients as well as familiar with their cultural values. Schools and training programs cannot passively wait for these individuals to appear and apply. Recruitment of bilingual students and practitioners is often necessary in all positions ranging from undergraduate programs to master's and doctoral programs to professional mental health staff.

It is also important for therapists to recognize that some of our words and concepts from different evidence-based models and other theoretical orientations may be understandable in English, but may not translate easily into other languages. This may lead to confusion when translations are made. For example, a young clinician working as a multisystemic (Henggeler & Borduin, 1990; Henggeler & Santos, 1997) therapist discovered through trial and error that he had to translate the word behavior in different ways depending on the dialect of Spanish that his clients spoke. At times, even the Spanish translations of these words were not easily understandable depending on the educational level of the client or the parent. This type of situation can occur for therapists working with immigrant clients from many different ethnic backgrounds who may not be fluent in English. In these situations, it is important that therapists are cautious about the use of jargon and technical terms.

Working with Asian Clients and Families

While displaying some similarities, Asian clients are diverse in terms of country of origin (China, Japan, Korea, the Philippines, Cambodia, Laos, Indonesia, and Vietnam, among others), language and dialects, history, political experiences and viewpoints, socioeconomic level, immigration experiences, and cultural and religious or spiritual practices (McGoldrick et al., 2005). (The experiences of South Asian clients including Indian, Pakistani, and Bangladeshi are somewhat different and will be discussed in a separate section below.) There are also often major differences in acculturation, even within the same family.

Much of the multicultural literature on Asian clients and families has focused on recent immigrants from traditional cultural backgrounds. As is the case with many African American and Latino clients, close family involvement is common among many Asian clients. In order to treat these clients, it is essential to understand the cultural and family experiences that may have shaped their lives. Lee (1997) and Lee and Mock (2005) have identified five different types of Asian families that may help clinicians to have a better understanding of their clients from these backgrounds. Although originally developed to describe Asian clients and families, we have found these distinctions to be helpful in our work with clients from other cultural backgrounds and ethnicities who share an immigrant background.

The first type of family is the *traditional family*. Lee and Mock (2005) have described these:

> Traditional families usually consist entirely of individuals born and raised in Asian countries. They include families from agricultural backgrounds, recent arrivals with limited exposure to Western culture, unacculturated immigrants who are deeply steeped in their home culture at the time of immigration, and families who live in ethnic Asian communities (e.g., Chinatown, Little Saigon, Korea town, Japan town), having limited contact with American mainstream society. Tending to be elders, these family members hold strong beliefs and traditional values and regularly speak in their native languages and dialects. (pp. 275–276)

Many of our clients in mental health centers are from the second type, *families in culture conflict*. The conflict may manifest between parents and children or between spouses at different levels of acculturation:

> These families have either American-born children or children who were quite young when they arrived with their parents more than a decade ago. The family system usually experiences a great deal of cultural conflict between acculturated children and traditional parents and grandparents. Intergenerational conflicts and role confusion in which, for example, parents are reliant on their children to communicate with others in English are common problems. Some families have conflicts because one spouse is more acculturated than the other. For instance, a husband may have lived in the United States for many years and eventually marries a wife from the home country who is not familiar with American culture. (Lee & Mock, 2005, p. 276)

The third type, *bicultural families*, are often quite different culturally in terms of education, urbanization, and socioeconomic status, and are often bilingual or multilingual. These clients frequently may have privileged backgrounds and may not face some of the same adjustments as the two types of families described above:

Bicultural families consist of well-acculturated parents who grew up in major Asian cities and who were exposed to urbanization, industrialization, and Western influences. Many came to this country as young adults. Some were born in the United States but raised in traditional families. These parents often hold professional jobs, come from middle- or upper-class family backgrounds and are bilingual and bicultural. . . . These families typically do not live within their own ethnic neighborhoods. (Lee & Mock, 2005, p. 276)

Many of the fourth types of clients, described as part of *Americanized* or *highly acculturated families,* have grown up in the United States in White, middle-class communities. Some may identify as "American" and may have no connection to the Asian part of their roots or identities:

Some Asian families have become highly acculturated, adopting largely mainstream American ways. They usually consist of parents and children born and raised in the United States. As generations pass, the roots of traditional Asian cultures slowly recede, and individual members may not express interest in or make any effort to maintain their ethnic identities. Families communicate in English and may even adopt a more individualistic and egalitarian orientation. In many ways, they stress the American aspects of their identities and may not identify with their Asian roots or may do so only after deep consideration and exploration. (Lee & Mock, 2005, p. 276)

The fifth and final type of client comes from what Lee and Mock (2005) have called *new millennium families.* Lee (1997), in a prior work, referred to many of these families as *interracial families*:

As testimony to dynamic changes in cultural identity, new millennium families may be described as those going beyond any prior set norms or standards. Members of these families may call into question prior cultural expectations and are forging new identities. Lee (1997) previously described these families as "interracial families," noting the increasing number of multiracial Asian American families and interracial relationships, especially among Japanese, Filipino, Chinese, Vietnamese, and Korean Americans. Some multiracial families are able to integrate their multiple cultures with a high degree of success. Others may experience clashes in values, conflicts in communication styles, differences in managing societal pressures, and identity confusion. (p. 277)

As Asian clients come from such diverse family environments and may present with different issues, it is important for therapists who are working with clients individually to be able to assume the asking stance (Cave, as cited in Salerno et al., 2007, 2008b), described above, and inquire about their family and cultural backgrounds. In one case, for example, a young Asian man was referred to a clinician at a hospital-based outpatient clinic for individual therapy. Because of his Asian appearance, the therapist assumed an immigrant background. When she asked where he was from, he responded, much to her surprise, "San Francisco." Undaunted, the therapist persisted, and said, "Yes, and where were your parents and grandparents from?" To her further surprise, her client revealed that his family had lived in the San Francisco area since his great-grandparents emigrated from Japan. He had been born in San Francisco and later moved with his family to a middle-class White suburb and maintained no conscious connection to Japanese culture. His experience was an illustration of the fourth type of family discussed above—*Americanized* or *highly acculturated.*

The following case illustrates some of the challenges faced by a therapist working with a Chinese American man from a traditional family who was experiencing a number of culture conflicts with his parents and grandparents.

David Wong, a 19-year-old Chinese American college student, was referred by his academic advisor to the university counseling center. His advisor was concerned because David, who had previously been an excellent student, was now getting mediocre grades. He was also experiencing a great deal of anxiety about declaring his major—a decision that had to be made as he was at the end of his sophomore year. At the counseling center, David was referred to Mary, a 28-year-old White female psychologist.

In the first session, Mary focused on joining and establishing therapeutic rapport with David. He explained that he was embarrassed at having been referred for counseling. He felt a great deal of embarrassment at his declining grades and was afraid that he would bring shame to his parents and other family members. Mary encouraged David to tell her about his family and their expectations of him. David explained that his parents had moved from China to Hong Kong before he was born. His family came to America when he was 3 in order to make a better life for him and his newborn sister. They had always been focused on their children's education and had made many sacrifices for them. When Mary explored their expectations further, David became anxious and explained that his family wanted him to become a doctor or an engineer in conformance with the cultural norm that he be a "model minority." David hated science but received excellent grades until the courses became more difficult. He described himself as a "failure" and he talked about bringing shame on his family because he could no longer achieve the "A's" that his parents expected.

When Mary asked what subjects David had enjoyed most in college, he seemed uncomfortable at the question and answered, "I don't know." Later in the session, he described his love of art and his desire to paint, but he quickly added that pursuing this interest would be totally unacceptable to his family.

At the end of the session, Mary asked David what he thought about the session. He responded that he was not sure and asked her what he should do. The therapist responded that they could discuss this together and explore what he wanted to do. David did not return for a second session, however, and attempts to contact him were not successful.

David's dilemma is a common one for Asian college students. Their families, particularly their parents, have sacrificed a great deal to come to this country to give their children educational opportunities. In return, parents expect respect, obedience, and filial piety (Lee & Mock, 2005). The possibility of not fulfilling parental expectations can result in shame and loss of face, not just for the young man or woman but also for his or her parents and entire family.

Working with Gay and Lesbian Asian Clients

The cultural imperative not to cause one's family loss of face and shame can also lead to serious consequences for some Asian clients. The following case illustrates how these issues led a gay adolescent to become suicidal.

Mark Mun, a 17-year-old Korean male adolescent, was attending one of the top high schools in his city. His grades had been good during his first 2 years, but during his junior year they had begun to decline. Throughout the year, his teachers and fellow students had noticed that he seemed depressed and withdrawn. In January of that year, he attempted suicide by taking an overdose of pills. His parents found him in his room and called an ambulance. He was rushed to the hospital and, after medical treatment, was admitted to the inpatient adolescent psychiatric unit. Initially, Mark was withdrawn and guarded. His assigned therapist, Matt, was a young White male. Matt took his time and joined and established therapeutic rapport with Mark. They talked about the things that were most important to Mark and, as they developed trust, they began to discuss the reasons for his suicidal gesture.

Mark's parents had sacrificed a great deal to move to this country and to provide a good education for Mark and his younger brother and sister. Neither of his parents had much education in Korea and spoke little English. Nonetheless, Mark explained that they had high expectations for him, such as going into the sciences, getting a great job, marrying a Korean woman, and caring for his parents and grandparents as they aged. He explained to his therapist that he felt he owed his parents filial piety, respect, and obedience because of all of their sacrifices for him.

Then Mark revealed a major secret to Matt that he had told no one else. He was gay and, prior to his hospitalization, he had just broken up with his first male lover. He explained that he and his partner, a senior at his high school, had kept their relationship secret from their families and everyone at school. Mark cried as he explained to his therapist the shame and loss of face he would bring to his parents and family if they learned he was gay. In addition to the violation of cultural norms, his parents were churchgoing Christians and their minister preached against gay relationships. He was afraid that if he told his parents that he was gay, they would not only reject him but would be destroyed.

Matt knew a Korean American psychologist in private practice and consulted with him about the cultural issues involved. He confirmed the issues of shame and loss of face that were so important for people in this culture. Matt was torn because the average stay on the acute inpatient unit was about 1 to 2 weeks (dictated by the real-world demands of managed care guidelines) and it was standard practice to invite the family in for therapy sessions and to begin to discuss discharge plans that, given Mark's status as a minor, would involve his parents. When Matt apprised Mark of this standard procedure, his client became agitated. He was concerned that the therapist would tell his parents about his sexual orientation and that they would reject him.

The Korean American psychologist offered to do a consult with Matt and Mark. During that session, Mark again emphasized that knowledge of his sexual orientation would cause great shame and loss of face for his parents and would "destroy" his relationship with them. He was thus unwilling to discuss these issues with his parents in the family session at the hospital. With this in mind, the psychologist and Matt discussed with Mark the possibility of his continuing to work with the psychologist in outpatient treatment after his discharge in the coming week. The psychologist attended a final family session with the parents before Mark's discharge and was able to join with them about their concern that his grades for the school year might be impacted by his depression, suicidal gesture, and the hospitalization. They agreed that Mark would continue to see the psychologist when he was released from the hospital. At the psychologist's request, they also agreed to come in for family sessions regularly.

Mark continued in outpatient treatment with the psychologist. During his senior year of high school, Mark discussed his conflict between his sexual orientation and his family's cultural values. The therapist had a number of family therapy sessions with Mark and his family that focused primarily on their concerns about his academic work. The psychologist joined with Mark's parents around their concerns about his academic achievement, an issue that he knew was primary for many Korean parents. Mark's grades began to improve and he completed college applications. His depression lifted, and he had no further suicidal ideation.

Mark explored his options about whether to reveal his sexual orientation to his parents or family members. He was concerned about them, but role-played with his therapist different ways to tell them if he decided to do so. Despite his continued ambivalence, after 1 year of outpatient treatment Mark agreed to have a discussion with his parents about his sexual orientation in a family session with the psychologist present and participating. His parents were stunned and angry, and refused to accept Mark's sexual orientation or to discuss it with him any further. They refused to return for family therapy sessions despite repeated attempts to schedule meetings. In all future interactions, they acted as if the disclosure had never been made. Mark shared with the psychologist that his parents had experienced loss of face and intense shame by the discussion of his sexual orientation in the presence of the psychologist, a reaction that the psychologist had anticipated might occur and had discussed with Mark before the family session.

Mark's status in his family improved when he received acceptance to a prestigious Ivy League university. This achievement delighted his parents. He made the decision to attend and to explore his sexual orientation and relationships with men while in college. The psychologist helped him to arrange a referral to a therapist at the counseling center at his university and Mark continued in treatment throughout his college years. Mark also decided that there were many reasons for him to respect his parents' wishes and retreat from any discussions with them about his sexual orientation. Filial piety, respect for his parents, and family loyalty were important values in his culture. His family was essential to him. He talked openly about not wanting to bring shame upon his parents or family members. Throughout his college years, he kept his relationships with men a secret from his family—the price he felt he had to pay in order to continue to relate to and engage with them.

This case presents a number of complex treatment issues that are common in work with clients from traditional Asian families. Connection and loyalty to the family is an important cultural value. In addition, Liu and Chan (1996), in their discussion of treatment issues with lesbian, gay, and bisexual Asian Americans, state:

> Exploring sexuality in relation to LGBAAs [lesbian, gay, and bisexual Asian Americans] can be a challenge, since a cultural prohibition surrounds the entire topic. Same-sex sexual behavior, awareness, and identification are shrouded in secrecy, stigma, and sometimes overwhelming power of cultural expectations. In East Asia, homosexual

activity is almost universally "underground" and is rarely disclosed to society at large. (p. 137)

Consistent with his Asian cultural values, Mark was loyal to his parents and family and was afraid that the process of coming out to them would result in a loss of face for the entire family. He also feared their rejection—a fate he felt both inevitable and intolerable.

The question of whether to come out to family members, particularly parents, can cause major conflicts for LGB Asian youth. Liu and Chan (1996) have found that Asian gay and lesbian clients from more acculturated families are more likely to come out to their families. They have indicated that although families may initially reject the children, continued contact may eventually lessen opposition from parents.

Other clients of Asian heritage, like Mark, who are from traditional families, may "often feel caught between East Asian and Western influences and may have difficulty integrating their LGB identities with their ethnic identities" (Liu & Chan, 1996, p. 144). These clients may make the same choice Mark did, and "keep their LGB social, romantic, and sexual world completely secret and separate from their families and their East Asian community" (Liu & Chan, 1996, p. 144).

The issue of secrecy can present a complex dilemma for therapists. Those who follow Western psychological values may consider that their objective is to help clients to open up secrets and, thus, to come out to their families. This may seem to be an unsatisfactory option to some clients. Others, like Mark, may make the attempt to come out and then retreat when confronted by their family's discouraging response. Despite his misgivings, Mark, with his therapist's help, came out to his family, but after their initial anger they chose to ignore his disclosure. He found a solution that worked for him—by keeping his gay sexual orientation and relationships separate from his family, he could maintain his close ties with them and his culture.

Many therapists have struggled when clients make the decision not to disclose their gay sexual orientation or same-sex partner to their family. Although it is certainly not an ideal resolution, it is important for clinicians to recognize that for some Asian clients from traditional families, secrecy and living a double life may be the only alternative acceptable to them.

The dilemma that Matt, the therapist on the acute inpatient unit, felt when confronted with his client's adamant refusal to disclose to his parents that conflicts over his sexual orientation and his fears about his family's response had led to his suicidal gesture, also represents a major challenge. The therapist on the inpatient unit worked to connect Mark to a Korean outpatient psychologist who would continue to work with him after discharge. It took almost a year of such outpatient treatment before Mark could raise this issue with his parents. In the real world, this luxury of the time necessary to resolve such complex and culturally laden issues is often not available given that the mental health system is so dependent upon insurance company reimbursement schedules. An acute inpatient hospital stay of 7 to 14 days would hardly have allowed Mark to resolve his struggle with the conflict over disclosing his sexual orientation given his parents' cultural values and his concerns about causing them shame and loss of face.

Working with Asian Indian Clients and Families

Clients from Asian Indian families present with many similar issues to those of East Asian clients discussed above. There are, however, major differences in terms of history, culture, immigration patterns, skin color variations, expectations of arranged marriages, social, economic, and religious or spiritual beliefs (Almeida, 2005; Nath, 2005; Pillari, 2005). India is a diverse country, with "18 official languages, including English, and about 1,652 mother tongues/dialects" (Pillari, 2005, p. 395). There are also a wide range of religious practices including Hindu, Sikh, and Muslim. Similar to the different types of Asian family backgrounds mentioned above, Indian clients vary greatly in terms of their level of acculturation in the United States, caste, and socioeconomic class. As Pillari has indicated, in India it is common for large extended families to live in the same home or close by. As families have migrated to the United States, they often gravitate to smaller households, frequently either restricted to the nuclear family or including a few extended family members.

One issue that has been complicated for Indian clients in the United States has been the cultural expectation of the arranged marriage (Almeida, 2005; Pillari, 2005; Rathor, 2011). In traditional Indian society, marriage is considered a union of two families rather than two individuals. For generations in India, families have chosen spouses for their children based on relationships with and knowledge of other families in their community. In America, serious family issues may arise, particularly if adult children fall in love with someone who is not from the family's religious or cultural group or caste, or is not Indian. This can lead to major problems and critical mental health issues. The case below illustrates this dilemma.

Priya, a 28-year-old Hindu Indian woman, entered treatment at the encouragement of her former college roommate when she became depressed and withdrawn. Initially, she was embarrassed about entering therapy and was concerned about others finding out because of the stigma in her community. Her therapist, Angela, was a White woman with little exposure to Priya's culture. Angela was open and warm and was able to join with Priya and help her to begin to trust the therapist.

Gradually, as the therapeutic relationship grew, the following story emerged. Despite Priya's academic achievements and career as a pharmacist, she felt that she had let her family down. Priya explained that in her culture, she was already older than the average bride and she was receiving a lot of pressure from her parents and family members to marry. Her parents, both medical doctors, had come to the United States originally to attend college. They were acculturated and had raised Priya with a mixture of Indian and United States mainstream values. They considered themselves progressive and would allow Priya to choose her own husband, as long as he was Indian and Hindu. They had indicated that if she did not choose a husband who met these criteria by her 29th birthday, they would arrange a marriage for her in India.

Priya's dilemma was that she had fallen in love with a colleague, Andrew, a White American pharmacist. She had kept their 2-year relationship a secret from her family. She was sure that her parents would object if she chose to marry him. As Priya's therapist, Angela struggled to understand the cultural expectations that Priya was experiencing. She encouraged Priya to explain her relationship with her parents and their expectations of her. Priya related that she was the oldest daughter. Her sister was 4 years younger and the family expected Priya to marry before her sister. Priya had begun to feel greater anxiety in response to her parents' pressure. They had contacted family members still residing in India to discuss an arranged marriage for her. Her father had even proposed putting an ad in an Indian newspaper or putting an ad on an Indian Internet site. These actions had upset and embarrassed Priya.

Using a motivational interviewing decisional balance strategy (see Chapter 6), her therapist helped Priya to clarify her options and to look at the pros and cons and consequences of each possible choice. The therapist offered to see Priya with her family to discuss the issues, but Priya was horrified at the possibility and refused to have a family session. The therapist also helped Priya to role-play possible scenarios with her parents. Together, they constructed a family genogram or family tree and the therapist explored whom she might discuss this with in her family or extended family. Priya identified a 25-year-old female cousin, a medical resident.

In her discussion with her cousin, Priya learned that Priya's parents had already been in contact with a family from their hometown in India about arranging a marriage between Priya and their son. Priya panicked and indicated that she felt she could no longer avoid talking with her parents lest they actually arrange this marriage for her. She went to their home for dinner and raised the issue. With a great deal of anxiety, she told her parents about her relationship with Andrew and also told them that he had asked her to marry him. Initially, her parents were angry with her. There was a lot of tension over the next few weeks. She talked through her experience with her therapist and expressed her depression over the conflict with her parents. She had a phone conversation with her mother in which they both cried and Priya explained how scared she was about the idea of an arranged marriage to a total stranger.

Priya continued to see Andrew. In April of that year, Priya became pregnant. She and Andrew decided to marry and raise their child together. They had a civil ceremony at city hall, after which she called and notified her parents. They were furious and refused to see her. With her therapist's support, she sent them the announcement when the baby was born along with a picture of their newborn grandson. A week later, her mother called. The door had been opened. It took 6 more months before Priya could convince her parents to come and see the baby. Although things had not been resolved fully, Priya's depression had lifted and she had begun to feel more hopeful. She completed her treatment 2 months later.

This case illustrates one of the challenges for young men and women whose families have emigrated from India. Despite Priya's parents' education in the United States and acculturation, they were insistent that she marry a man from a Hindu Indian background. Rathor (2011), in a qualitative research study interviewing Hindu Indian women between the ages of 25 and 35, discovered that Priya's dilemma is quite common. In fact, traditional families will insist on arranging a marriage with the two young people frequently not meeting one another until shortly before the ceremony. Priya's parents considered themselves "progressive" because they were willing for her to find her own husband with the only stipulation being that he be Indian and Hindu, before they would intervene. In Rathor's study, Hindu Indian women described themselves as "born to be a bride" (p. 39). They explained that many Indian parents often experience a great deal of pressure from their own extended families to arrange a marriage for their daughters at a relatively young age (approximately ages 22 to 25, following college) because of concerns about childbearing. Men receive similar pressure but, without the biological imperative of childbearing, they may be given more leeway in terms of age. Nevertheless, by their mid to late 20s, both men and women may experience family anxieties about the issue of the arranged marriage. Family members, particularly parents, may experience a great deal of shame in their extended families and communities if their children are not successfully married by their late 20s.

Conclusion

As this chapter has discussed, clinicians in the real world today will experience clients from a wide range of diverse cultural, ethnic, racial, religious, and socioeconomic backgrounds. They may also encounter clients of lesbian, gay, bisexual, and transgender sexual orientation. Therefore we emphasize throughout this book the importance of assuming an asking stance (Cave, as cited in Salerno et al., 2007, 2008b) with clients in which we do not assume that we "know" our clients' cultural values or beliefs, but convey a respectful curiosity about their values and backgrounds.

As Boyd-Franklin (2003) has indicated, it is important to avoid stereotyping our clients. While some cultural knowledge of clients from different backgrounds may be helpful, it is virtually impossible for clinicians to obtain in-depth cultural knowledge about clients and families from all ethnic and racial backgrounds. Boyd-Franklin uses the metaphor of the camera lens (described above) to remind us that we have to adjust the lens for each new client or family. Exploring with clients the built-in supports, strategies, and barriers associated with family and culture can set the groundwork for meaningful treatment. Seeking knowledge about our clients' culture and values through various resources and consultation may help us to better understand their cultural world view, as it applies to their lives and treatment. Much like adjusting the camera lens, however, this knowledge can then be discarded if it is found not to be relevant to our clients' or families' experiences. Through curiosity, flexibility, and a continuous asking stance (Cave, as cited in Salerno et al., 2007, 2008b), we can come to better understand and meet the needs of our diverse clients in the real world, who do not fit neatly into the box of stereotype, but instead present as multifaceted and heterogeneous across a number of domains.

PART II

Core Mediational Processes

CHAPTER 4

Joining and Establishing
the Therapeutic Relationship

Introduction

There is often an emphasis on pathology in the mental health field (Chapin, 2011; Walsh, 1998). Our emphasis throughout this book and in our own work has been on strength-based approaches and competency-based interventions (Brun & Rapp, 2001; Chapin, 2011; Nissen, 2001; Rapp, 1998). These approaches focus on the resiliency of clients (Masten, 2001; Saleebey, 2000; Walsh, 1998, 2006). The challenge for many clinicians involved in real-world practice has been that clients do not present first with their strengths; they present with their problems. Therefore, it is incumbent on the clinician to recognize the strengths of each client and to be able to verbally validate these strengths. Also, as we have discussed throughout this book, another challenge in this work has been that many clinicians have been trained to work with clients who want therapy (Boyd-Franklin, 2003). This can be a disadvantage in working with clients who may not have been self-referred or who may have been mandated to attend therapy. With these concerns in mind, this chapter presents the first core mediational process—joining and establishing a therapeutic relationship.

This chapter begins by examining the importance of joining and establishing a therapeutic alliance for treatment outcome. We will distill some of the more critical elements in achieving a strong working alliance and will examine factors including therapist empathy, positive regard and affirmation, genuineness and authenticity, and attitudes and values. The use of mindfulness by the therapist as a way of staying present in the relationship will also be discussed. In this chapter we highlight the importance of taking a strength-based approach in joining with a client or family and discuss the importance of emphasizing the client's resilience in the initial stages of treatment. Finally, we end with a discussion of the difference between empowering a client and advocating on his or her behalf, and the impact that this can have on setting the parameters of the therapeutic relationship and on a client's self-efficacy.

Joining and Establishing the Therapeutic Alliance and the Therapeutic Relationship

Joining, a term that is common in the family systems literature, refers to the initial stage of therapy in which the clinician establishes therapeutic rapport with the client or family (Boyd-Franklin, 2003; Boyd-Franklin & Bry, 2000a; S. Minuchin, 1974). On a basic level, Haley (1976) described this process as a social stage in which the therapist gets to know the client or family before problems are discussed. It is not just important in the initial phases of therapy but can be helpful throughout the treatment process. Boyd-Franklin and Bry (2000a) encourage therapists through the statement "When in doubt, join." They argue that therapists may make the mistake of assuming "buy-in" from their clients and "getting down to business" too quickly in the first session (p. 39). They note that the first session might be spent in getting to know the client(s) and helping them to feel comfortable in the presence of the therapist. These clients initially may not see therapy as a vehicle for change or enter the treatment process with a readiness to take action to solve their problems. This chapter provides an overview of the process of building a therapeutic relationship. For some clients who are new to therapy, the initial stages can also help them to understand the process of therapy and how it can help. (In Chapter 5, we discuss the process of psychoeducation and recovery principles in psychotherapy with all clients.) McKay and Bannon (2004) provide an excellent overview of strategies for engagement of families including changes to clinic intake procedures, training for staff on engagement from first contact, and including input from those served into the development of policies and procedures (Gopalan et al., 2010; McKay & Bannon, 2004).

This chapter's premise is consistent with Prochaska and DiClemente's transtheoretical stages of change model (Prochaska & DiClemente, 1982; Prochaska, DiClemente, & Norcross, 1992). They argue that therapists often make the mistake of assuming that the client is committed to using therapy to produce behavioral change. This can lead therapists to plunge into interventions that focus on action and behavior change when a client is still at the *precontemplation* level and has not yet acknowledged that there is a problem (see Chapter 6).

The issue of joining with the client in the beginning of therapy is important in establishing the therapeutic alliance and building the therapeutic relationship. As we have emphasized throughout this book, research has repeatedly shown that the establishment of the therapeutic relationship is one of the most important variables in treatment outcome, regardless of the theoretical orientation of the clinician or the treatment modality (i.e., cognitive behavioral, psychodynamic, humanistic, family systems, group dynamics, etc.; Norcross, 2011a). Gaztambide (2011), in his review of research on the therapeutic alliance within treatment, reinforces these observations:

> After decades of ongoing controversy and research, the therapeutic alliance remains one of the most robust predictors of outcome in psychotherapy research, regardless of treatment modality or theoretical orientation (Horvath & Bedi, 2002; Horvath & Symonds, 1991; Martin, Garske, & Davis, 2000, Orlinsky, Grawe, & Parks, 1994). Complementing this finding are an increasing number of studies examining the relationship between symptom improvement and the strength of the therapeutic alliance, concluding in turn that development and growth of the alliance precedes as well as predicts symptom improvement (Baldwin, Wampold, & Imel, 2007; Crits-Christoph, Connolly-Gibbons, & Hearon, 2006; Crits-Christoph et al., 2011; Klein et al., 2003; Norcross & Wampold, 2011; Zuroff & Blatt, 2006). Furthermore, clinicians who establish stronger alliances earlier in treatment, and are able to maintain them, show better outcomes than therapists whose alliances with their clients are not strong (Baldwin et al., 2007; Klein et al., 2003). (p. 1)

These findings confirm the long-held belief in the mental health field that establishing a positive therapeutic relationship between the clinician and the client is central to therapeutic outcome. Norcross (2011a), in the second edition of his book *Psychotherapy Relationships That Work,* provides meta-analyses of numerous research studies that draw the conclusion that clearly a positive therapeutic relationship is essential to therapeutic success. Norcross and Lambert (2010) argue that "The therapeutic relationship accounts for why clients improve (or fail to improve) as much as the particular treatment method" (p. 1). They also state that "efforts to promulgate best practices or evidence-based practices (EBPs) without including the relationship are incomplete and potentially misleading" (p. 1). Consistent with the work of Norcross (2011a), numerous researchers have provided meta-analyses of the importance of therapeutic alliances in many forms of psychotherapy and have found similar results in child and adolescent psychotherapy (Shirk & Karver, 2011), couple and family therapy (Friedlander, Escudero, Heatherington, & Diamond, 2011), and in group therapy (Burlingame, McClendon, & Alonso, 2011).

Horvath, Del Re, Flückiger, and Symonds (2010, 2011), in their meta-analytic review of the concept of therapeutic alliance in individual psychotherapy, found that the core consensus of many definitions of therapeutic alliance was that "the alliance is an emergent quality of partnership and mutual collaboration between therapist and client" (Horvath et al., 2010, p. 5). They argue that the establishment of this therapeutic alliance is not separate from the techniques that the therapist implements, rather that "It is influenced by and is an essential, inseparable part of everything that happens in therapy" (p. 5). Since clients and therapists may view the therapeutic alliance in different ways, they recommend that clinicians monitor the client's experience of this alliance throughout therapy (Horvath et al., 2010, 2011). Specifically they note that a crucial element in establishing a strong therapeutic alliance is the ability of the therapist to learn to respond nondefensively to a client's anger or resistance to therapy (Horvath et al., 2010, 2011). (See Chapter 3 on the issues of cross-racial and cross-cultural treatment, as well as the employment of motivational interviewing techniques in Chapter 6.)

 Cognitive and cognitive-behavioral therapists and researchers have also addressed the importance of the therapeutic relationship and its collaborative nature (J. S. Beck, 2011; Meichenbaum, 2008). For example, Young, Rygh, Weinberger, and Beck (2008), in their chapter on "Cognitive Therapy for Depression" in Barlow's (2008) book on evidence-based treatments, address the importance of the collaborative relationship:

> Basic to cognitive therapy is a collaborative relationship between the patient and the therapist. When therapist and patient work together, the learning experience is enhanced for both, and the cooperative spirit that is developed contributes greatly to the treatment process. (p. 266)

Because of the importance of this relationship to the treatment process, Young et al. (2008) have emphasized the interpersonal qualities of the therapist that may contribute to this alliance:

> Because collaboration requires that the patient trust the therapist, we emphasize those interpersonal qualities that contribute to trust. As noted earlier, warmth, accurate empathy, and genuineness are desirable personal qualities for the cognitive therapist, as well as for all psychotherapists. . . . The therapist should be able to communicate

both verbally and nonverbally that he or she is sincere, open, concerned, and direct. (p. 266)

Experienced therapists from cognitive-behavioral (J. S. Beck, 2011, Meichenbaum, 2008), psychodynamic (McWilliams, 1999, 2004, 2011), family therapy (Boyd-Franklin, 2003; Minuchin, 1974; Nichols, 2011), and group therapy (Yalom & Leszcz, 2005) approaches will all recognize these characteristics as desirable ones to nurture in a therapist. Unfortunately, with real-world pressures for short-term treatment and productivity requirements, some new therapists may focus more on learning interventions than on developing the person of the therapist (Aponte, 1994a).

Empathy and the Therapeutic Relationship

Carl Rogers (1980) defined empathy as "the therapist's sensitive ability and willingness to understand the client's thoughts, feelings and struggles from the client's point of view" (p. 85, as cited in Elliot, Bohart, Watson, & Greenberg, 2010, p. 13). In addition, he emphasized it as the "ability to see completely through the client's eyes, to adopt his frame of reference . . . entering the private perceptual world of the other . . . being sensitive, moment by moment, to the changing felt meanings of which he or she is scarcely aware" (p. 142, as cited in Elliott et al., 2010, p. 13).

Therapist empathy has been found to be a crucial indicator of treatment outcome. In their meta-analysis of the relationship between therapist empathy and client success, Elliott et al. (2010; Elliott, Bohart, Watson, & Greenberg, 2011) found that empathy consistently predicted treatment outcome across different theoretical orientations and treatment formats (e.g., individual, group), regardless of levels of client problem severity. These authors also noted that these effects were strongest in both client- and observer-rated empathy. Interestingly, empathy also predicted better outcomes for less experienced therapists (Elliott et al., 2010, p. 13).

Based on their meta-analytic review of empathy, Elliot et al. (2010) recommend the following:

- It is important for psychotherapists to make efforts to understand their clients' experiences and to demonstrate this understanding through responses that address the client needs as the client perceives them.
- Empathic therapists do not parrot clients' words back or reflect

only the content of those words; instead they understand overall goals and moment-to-moment experiences.

- Empathic responses can take many forms, including straightforward responses that convey understanding of the client experience, but also responses that validate the client's perspective, that try to bring the client's experience to life using evocative language, or that aim at what is implicit but not yet expressed in words.
- Therapists should neither assume that they are mind readers nor that their understanding of the client will be matched by clients feeling understood.
- Finally, because research has shown empathy to be inseparable from the other relational conditions, therapists should seek to offer empathy in a context of authentic caring for the client. (p. 13)

Thus, research has confirmed what Carl Rogers first presented in the 1950s—that is, that empathy for the client is an essential factor in establishing a positive therapeutic relationship between therapist and client and that it can have a significant impact on successful treatment outcomes (Rogers, 1951, 1980). The following case illustrates these issues.

Leonard, a 45-year-old African American man diagnosed with schizophrenia, arrived at his initial appointment with the therapist upset and angry. He proceeded to express extreme anger at anyone from his mother, his siblings, to the crossing guard on the street who he felt treated him with disrespect. He then complained that he had to wait an extra 5 minutes before he was seen today, and accused the therapist of only caring about her paycheck. The therapist initially felt fearful, threatened, and defensive and had the compulsion to set limits, defend herself, and effectively silence Leonard. However, she recognized the importance of establishing a relationship with the client and intervening in a way that would validate and empathize with Leonard's experience. She stated, "I get the sense that you often feel misunderstood and not taken seriously." Leonard felt heard by this statement and, as a result, participated more calmly in the session.

Positive Regard and Affirmation

Farber and Doolin (2010, 2011), in their meta-analytic review of the issues of positive regard and affirmation, drew their initial definition of these factors from the seminal work of Carl Rogers (1951):

Carl Rogers (1951), the founder of client-centered therapy, did not believe that a therapist's neutrality, dispassionate stance, or intellectual understanding could facilitate a client's growth, no matter how astute the interpretations. Instead, he believed that treating clients in a consistently warm, supportive, highly regarding manner would enable them to grow psychologically and to reduce their suffering. Rogers' notion of positive regard is embodied in two questions he posed: "Do we tend to treat individuals as persons of worth, or do we subtly devaluate them by our attitudes and behavior? Is our philosophy one in which respect for the individual is uppermost?" (p. 20). This caring attitude has most often been termed positive regard, but early studies and theoretical writings preferred the phrase _nonpossessive warmth_.

In his famous filmed work with Gloria (Shostrom, 1965), Rogers struggled to find a single phrase to illuminate this concept. It is, he said, "Real spontaneous praising; you can call that quality acceptance, you can call it caring, you can call it non-possessive love. Any of those terms tend to describe it." (Farber & Doolin, 2010, p. 17)

In their meta-analysis of 18 studies on positive regard, Farber and Doolin (2010) found that positive regard was a significant part of establishing the therapeutic relationship and effected client outcome. One interesting finding of their meta-analysis was the indication that "Positive regard may be especially useful in situations where a nonminority psychotherapist is working with a racial/ethnic minority client" (p. 18; see Chapter 3). Not surprisingly, Farber and Doolin (2010, 2011) also discovered that it is important for therapists to share their positive feelings and to communicate them directly to clients. Research shows that the belief that their therapists cared about them seemed to have been particularly crucial when clients were experiencing stress in their lives. This is evident in the following case.

Marylin, a 37-year-old White woman with a long history of depression, isolation, and abusive relationships, came to a session after about a year of therapy feeling particularly down and hopeless about the future. She expressed doubt about the future and her capacity to withstand her painful experiences. The therapist tuned into his own feelings of discouragement and checked the urge to talk Marylin out of her depressive experience. Rather, he reflected on their relationship and offered, "I hear that you are really down and feel defeated. Can I offer you some feedback? I've watched you over the last year battle through in ways that I can't help but admire. You've committed to the therapy process, even when it felt hard to engage in it, and you have taken steps in your life that are nothing short of courageous. The proof for this, Marylin, is that you are sitting here, telling me how much you are struggling, and yet you came today and had enough trust in this relationship to share something that feels really hurtful."

Genuineness and Authenticity

Another important aspect of the therapeutic relationship is the "mindful genuineness on the part of the therapist, underscoring personal awareness as well as authenticity" (Kolden, Klein, Wang, & Austin, 2010, p. 12). The therapeutic relationship may be a unique one for some clients. Some do not experience many genuine relationships in which they feel accepted and valued. Kolden et al. discuss the importance of congruence in the relationship between the therapist and the client. They state that "An effective therapist *models* congruence. This may involve self-disclosure as well as sharing of thoughts and feelings, opinions, pointed questions, and feedback regarding client behavior. Congruent responses are honest; they are not disrespectful, overly intellectualized or insincere" (p. 13). With this in mind, it is important that therapists remain emotionally honest with their clients without being heavy-handed or critical in their responses. Many of these qualities of the therapeutic relationship are consistent with mindfulness concepts discussed below. The following case illustrates many of these concepts.

Luis, a 34-year-old Latino firefighter, was among the first responders to the World Trade Center site on 9/11. Since the tragedy, Luis had been experiencing PTSD [posttraumatic stress disorder] symptoms in the form nightmares, flashbacks, numbing, and hypervigilance. Luis entered treatment after he felt the need to leave his squad and retire due to his symptomatic experience and being constantly triggered by his environment. In a particularly powerful session, Luis demanded to know from the therapist when he was going to feel better, and expressed frustration with his continued symptomatic experience despite his leaving the force in order to get away from triggers. The therapist felt caught between wanting to assuage Luis's anxious attempt for control with the reality of the uncertainty inherent to the healing process. The therapist couldn't help but feel a sense of hopelessness and used that experience to connect with Luis and deepen the work. "Luis," he offered, "I can feel how excruciatingly painful this is for you. I too relate to your desire and need to have immediate answers. The truth is, I wish I could give you immediate answers, but I can't. What you experienced on 9/11 was unimaginable, and I don't think anybody can make sense of it. I can't immediately take away your pain. What I do know, is that I am willing to sit with you and go through this process with you. I am confident that you can achieve some sense of peace and resolution." ✗

Attitudes toward Clients
and the Clinician's Relational Stance

Madsen (2007) argues that the attitudes that therapists hold toward their clients and the relational stance that they maintain are two major factors in successful therapy. In addition to all of the factors discussed above, the respect for clients and the hope that therapists bring to the therapeutic relationship are also powerful factors for change (Meichenbaum, 2008). Although his work has focused on collaborative therapy with multistressed families, his approach is relevant for the development of all client–therapist relationships. Madsen encourages clinicians to assume a relational stance of an appreciative ally:

> The stance of an appreciative ally is characterized by the active cultivation of respect, connection, curiosity, and hope. Four commitments that support the development of an allied stance include striving for cultural curiosity and honoring [client and] family expertise, believing in possibilities and building on [client and] family and community resourcefulness, working in partnership and fitting services to [clients and] families, and engaging in empowering processes and making our work accountable to clients. These commitments help us to maintain this type of relational stance. Our relational stance reflects "how we are" with clients. (p. 44)

Madsen (2007) argues throughout his book that the installation of hope and the ability to see the hope inherent in the client's situation is one of the greatest gifts that a therapist can provide. His work offers a conceptual and clinical framework for understanding the difficulties that our clients face in "nonblaming nonshaming ways" (p. 46). He encourages a collaborative assessment process with clients that focuses on strengths and resourcefulness. He states that throughout the process of therapy,

> it is important to keep in mind that the attitude with which we conduct assessments is a powerful intervention (Madsen, 1998). It is important that we conduct assessments in a friendly, positive atmosphere, that we use normal everyday language, that we maintain a hopeful view of clients and families, that we acknowledge their expertise on their lives, and that we attempt to put ourselves in their shoes and conduct ourselves in ways in which we would want others to treat

us. Finally, it is important to keep in mind the honor and privilege of
★ being allowed to enter people's lives. (p. 86)

It is this relational stance, coupled with the factors discussed above, that
create the foundation for a positive therapeutic relationship as illustrated
in the case below.

Carl, a 27-year-old White male and recent graduate from an MSW program, was working in a community mental health center serving a primarily
African American client population. He was assigned to work with an African American family consisting of a 38-year-old father, a 28-year-old stepmother, and four children ranging from 4 to 16 years of age. In their first
session together, the father looked at Carl with apprehension and stated,
"Are you going to try and tell me that you can help my family? I need some-
body who's going to be able to understand us." Carl was taken aback and
felt the need to justify his abilities as a therapist. However, rather than being
defensive, Carl decided to approach the father from the position of an ally.
"You know what, you are right. There is a lot I don't know about your
family and the things that you have encountered. In fact, I'd be doing you a
disservice if I didn't own up to this at the outset. My role here is to pair up
with you, hear your story, so we can figure out, together, how to help you
and your family move forward in a way that is best for you."

Mindfulness and the Therapeutic Relationship

Within the last 10 years, there has been a growing interest in the role of
mindfulness in establishing the therapeutic relationship. (See Chapter 8
for a more extensive discussion of the use of mindfulness and acceptance
principles and practices.) Hick (2010) and Hick and Bien (2010) have
argued that mindfulness practice can be used as a vehicle for training
mental health professionals to "cultivate empathy and compassion and
develop a sense of presence or listening skills" (p. 4). Hick has described
mindfulness as "focusing attention, being aware, intentionality, being
non-judgmental, acceptance, and compassion" (p. 5). Within the therapeutic relationship, mindfulness is seen as a "way of paying attention
with empathy, presence, and deep listening that can be cultivated, sustained and integrated into our work as therapists" (p. 5). Some authors
have encouraged therapists to learn and develop their own mindfulness
meditative practice in order to help them with this process (Gehart &
McCollum, 2010; Hick, 2010; Hick & Bien, 2010; Shafir, 2010).

Others have taught mindfulness practices with nonmeditative
mindfulness-based exercises (Wilson & Dufrene, 2010). Dialectical

behavior therapy (Linehan, 1993; Linehan, Cochran, & Kehrer, 2001) and acceptance and commitment therapy (ACT) (Hayes & Smith, 2005; Hayes, Strosahl, & Wilson, 1999, 2011; Hayes et al., 2004) are both examples of nonmeditative mindfulness approaches. (See Chapter 8 for a more in-depth discussion of these mindfulness and acceptance principles and practices.) Mindfulness has been proven effective in helping mental health providers to establish effective therapeutic alliances and relationships with their clients (Bachelor & Horvath, 1999; Kabat-Zinn, 2005). Bowen et al. (2011) and Marlatt et al. (2008) have utilized a mindfulness approach in helping therapists treat addiction. Moore (2009), in her description of the value of mindfulness as a part of training service providers, makes the following observation:

> One of the main messages of the training was the encouragement of care providers to be more present and egalitarian in their relationships to clients—in order to experience more fully the pain of the people they serve in order to better understand them and the underlying message of their client's suffering. When a person is genuinely empathized with, that person feels more fully understood and met in the therapeutic relationship. They feel seen and that in itself is very therapeutic. (p. 2)

One aspect of Carl Rogers's (1957) model was based on the notion of the therapist's role of providing unconditional positive regard to clients. This nonjudgmental therapeutic stance is also central to a mindfulness-based approach to clinical work. Bien (2010) has described this clinical approach as being "warm and accepting, kindly and compassionate without being possessive and without conditions that the client must meet to merit such attention" (p. 40). This is an extremely important concept because one of the traps that therapists can sometimes encounter is the tendency for the clinician to become more invested in change or a particular decision than the client. Therapists are human; they can become frustrated and demoralized if they work with clients toward a particular goal and then the client has a setback or refuses to continue. Bien points out that therapists who feel compassion for their clients must be willing to allow them freedom of choice "including the freedom to make bad choices" (p. 46).

New therapists may begin to feel that they are responsible for change and growth in their clients. This can become a prescription for burnout (see Chapter 15). Some therapists in the course of their work distance from their clients or become indifferent in order to protect themselves from what they feel is the burden of being responsible for someone else. Bien (2010) addresses this dilemma through a mindfulness approach:

rception, however, this is ineffective. It is ineffective because
ice is not a therapeutic stance. But I think it also doesn't
ause when we become indifferent, our clients' difficulties
ɔme an irritation. But if we cultivate equanimous compassion, we
become large enough to take in the client's distress without suffering
because of it ourselves. Because of equanimity, we see clearly that we
cannot control the 40% of the variance accounted for by factors outside of therapy (Lambert, 1992). Deep acknowledgment and acceptance of this reality offer the possibility of both greater peace and an
enhanced ability to be present.

It may also make us more effective. By being mindful, by practicing kindness, compassion, joy, and equanimity, we may enhance our
capacity to be concerned and present without overidentification. . . .
(p. 48)

Equanimity on a basic level is our ability to let go and allow our
clients to chart their own course and make their own difficult decisions
(Bien, 2010). Chapter 8 explores this and other aspects of mindfulness
and the therapeutic relationship in more detail. In addition, in Chapter 15, we explore the therapist's ability to be connected to our clients
through our empathy and compassion without overidentification, which
can lead to compassion fatigue and burnout over time (Dass-Brailsford,
2007). This ability can be an essential component in clinician self-care
and should be an important part of all training programs. Unfortunately, this important element is often neglected or overlooked entirely
in the training of therapists and counselors in all of the mental health
disciplines. It is certainly mentioned as important but young therapists
need to be given the tools to create this balance in their work. (See Chapter 8 for a discussion of this and of the process of mindful listening
[Shafir, 2010].)

Strength-Based Approaches
and Competency-Based Interventions

As stated above, there has been a shift from the more pathology-focused
emphasis in the mental health field to a strength-based and competency-
based approach (Barnard, 1994; Walsh, 1998). This has also been evident across modalities of treatment and theoretical orientations (Brun &
Rapp, 2001; Nissen, 2001). This approach has been based on the human
capacity to demonstrate strengths even in the midst of adverse situations (Walsh, 1998, 2006). As noted above, the strength-based model
is particularly important because many clients do not present first with
their strengths; often it is their problems that command our attention

(Walsh, 1998, 2006). For example, many ethnic minority clients living in poor communities may be overwhelmed not only by their own personal or family problems but also by systemic issues such as poverty, homelessness, substandard housing, unsafe neighborhoods, violence, gangs, racial profiling by the police, unemployment, and so on. With this is mind, it is crucial that therapists learn to recognize personal, familial, cultural, and community strengths and to label and verbalize them for our clients (see Chapter 3).

The National Alliance on Mental Illness (NAMI) and the Family Alliance on Mental Illness (FAMI) have worked to explore the experiences, strengths, and resiliency of clients with various levels of serious mental illness. These organizations have worked to help these clients lead normal lives and obtain the assistance that they need to do so. NAMI has also worked to help family members to understand the realities that the client may face and provide psychoeducation about mental illness. The organization offers concrete resources to clients and family members in the form of educational pamphlets—available on the NAMI website *(www.nami.org)* and a family tool kit to help family members understand the system, client needs, and their rights *(www.naminys. org/family-toolkit)*.

A number of high-profile individuals in the mental health field have, in fact, revealed their own struggles with these illnesses in order to help others feel hope and as a testament to the resiliency of persons with these conditions. One example of this was the courageous disclosure of Dr. Marsha Linehan, a renowned therapist and researcher who developed dialectical behavior therapy (DBT), an evidence-based treatment approach for patients with borderline personality disorder, many of whom have had serious suicidal ideation, attempts, and gestures, and experiences of self-harm (Linehan, 1993). Recently, Linehan returned to her hometown for a presentation at an inpatient hospital where she had been hospitalized as an adolescent and revealed that she also suffered from borderline personality disorder (Carey, 2011). Her own personal journey, strengths, and desire to help those who suffered in similar ways led her to her life's work.

These strengths often remain hidden. In an article in the *New York Times*, Carey (2011) observed:

> No one knows how many people with severe mental illness live what appear to be normal, successful lives, because such people are not in the habit of announcing themselves. They are too busy juggling responsibilities, paying the bills, studying, raising families—all the while weathering gusts of dark emotions or delusions that would quickly overwhelm almost anyone else. (p. 1)

In this article Carey (2011) quotes Elyn R. Saks, a professor at the University of Southern California School of Law who has written a book titled *The Center Cannot Hold: My Journey through Madness*, about her own challenges with schizophrenia. Saks states:

> There's a tremendous need to implode the myths of mental illness, to put a face on it, to show people that a diagnosis does not have to lead to a painful and oblique life. . . . We who struggle with these disorders can lead full, happy, productive lives, if we have the right resources. (as cited in Carey, 2011, p. 2)

Carey further observes:

> These [resources] include medication (usually), therapy (often), a measure of good luck (always)—and, most of all, the inner strength to manage one's demons, if not banish them. That strength can come from any number of places . . . former patients say: love, forgiveness, faith in God, [or] a lifelong friendship. (2011, p. 2)

It is important for new clinicians as well as those who are experienced to read these accounts of personal strengths and supports that have allowed persons with mental illness to live productive lives. As we demonstrate throughout this book, the therapist is often the "container of the hope" for our clients. Training programs that only prepare clinicians to diagnose and treat clients with mental illness without sharing the personal stories of strength and resiliency may deprive these therapists of a central ingredient that is essential for our work—hope (Carey, 2011).

Focus on the Resiliency of Clients and Families

The focus on strength-based approaches has led to an interest in the resiliency of clients and families in the mental health field. Walsh (1998) gives the following definition of resilience:

> Resilience can be defined as the capacity to rebound from adversity strengthened and more resourceful. It is an active process of endurance, self-righting, and growth in response to crisis and challenge . . . the qualities of resilience enable people to heal from painful wounds, take charge of their lives, and go on to live fully and love well. (p. 4)

A client's or family's belief system or worldview can be central to their ability to be resilient and mobilize their strengths to overcome adversity:

> Belief systems are at the core of [client and] family functioning and are powerful forces in resilience. We cope with crisis and adversity by making meaning of our experience: linking it to our social world, to our cultural and religious beliefs, to our multigenerational past, and to our hopes and dreams for the future. (Walsh, 1998, p. 45)

Given this reality, it is important that therapists be open to learning their clients' belief systems and recognizing that they may be different from their own. This might also include spiritual beliefs (Boyd-Franklin & Lockwood, 2009; Walsh, 2009). Chapter 3 also addresses this process for clinicians who are working with clients from diverse socioeconomic, cultural, ethnic, racial, and religious groups.

Emphasis on positive outlook (Walsh, 1998) and learned optimism (Seligman, 1990; Seligman & Csikszentmihalyi, 2000) have been recognized by researchers and clinicians as contributing to resilience. Walsh (1998, 2006) discusses the ways in which a positive outlook can help clients and families to overcome adversity. She also emphasizes the process of sustaining hope, which allows resilient individuals and families to look toward the future and hold on to future hope and possibilities for themselves and even their children.

Clinicians can contribute to this process by being the container for the hope during times when clients, families, and other practitioners, agencies, or systems may have given up on a client or family (see Chapter 12). The following case illustrates this.

The Barkeley family, originally from Jamaica in the West Indies, consisted of a 45-year-old mother who was diagnosed with bipolar disorder and had a history of not taking her medication, a 16-year-old daughter who had stopped going to school 3 months previously, a 13-year-old daughter who was engaging in cutting, an 11-year-old daughter who was recently hospitalized due to suicide risk, and the mother's boyfriend who, despite numerous attempts at engagement, had not yet come to any sessions at the clinic. This family was often discussed in the community mental health center's weekly staff meeting, as each child and the mother had her own therapist. After a period of time in which one family member would be discussed at a meeting with no forward movement, it was suggested that one therapist begin to work with the whole family as a unit. The case was assigned to a young therapist who had recently completed training at a local family therapy training institute. The therapist was told by the agency director and the other therapists working with the family not to expect the family to be responsive to any interventions.

When the therapist called the home to schedule the first appointment, she reached the mother and engaged her in a 10-minute phone conversation about the hard work that the family members had been doing individually, and the courage they were exhibiting in agreeing to try something new and be seen as a family. The therapist asked the mother if she had any questions about family therapy and emphasized the importance of all household members attending the first session. The mother stated that she would never be able to get her boyfriend to attend the appointment, that he did not believe in therapy, and that, since he had returned from jail, he had been angry and commonly yelled at her daughters. The therapist offered to reach out to the boyfriend herself. The mother eventually responded, "Don't worry, I'll get him there."

The boyfriend ended up accompanying all family members to the first family session. As they filed into the session room, they were in the process of having an argument about being late due to dinner taking longer than planned. The boyfriend was yelling at the mother, who was in turn yelling at her daughters. Rather than get pulled into the family argument, the therapist inquired as to what the boyfriend had made for dinner. The boyfriend had talked about making pernil. The therapist then asked if the boyfriend cooked often, to which he responded yes. The therapist asked what his specialty was, and the boyfriend replied oxtail stew. The boyfriend proudly stated that he had a recipe passed down from his grandmother and that he prepared it every Friday evening for the family. At the therapist's prompting, he went on to describe the intricacies of the recipe. While doing so, his back straightened and he smiled for a moment. The rest of the family members watched silently as the boyfriend took on a different public persona than they were accustomed to. After 15 minutes of engaging in such a dialogue, the therapist expressed a genuine appreciation for the family's ability to come together and have a family meal every Friday night. She pointed out that this quality in the family was just as important as any difficulties they had been experiencing. The conversation naturally turned to these struggles, with an emphasis on what they hoped to achieve together and how they might carry over their commitment to the family meal and their desire to move forward as a family.

Empowerment versus Advocacy and Helping

As we have noted, many counselors and therapists enter the mental health field with a basic desire to help others. Others with genuine motivation for social justice see their role as primarily advocating on behalf of their clients in many of the multisystems that impinge on their lives (courts, welfare department, child welfare or child protective services, schools, police, health and mental health facilities; see Chapter 11). This can be important initially particularly for therapists who are working with clients who are poor and who experience intrusion into their lives by many of these agencies. While both helping and advocacy are valuable initial goals and may help to strengthen the early therapeutic alliance, it can be problematic if the therapist stops at one of these levels. It is important that the counselor move beyond these approaches to the ultimate goal of empowerment (Boyd-Franklin & Bry, 2000a).

As Boyd-Franklin and Bry (2000a) have demonstrated, many beginning therapists, when faced with clients and families with multiple problems, feel that it is their job to "fix or solve these problems" (p. 42). Although their work was originally addressed to family therapists, it is relevant for all clinicians and counselors. They state:

> Although this approach to addressing urgent problems may be an excellent joining technique in the initial treatment process, it should not constitute the only method by which the therapist engages with the [client or] family. It is important to impart to [clients or] family members the tools that will empower them to interact effectively with other systems and begin to find their own solutions. With this in mind, [clinicians and] family therapists must learn to give the credit to [clients and] family members for the changes they make and not to take credit for themselves (Berg, 1994; Minuchin, 1974). Helping, if it continues for too long, may create a dependency on the [clinician or] family therapist or worker that is not healthy or helpful for the [client or] family in the long run. (p. 42)

With this in mind, clinicians should repeatedly ask themselves, "Am I doing too much for my client(s)? Is this something that he or she could be empowered to do for him- or herself?" Clearly, advocacy also has its place. It may be appropriate for a counselor or therapist to accompany clients to court or to go with them to a child study team meeting in their child's school. As much as possible, however, it is empowering for the clinician to role play with their clients a strategy that they might use in giving their own testimony and emphasizing their view of both the problem and the solution. The case below illustrates the difference in these approaches.

Ms. Brown, a young African American foster mother, was referred for therapy after she made the decision to adopt her foster daughter, Aliyah (age 7), who had lived in her home for the last 3 years. Ms. Brown had been told that Aliyah's biological mother was "strung out on drugs" and that there were no biological extended family members able to raise her. The case worker informed her that they were in the process of "terminating the biological mother's parental rights." Ms. Brown was uncomfortable with this because Aliyah frequently talked about her mother and expressed hope that her mother would visit on her birthday or during the holidays. As the Christmas holidays approached, Aliyah began acting out at home and in school. During the holidays, Aliyah's mother did not appear. In January, Aliyah returned to school and was unable to focus or concentrate and felt increasingly angry and disappointed. Finally at the end of the first week in January, she pulled the fire alarm in the school and ran out of the building. She was suspended indefinitely from school.

During this time, Ms. Brown became concerned about Aliyah and she was worried that she might lose her job because she had no one to take care of Aliyah during the day while she was out of school. Ms. Brown raised these concerns with her therapist. She was feeling overwhelmed and defeated by these events. Her therapist asked if she would be willing to call a meeting of all of those who might be able to help with this problem. Ms. Brown responded that she was desperate and was willing to try anything. Together, they made a list of all of the agencies involved (i.e., the school, child protective services, etc.). With the therapist's support, Ms. Brown called the principal, the child's guidance counselor, and the child protective service worker and her supervisor, to schedule a meeting. The therapist, a psychology intern, also requested that her supervisor, a program administrator, attend the meeting.

The therapist asked Ms. Brown to make a list of the concerns that she had and the types of help that she needed. They role-played and rehearsed Ms. Brown taking control of the meeting and asserting her concerns for Aliyah. When the meeting was held, Ms. Brown took the leadership role with her therapist's support. She first raised concerns about Aliyah's schooling, as she had been out of school for 2 weeks. The guidance counselor explained that Aliyah's behavior problems had become very serious and that they were referring her to the child study team for testing but that this process took time. Ms. Brown explained that she could no longer afford to miss work and was concerned about the amount of school work that Aliyah was missing. The therapist's supervisor, in response to the impasse in the room, suggested that Aliyah be considered for the day treatment program at the community mental health center, where her behavior problems and feelings of loss and abandonment by her mother could be addressed.

Ms. Brown was relieved and was encouraged to raise another serious concern. Although she wanted very much to adopt Aliyah, she had observed that she was attached to her biological mother and would be likely to "go ballistic" if her mother's parental rights were terminated. With this in mind, Ms. Brown stated that she felt that it was in her child's best interest not to have her biological mother's parental rights terminated. She asked her child welfare worker if she would be able to be a permanent foster mother for Aliyah. Initially, her child welfare worker responded that the law was such that if a child had been in foster care for 2 years (as Aliyah had), steps must be taken to either return him or her to the biological parent, an extended family member, or to terminate that parent's parental rights and free the child for adoption. The child welfare worker then turned to her supervisor who recalled that, in rare circumstances, the family court judge had allowed permanent foster care if it was deemed to be in the best interest of the child. At her suggestion, Ms. Brown agreed to write a letter to argue for this unusual solution. The school officials and therapist also offered to write their own letters on Aliyah's behalf.

Over the next month, the therapist worked with Ms. Brown on her letter and encouraged Ms. Brown to keep after the other parties to obtain their written support. She also accompanied Ms. Brown to the court hearing, where Ms. Brown eloquently stated her concerns. The judge was persuaded and Ms. Brown was allowed to keep Aliyah as a permanent foster child without parental rights being terminated.

At the end of the school year, Aliyah's behavior in the day treatment program had significantly improved. Family therapy also continued and she was doing much better at home. The therapist at the end of the year asked if Ms. Brown would like to have one more multisystemic meeting with the treatment team, the school officials, and the child welfare worker to discuss plans for Aliyah's return to her regular school. It was clear that empowerment had occurred when the day before the meeting, Ms. Brown e-mailed everyone her agenda for the meeting.

This case is an excellent example of the differences between helping, advocacy, and empowerment. Rather than taking over and helping or advocating for this client, the therapist chose to take a back seat and play a supportive role, empowering Ms. Brown to demonstrate her ability to advocate for herself and for Aliyah. This empowerment, in the long run, will be far more useful to Ms. Brown. For example, she encouraged Ms. Brown to call and schedule the meeting with the agencies and services involved; and she role-played with Ms. Brown the items that she would discuss in the meeting. By the end of that treatment, Ms. Brown was confident in her ability to successfully navigate the complex child welfare system on her child's behalf. Her therapist was able to bear witness and validate Ms. Brown's strengths in these areas.

Conclusion

The effectiveness of clinical technique hinges upon the establishment of a meaningful, authentic relationship. The elements that are critical to joining and establishing a therapeutic relationship rest upon the clinician's ability to approach each person with dignity and respect, to honor his or her strengths and competencies, and to mindfully make humanistic contact with his or her clients. With each new client or family, empathy, genuineness, positive regard, and authenticity are critical in the joining process. Mindfulness and a strength-based approach can help therapists establish a relationship with a client that is based on compassion, understanding, and resiliency. Finally, empowering clients to take control of their lives and to find solutions to their problems that are consistent with their values represents an important stance for the therapist to take in supporting clients to achieve their goals.

CHAPTER 5

Psychoeducation and Recovery Principles in Mental Health Services

Introduction

Among the more compelling trends in the field of mental health is the use of transparency, collaboration, hope, optimism, resilience, and finding meaning through adversity in treatment. Clinical best practice dictates that clients, as they enter therapy, should be met with a perspective that respects their personal choice, preferences, and rights to satisfying relationships, education, employment, and personal fulfillment. Clinical work that is infused with psychoeducation (i.e., providing information and knowledge to promote a client's increased awareness and choice) and recovery principles (i.e., inspiring the client to tap into individual strengths, competencies, values, traditions, and resources in overcoming adversity) lays the foundation for a client to assume an active role in his or her treatment efforts. It is for this reason that we have chosen the combination of psychoeducation and recovery principles as the second core mediational process.

This chapter begins by providing an overview of the need for psychoeducation and the use of recovery principles in treatment today. Next, the concept of recovery and its role within the mental health field will be explored. Finally, we discuss how psychoeducation can be used to inform clients and their families about psychological conditions and empower them to make choices in treatment that are consistent with their values.

95

The Need for Psychoeducation and Recovery Principles

The following example illustrates the need for psychoeducation in the treatment process. Imagine that your physician tells you that you have congestive heart disease. She offers you no information about what the disease entails, life expectancy, or details regarding treatment options. She hands you a card with a specialist's name and tells you to meet this person next week at 3:00 P.M. This approximates how those struggling with mental health problems often experience service delivery, where there continues to be a lack of transparency about the nature, etiology, treatment options, and the course of recognizable symptoms and common challenges people often face when struggling with mental health problems. Treatment that lacks psychoeducation further supports an existing stigma regarding mental health problems in our society. Just as an individual with heart disease would expect his or her cardiologist to be well versed in and communicate the most up-to-date scientific literature and protocols related to his or her condition, a mental health client should be able to expect his or her therapist to afford them the same treatment standard. When this does not occur in the field of mental health treatment, client feelings of shame, self-doubt, and alienation that often emerge alongside symptomatic experiences can be reinforced.

In mental health settings, clients often encounter treatment where they are subjected to the arbitrary, random theoretical orientation of the practitioner. For example, a 42-year-old male presenting at a mental health clinic with depression could be treated from a psychodynamic, cognitive-behavioral, gestalt, or family systems approach, depending on the theoretical orientation of the therapist to whom he or she is assigned. Additionally, this client may not even know that his or her therapist utilizes a psychodynamic or cognitive-behavioral perspective or that there are other options, much less what these options are.

There is a growing, scientifically based literature that can significantly inform diagnosis and treatment. It is the mental health professional's responsibility to verse him- or herself with this literature and make it available to clients in order to promote choice and transformation. The empowering nature of education and normalization can reduce stigma, promote a client's active participation, and afford the client the opportunity to contextualize his or her experience within a broader recovery framework. Recovery and psychoeducation represent a powerful pairing of theoretically sound principles and interventions that can foster transparency, hope, and optimism.

Recovery is a word that has evolved over the years. William Anthony (1993) defines it as a deeply personal, unique process of changing one's attitudes, values, feelings, goals, skills and/or roles. It is a way of living a satisfying, hopeful, and contributing life even with limitations caused by the illness. Recovery involves the development of new meaning and purpose in one's life as one grows beyond the catastrophic effects of mental illness. (p. 17)

The use of psychoeducation and recovery principles in treatment is a core mediational process because it affords individuals the opportunity to partner with clinicians in proactively reframing their symptomatic struggles, making room for action, and establishing an identity apart from mental illness. For instance, a 32-year-old female client with a long history of mood swings, impulsivity, suicide attempts, depression, and fractured relationships is diagnosed as having bipolar disorder. In a treatment session at a local mental health clinic, her therapist and psychiatrist discuss the existing knowledge, treatment, and course of bipolar disorder, while the client is encouraged to compare this knowledge to her own experiences. As the client is empowered to contextualize the knowledge she is being given by her treatment team, she realizes that up until this point, her whole life has been lived in reaction to the constant mood swings, depression, fragmented relationships, and low self-esteem she experiences. This realization enables her, perhaps for the first time, to reestablish an identity separate from her illness.

The power of a psychoeducation and recovery-oriented perspective is that it allows the client to integrate and utilize the requisite knowledge to become a proactive partner in his or her own recovery. Far too often clients are unaware of what they are being treated for. They may see their therapist, visit their psychiatrist, and take their medication without really understanding the reasons why they are engaging in these treatment activities. By providing clients with reputable psychoeducational information and assisting them in better understanding what it is that they are collaborating with their therapist to address, clients are given an increased opportunity to expand their identity beyond their illness and to establish meaning in their lives. The following case example illustrates the degree to which psychoeducation can empower a woman with chronic depression.

Marie, a 28-year-old Italian American woman, presented with a long history of major depressive episodes characterized by long periods of staying in bed, isolation, hopelessness, and low motivation. In the first session she reported a history of dissatisfying treatment experiences and noted that she had taken a long break from therapy. However, she was ready to give therapy another try because of increased stress and unhappiness at work and home. She complained that life was passing her by, that she was tired of feeling stuck, and that she felt unable to sustain friendships and intimate relationships.

After meeting with Marie for a few sessions, it became increasingly clear to the therapist that Marie suffered from depression. The therapist then began to talk with Marie about her illness. After providing information about the etiology, symptoms, and treatment options regarding depression, the therapist engaged Marie in a dialogue that provided her an opportunity to take a look at her experience in relation to this information. The two discussed how Marie's family and cultural background influenced how she thought about and judged her depression.

Marie responded positively to the therapist's attempts to integrate information about her diagnosis with her culture, values, and identity as a person. The therapist normalized her depression and pointed out that depression is a real and recognized medical condition that is highly treatable. The therapist noted that just as someone diagnosed with diabetes is encouraged to learn about and develop strategies for managing his or her condition, someone with depression would also benefit from doing the same. The therapist then discussed treatment options with Marie, and the two talked about cognitive-behavioral therapy, medication utilization, diet, exercise, and stress reduction.

As a way to help Marie to externalize her experience of the disorder, rather than blame herself for her illness, the therapist asked her to consider what a typical person with major depression would say to him- or herself. Marie responded by saying that there would likely be a running tape of a voice saying "you're a failure, life is not worth living, why bother, and so on." The therapist then asked Marie to consider—if that person were not educated about depression, including its symptoms and the number of people who suffer from it—whether she would mistake those statements as innate truths about herself? Through this conversation, Marie began to develop a more externalized view of her depressive symptoms and to reclaim her identity, apart from them.

Over a series of sessions, Marie conveyed that this was the first time that she had ever experienced the treatment process in this way. She described past treatments as focusing on personal insight without contextualizing the diagnosis as only one part of her life. She expressed feeling like a failure in the past for not being able to overcome her depression based on the insights that she had acquired. She would repeatedly convey frustration at herself for not being able to utilize this insight to move forward in her life. By co-creating a definition of depression grounded in personal experience and clinical science, she began to adopt a more empowered stance toward her recovery process.

Marie was struggling with feelings of shame regarding her emotional difficulties. She had never been afforded an opportunity to educate herself about depression and grew up in an environment where feelings such as hers were characterized as weak, lazy, and experiences that she should just "get over." Stigma remains a prominent issue and the field of mental health continues to struggle to reconcile advanced clinical science with outdated societal views of mental illness. The transformative potential of psychoeducation is of such great import that it is necessary to include it alongside recovery as one core mediational process, as true recovery does not occur without a contextualization of one's experience in a well-established and well-researched knowledge base.

Recovery

The 2005 National Consensus Statement on Mental Health Recovery from SAMHSA defines mental health recovery as "a journey of healing and transformation enabling a person with a mental health problem to live a meaningful life in a community of his or her choice while striving to achieve his or her full potential" (Substance Abuse and Mental Health Services Administration, 2005, p. 1). Deegan (1990) has indicated that "Those things that raise our self-esteem and make life worth living are vital to recovery."

Recovery is a principle that has taken on an expanded meaning over the last several years, particularly as it relates to mental health (Ralph & Corrigan, 2005). While it had initially been associated with addiction (Kelly & White, 2011) and 12-step programs, it is now widely applied across all mental health domains and is systematically shifting the paradigm from pathology to one that includes the "lived experience of moving through and beyond the limitations of one's disorder" (W. White et al., 2005). There is also a growing literature in the mental health field that includes personal narratives from individuals with mental illness concerning their own recovery processes (Basset & Stickley, 2010; Slade, 2009).

A key idea in recovery is that life is richer for having overcome the added challenges associated with living with a mental illness (Ralph & Corrigan, 2005). While living with a mental illness involves pain, it also involves the development of internal capacities that otherwise would not be developed without the experience of overcoming adversity. Suggestive in this notion is that there is always a silver lining, and it is the mental health professional's responsibility to create a framework where hope and resiliency can be realized (Ralph & Corrigan, 2005).

There are a few component parts that support this process. First is the notion of hope (Meichenbaum, 2008; Ralph & Corrigan, 2005). Like Marie, many people enter treatment feeling hopeless, alienated from themselves and from others, and confused about what they are feeling and why they are having the experiences they are having. They are often unaware that their experiences are consistent with a known biomedical condition that can be treated. Anthony (1993) states that the introduction of the belief that one can get better goes a long way to fuel the recovery process. Providing clear, concise information about treatment options in a transparent way sets the stage for cultivating the idea that one can develop meaning and live a fulfilling life.

Through psychoeducation and the establishment of a recovery-oriented framework, practitioners can begin to foster acceptance of mental illness that promotes a proactive stance in relation to treatment and recovery (Hayes et al., 2004; Ralph & Corrigan, 2005). For example, medication is widely recognized as an essential and critical part of mental health recovery for many biologically based mental illnesses. However, people often resist the idea of medications due to the stigma often associated with taking them. The framework of transparency, hope, and education can begin to nurture a relationship to one's illness in which medication is experienced as something to utilize in order to move forward in one's desired direction. Just as someone with diabetes utilizes blood sugar ratings and insulin regulation to stay on a wellness path, a person struggling with serious mental illness can and in many cases should utilize medication in the service of wellness. For example, Deegan (1990, 1992) has introduced the idea of utilizing medications versus complying with medications. This is best accomplished in the context of supportive and transparent relationships with mental health professionals, including psychiatrists, where an ongoing dialogue regarding stigma, side effects, and other challenges are addressed.

As White et al. (2005) have noted, recovery and treatment are not the same. "Treatment encompasses the way professionals intervene to stabilize or alter the course of an illness; recovery is the personal experience of the individual as he or she moves out of illness into health and wholeness" (p. 235). Therefore, within the context of recovery, treatment must be a partnership where "appropriate, effective medication and a wide range of services tailored to [the client's] needs" is utilized to support the person's path to recovery.

Therefore, also central to recovery is the exploration, clarification, and ultimately the realization of one's values and personal life goals (Deegan, 1992). Values serve as anchors in the change process. They are the things that give life meaning and propel one toward wellness. Before treatment, many people feel trapped, defined by, and in a constant state of reactivity to their mental illness. With treatment and a recovery-oriented framework, individuals can begin to live life in the service of their values and goals rather than in response to their symptoms. For example, whereas someone with depression might initially see him- or herself as worthless and no good, after going through treatment and entering into recovery, he or she can learn to recognize these thoughts and feelings as symptoms. Here, the integration of psychoeducation and recovery-oriented principles can drive a wedge between the person and the symptom, thus creating more space and flexibility to pursue his or her values and goals (Hayes, Strosahl, & Wilson, 1999, 2011).

when you become feelings "not good"

Marie, from the case above, reentered treatment feeling trapped in a reactive cycle with her depression symptoms. She was in a sort of psychological paralysis and felt yoked to her depressive experience. She had little differentiation between herself and her symptoms. And it was not until this recovery-oriented framework was introduced that she began to see the separation between her innate self and her depression. This set the stage for Marie to take a closer look at what was important to her and how she was going to move on with her life, as this separation allowed for increased psychological space to spend a few sessions focused on her values. She began to understand that while she could not control the neurophysiological aspects of her depression, she could begin to modify the way she related to her depression. *modify her relationship to it*

If Marie's depression was going to exist within her, and she might have to live her life experiencing some periods of depression, the focus became how exactly she was going to do this. The therapist engaged Marie in a discussion about what qualities she wanted to exemplify, and what gave her life meaning. He asked her to think about her 80th birthday party, and if people were going to stand up and recognize her life's accomplishments, what would she want them to say? (Hayes, Strosahl, & Wilson, 1999, 2011). What did she want her life to stand for? Marie found herself saying that she wanted to be a good friend; she wanted to remain true to the morals she was taught growing up; she wanted to be seen as someone who connected with her community. Marie began to understand that no matter how severe or strong her depression was, nothing could rob her of the ability to move in the direction that she wanted to move. The therapist contextualized this discussion by stating that recovery was not a straight line (Ralph & Corrigan, 2005), that there might be times when the depression reasserted itself, and that recovery was a constant reorienting toward the direction of personal values and goals (Hayes, Strosahl, & Wilson, 1999, 2011).

Values exploration, the recontextualization of suffering, education, and the installment of hope are best cultivated in a spirit of transparency.

In order to deliver true recovery-oriented treatment, we as clinicians must be comfortable with providing psychoeducation, with seeing the person as he or she really is, and dialoguing with them about the treatment process. <u>Some of the difficulties regarding transparency are best exemplified when working with someone who is diagnosed with borderline personality disorder.</u>

There is a history in the field of mental health treatment that axis II diagnoses are not normally talked about in a transparent way with clients. Traditionally, there is a sense that this person has deficits and cannot understand the diagnosis. A true recovery-oriented framework would open and sustain a dialogue with this client about borderline personality disorder. For example, the clinician might discuss with the client that a person with a borderline diagnosis typically has difficultly managing intense emotions, struggles to sustain meaningful relationships, and harbors an intense fear of abandonment and rejection that may make sense in relation to the person's history (Linehan, 1993). The clinician might say that the condition is something that causes a lot of upheaval and instability in a person's life, that it can be painful, and that it can be difficult to make sense of these experiences, and most importantly that there is treatment for it, such as developing increased emotion regulation strategies, increased interpersonal relationship skills, and employing grounding techniques such as mindful breathing and positive self-talk (Linehan, 1993).

Transparency also features prominently in the treatment plan process. Often, even when clinicians try to be person centered, the tendency to rely on generic, universal categories is strong. For instance, examples of goals in outpatient mental health clinics can read as "Client will reduce frequency of depressive symptoms by 60%"; "Client will attend group each week," or "client will take medication as prescribed." Recovery principles challenge the treatment dyad to look beyond diagnosis and symptoms and address the client's goals in life. For example, although a person may still experience some symptoms of depression, he or she may decide to go back to school, and treatment would focus on how to do this.

Sometimes mental health providers are surprised when they realize a client's true goals and values. For example, a case conference was held in which a client in recovery from major depression and substance abuse met with his case manager, his therapist, his psychiatrist, and the substance abuse counselor from the client's residence (for individuals with dual diagnoses of serious mental illness and substance abuse). In his chart, this client's treatment plan goals were to reduce substance use, take his medication daily, and attend group. They were all talking and trying to figure out what this particular client needed to do. When the focus turned to the client, he looked at them dumbfounded and surprised everyone when he stated, "All I want to do is fix cars." This stopped the well-intentioned treatment providers in their tracks, and the tone of the discussion shifted to emphasize this client's own personal goals and values. By focusing on his goal of fixing cars, they were able to explore his love of this process and his early life experiences helping his father to fix cars. This led them to collaborate with the client to expand his treatment plan to include the possibility of job training in this area. This became the motivation that the client needed to address his addiction and his mental health issues.

Psychoeducation

Recent advances in the field of mental health suggest that there are biological determinants in major mental illnesses such as bipolar disorder, obsessive–compulsive disorder, panic disorder, major depression, and posttraumatic stress disorder (NAMI, 2012). These conditions are now seen as medical conditions that strongly interact with environmental stressors (McFarlane, Dixon, Lukens, & Lucksted, 2003). In light of this increased understanding, psychoeducation becomes critical in helping individuals make choices regarding their recovery. Education has been a part of mental health treatment since the early 20th century (Donley, 1911). Beck, in his formulations and research of the cognitive-behavioral therapy model, featured psychoeducation as a primary intervention (e.g., A. T. Beck, Rush, Shaw, & Emery, 1979). Psychoeducation has been known to reduce stigma (Lewisohn, Antonuccio, Breckenridge, & Teri, 1984) and psychoeducational models have been developed to recruit participants who might otherwise not seek treatment. Not all participants benefit from psychoeducation, particularly those who have concentration and cognitive impairments (Cuijpers, 1988), and the amount of information output from the treatment provider should be monitored according to the stress level, cognitive ability, and symptomatic severity of the client.

Consistent with the value placed on social and familial support in recovery-oriented services, McFarlane (2002) developed a multifamily psychoeducation model in which the main goal of treatment was to provide the client's support network with a clear understanding of the neurological mechanisms behind severe mental illness. The basic assumptions of this model include that families do not cause schizophrenia but can contribute to overall stress when trying to respond to it, that schizophrenia and schizo-affective disorders have a strong neurobiological basis to them, that "normal" life events can cause undue stress and erratic responses due to the disorders, and that medication is useful and should be utilized but is usually not sufficient by itself to bring about recovery (McFarlane, 2002). This model also strongly emphasizes ongoing clinical supervision in working with clients and their families. McFarlane's use of psychoeducation has been shown to have powerful positive results—preventing relapse and significantly reducing frequency of hospitalizations, while increasing utilization of medication and reducing substance use.

A primary aim of psychoeducation with a client about the nature of a mental health disorder is the externalization of symptoms. The goal of externalizing symptoms is to separate shame, stigma, and blame from the client's experience of the disorder. In McFarlane's model, both clients and family members work to increasingly shift blame away from the person and toward the neurobiological disorder (Jewell, Downing, & McFarlane, 2009). The potential for relief when blame is dispelled and reassigned away from the client is powerful. However, it should be noted that education should be delivered in the spirit of contextualism. In other words, one must honor the client's experiential field, frame the client as the expert on his or her experience, and couch educational information within consensus-driven scientific literature.

Psychoeducation, when paired with questions such as "How does this compare with your experience?" can serve to foster and encourage acceptance without the client feeling as though it is imposed upon him or her. Choice and empowerment are central to the clinically transparent nature of psychoeducation, in which medication and best-practice treatment options are also presented alongside the current scientific understanding of the client's illness. As an intervention, providing education is not about reducing someone to his or her diagnosis in a medical model, rather it involves utilizing knowledge as a way to reduce the significant barriers of shame and stigma and to achieve greater separation between his or her identity or innate selves and the illness process.

Another mechanism of action associated with psychoeducation is the establishment of a formalized, proactive, and holistic approach toward acceptance and wellness. The clinician, by providing information and the opportunity to contextualize collaboratively with the client, is attempting to invoke an understanding and appreciation of his or her struggles. Recall the woman discussed earlier in this chapter who, after being supplied with information about bipolar disorder, marveled at the extent to which she had identified with the manifestations of her mental illness. Through the process of externalization, clinical transparency, contextualization, and provision of medical information, the client is in the position to partner with his or her therapist on an individualized path to recovery.

Conclusion

Recovery-oriented clinical practice and psychoeducation go hand in hand. It is our responsibility, as mental health professionals, to create the conditions necessary for clients to ground themselves in reputable scientific information regarding their illness and treatment options and to foster a partnership in the service of change and wellness. This grounding process occurs in the context of transparency, partnership, empathic resonance, respect, and an appreciation for the value of the client's perspective.

As a way to shape this core mediational process, the acronym **HEROIC** can serve a guiding template for service delivery:

- Honoring the client as an expert in his or her experience. Above all, the client alone knows best his or her inner private experiences and pain, and has developed a repertoire of coping with these experiences. This set of coping skills is shaped by environment, culture, stigma, relationships, and past history of successes and failures, as well as an innate need to feel better. This must be honored above all else.

- Education regarding mental illness and treatment. Once the client's experience is honored and the client is invited into a partnership aimed at transformation and wellness, the door is opened for the client to receive information about the nature of his or her struggles. This information is provided in the context of respect and transparency.

- Recovery Orientation. People everywhere lead fulfilling lives alongside their mental illnesses. A recovery-based orientation illuminates the power by which personal preference, dreams, hopes, relationships, information, resources, and support can inspire change and the establishment of meaning. Recovery is not a straight line, and it looks different for each and every person.

- Integration and Contextualization. It is important not to impose any one understanding onto another person. The provision of education is not meant to pigeonhole a client into any one diagnostic category. Information is provided in the spirit of collaboration and curiosity, and encourages the client to examine new information in the context of his or her own experience and cultural background. Ultimately, integration will occur in the spirit of choice and empowerment and will expand a person's experience and understanding of him- or herself and others.

CHAPTER 6

Motivational Interviewing

Introduction

Many therapists are trained initially in treatment approaches that assume clients enter therapy voluntarily, are ready and motivated to work on their issues, and are committed to change. The challenge that all of us face in the real world is that many of our clients are not self-referred and some may be resistant to, or at least ambivalent about, therapy as a process of change. As a consequence, many therapists become overwhelmed when they encounter resistance on the part of their clients. The third core mediational process, motivational interviewing (MI), is one of the most useful models that we have found for addressing ambivalence and reluctance to change (W. R. Miller & Rollnick, 1991, 2002, 2013). This approach provides clinicians with an important framework to identify client readiness for change and with strategies to support the change process.

In this chapter, we begin with a brief description of MI. Next, we describe the "spirit of MI" (W. R. Miller & Rollnick, 2013), an important concept that presents the context and mind-set therapists should bring to the collaborative process with clients. Throughout the chapter, we describe the evolution of MI from its early connection with the transtheoretical stages-of-change model (DiClemente & Velasquez, 2002; Prochaska & DiClemente, 1982) to the separation and clear delineation between the two approaches (W. R. Miller & Rollnick, 2009, 2013). We then discuss the core concepts and intervention strategies of MI (W. R. Miller & Rollnick, 1991, 2002, 2013). More recent innovations are also discussed (W. R. Miller & Rollnick, 2013). We present the evolution of this approach because techniques from each of these stages have been helpful to us in our clinical work. The chapter concludes with a brief description of strategies for combining MI with other therapeutic modalities.

Overview of Motivational Interviewing

MI (Arkowitz, Westra, Miller, & Rollnick, 2008; W. R. Miller & Moyers, 2006; W. R. Miller & Rollnick, 1991, 2002, 2009, 2013) is an evidence-based treatment approach that has broad applicability in clinical work. Therapists often find themselves in clinical situations in which they feel tremendous pressure and responsibility for producing change in their clients. MI challenges the traditional notion of the therapist as the expert. It levels the playing field in the therapeutic relationship through its acknowledgment that the choice regarding whether to change rests ultimately with the client.

This model utilizes a guiding style, rather than directing or following (W. R. Miller & Rollnick, 2013), as clients are helped to move toward change. The focus shifts from an external force (i.e., the therapist) pushing the individual to an internal motivation for change. Thus, the client is put in dynamic tension with him- or herself rather than in a battle with the therapist.

This shift in the role of the therapist can be liberating for clinicians in that they are able to let go of the pressure to be "the expert" and their feeling of responsibility to solve all of their clients' problems. This model's recognition that many people are initially resistant to change, and that ambivalence—wanting to change but not wanting to at the same time—is a normal human condition (W. R. Miller & Rollnick, 2002, 2009, 2013), helps clinicians to become more able to tolerate clients' indecision and paralysis (W. R. Miller & Rollnick, 2002). It also helps therapists to be able to tolerate the inherent ambiguity and uncertainty that may be a part of clinical work. Imposing a change agenda on a client who is not ready can derail the change process and result in, for example, the client arguing against the clinician rather than moving in the direction of change. Collaboration between therapists and clients is one of the hallmarks of this approach (W. R. Miller & Rollnick, 1991, 2002, 2013).

The Spirit of Motivational Interviewing

Throughout this chapter we describe different aspects of MI as this model has evolved over time (W. R. Miller & Rollnick, 1991, 2002,

2013). First, it is important for therapists to understand the "heart and the mind" with which one enters the practice of MI (W. R. Miller & Rollnick, 2013). One thing that has remained consistent throughout this evolution has been the inherent "spirit of MI," which is composed of four interrelated elements: "partnership, acceptance, compassion, and evocation" (W. R. Miller & Rollnick, 2013, p. 15). Partnership implies an "active collaboration between experts" (p. 15). In MI, "the helper [or therapist] is a companion who typically does less than half of the talking" (p. 15). The therapist is a witness to the change process of the client.

The second element is a "profound acceptance of what the client brings" (W. R. Miller & Rollnick, 2013, p. 16). Acceptance involves "prizing the inherent worth and potential of every human being" (p. 17). It also entails "accurate empathy, an active interest in and effort to understand the other's internal perspective, to see the world through her or his eyes" (p. 18). The third component of acceptance involves "honoring and respecting each person's autonomy, their irrevocable right and capacity of self-direction" (p. 18). Finally, acceptance involves affirmation in which we not only seek and understand but also verbally acknowledge a person's strengths and efforts. This is important because many of our clients have experienced a great deal of criticism and censure in their lives.

Compassion, the third element, defined by W. R. Miller and Rollnick (2013) as "A deliberate commitment to pursue the welfare and best interests of the other" (p. 20), was added to the description of the underlying spirit of MI in the third edition of their book (W. R. Miller & Rollnick, 2013). When used correctly, this element is essential to the practice of MI; without it, MI can be misused as a series of techniques or as a way to manipulate clients.

The final element is the spirit of evocation. This challenges the deficit model, which presumes that a client is inherently lacking an ability or quality that only the therapist can provide. W. R. Miller and Rollnick (2013) make explicit that the spirit of MI

> starts from a very different strengths-focused premise, *that people already have within them much of what is needed,* and your task is to evoke it, to call it forth. The implicit message is "You have what you need, and together we will find it." From this perspective it is particularly important to focus on and understand the person's strengths and resources rather than probe for deficits. (p. 21)

Thus, MI provides therapists with a perspective that honors and respects our clients and defines the human aspects of our role in the change process.

Motivational Interviewing and the Transtheoretical Model (Stages of Change): Early Connection and Later Separation of These Models

W. R. Miller and Rollnick (1991, 2002) initially incorporated into MI the work by Prochaska and DiClemente (1982) and DiClemente and Velasquez (2002) on the transtheoretical model ("stages of change"). W. R. Miller and Rollnick (2013) have subsequently clarified the distinction between the two models and have stated that MI and the transtheoretical model are "kissing cousins who never married" (pp. 35–36). Nevertheless, we have found the stages-of-change model (in combination with MI) to be a helpful and empowering framework for clinicians. This model incorporates the concept of six stages of change: precontemplation, contemplation, preparation, action, maintenance, and relapse or recurrence (DiClemente & Velasquez, 2002).

Because with many clients the stages can fluctuate day to day or even hour to hour, we think these stages are best represented by a wheel (see Figure 6.1). In the precontemplation stage, a person is not yet ready to consider the idea of change (DiClemente & Velasquez, 2002; W. R. Miller & Rollnick, 1991, 2002; Prochaska & DiClemente, 1982). Persons in the precontemplation stage regarding a particular behavior may present as argumentative, hesitant to truly discuss the problem behavior, dismissive of attempts at support, or perhaps even hopeless (W. R. Miller & Rollnick, 2002). At this stage, a person can benefit from information and feedback to "raise his or her awareness of the problem and the possibility of change. Giving prescriptive advice at this stage can be counterproductive (Rollnick & MacEwan, 1991)" (W. R. Miller & Rollnick, 1991, p. 16; W. R. Miller & Rollnick, 2002).

In their work with clients in the precontemplation stage, DiClemente and Velasquez (2002) elaborate on the precontemplator's resistance to change. (Although W. R. Miller and Rollnick [2013], in a later version of the MI model, moved away from this concept of resistance and toward a more strength-based approach [discussed below], we have found DiClemente and Velasquez [2002] helpful to clinicians in understanding the different types of resistance to change that they may encounter and the different strategies for addressing these issues.) DiClemente and Velasquez have identified four qualities, or "four R's" that represent the distinct patterns displayed by those in the precontemplation stage who are still not ready to change. These "four R's include: reluctance, rebellion, resignation, and rationalization" (p. 204). According to their model, "*reluctant* precontemplators are those who, through lack of knowledge or perhaps inertia, do not

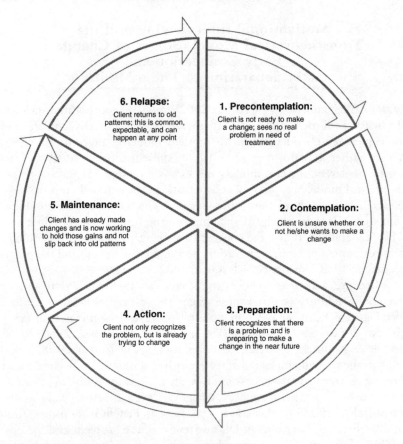

FIGURE 6.1. Stages of change. Based on Prochaska and DiClemente (1982).

want to consider change" (p. 205, italics added). For clients, who are "passively reluctant":

> Careful listening and providing feedback in a sensitive, empathic manner can be very helpful. . . . By allowing clients the freedom to make their own decisions, clinicians facilitate a situation where the possibility of change can be explored in a nonthreatening manner." (DiClemente & Velasquez, 2002, p. 205)

DiClemente and Velasquez (2002) make the following observation of the second group of precontemplators:

> *Rebellious* precontemplators often have a great deal of knowledge about the problem behavior. In fact, they often have a heavy investment in [maintaining] the behavior. . . . The rebellious precontemplator will

appear hostile and resistant to change . . . Motivational Interviewing provides a way of allowing rebellious precontemplators to express their strong feelings about change while at the same time directing their energy in a positive direction. For example, when a counselor agrees with the rebellious precontemplator that no one can force them to change, and in fact the counselor wouldn't dream of trying, it often diffuses the strength of their argument. (pp. 205–206, italics added)

The third type is the *resigned* precontemplative client. "Lack of energy and investment . . . is the hallmark of this person. These clients have given up on the possibility of change and seem overwhelmed by the problem" (DiClemente & Velasquez, 2002, p. 206). Many of these clients have attempted to change their behavior previously, but have been unable, despite repeated efforts, to prevent relapses into earlier patterns. For these clients, instilling hope and discussing what might get in the way of change is often helpful. Presenting change as a process in which relapse is common and should be viewed not as a failure but as a learning opportunity, can also serve to minimize a client's resignation and self-blame (DiClemente & Velasquez, 2002).

DiClemente and Velasquez (2002) describe the fourth pattern of precontemplation, *rationalization,* as someone who "often appears to have all of the answers," which can leave the clinician feeling "as though he or she is in a debate . . . " (p. 207). Here the authors suggest using empathy and reflective listening in working with these clients. In addition, they recommend using a decisional balance exercise in which the client is first asked to think through the good things about maintaining his or her current behavior. Acknowledging the "pros" of his or her behavior and the benefits or reasons why he or she keeps engaging in it, often opens the client up to then consider the cons of his or her actions. DiClemente and Velasquez warn clinicians, however, not to use the cons as "ammunition" against their clients or as combative arguments for change. Instead they suggest using them simply to help clients more fully understand and integrate their own experience of their behavior into their personal "change statements."

As the person becomes more willing to acknowledge the problem, he or she enters the contemplation stage. This stage is often characterized by ambivalence about change, that is, the person wants change but resists it (W. R. Miller & Rollnick, 1991, 2002). According to Miller and Rollnick (1991), "Ambivalence is accepted as a normal part of human experience and change, rather than seen as a pathological trait. . . . Reluctance to give up a problem behavior is to be expected at the time of treatment" (pp. 55–56).

DiClemente and Velasquez (2002) refer to contemplation, the second stage of the change process, as a "paradoxical stage" in which "clients are quite often open to information about the behavior and to exploring decisional balance considerations. It is also the stage where clients experience the most ambivalence . . . contemplation does not mean commitment" (p. 208). The key to this stage is to "assist the contemplator in thinking through the risks of the behavior and the potential benefits of change and to instill hope that change is possible" (p. 209).

The therapist's role at this stage is one of helping to "tip the balance in favor of change. . . . A counselor who launches into strategies appropriate for the action stage at this point is likely to engender resistance" (W. R. Miller & Rollnick, 1991, pp. 16–17). For instance, therapists often enter the treatment process ready to solve problems and approach the client armed with solutions and strategies. At the same time, the client is not always ready to find the solution from day one and, therefore, the clinician's action-oriented approach can backfire and undermine the treatment process by moving too quickly. In actuality, the client is more likely to move toward solutions when he or she has taken the time to grapple with ambivalence, and has undergone a process in which the pros and cons of taking action are considered and thought through (W. R. Miller & Rollnick, 2002).

The therapist's role in the contemplation stage requires a willingness to recognize and sit with the client's inner conflict between wanting and not wanting to change. When a therapist allows him- or herself to exist in this conflicted space without pushing his or her own change agenda, the client is likely to take ownership of the change process and acknowledge a need for change.

The case below describes this process.

Bobby, a 32-year-old Latino man diagnosed with bipolar disorder, constantly swayed back and forth between wanting to sustain recovery and the desire to experience the euphoric high associated with his manic swings. After the clinician empathically reflected back Bobby's ambivalence, the therapist invited Bobby to talk openly about the benefits experienced from not taking medication and experiencing manic episodes. Bobby spoke openly about his fears of crushing his creativity and about the wonderful artwork he produced while manic. He spoke about feeling more socially confident and less inhibited to connect with friends while in a manic state. He also spoke of his increased sexual prowess and the value he placed on sexual intimacy. The tone that the therapist used with Bobby was fundamentally different from Bobby's past experience with treatment providers who consistently urged him to take his medication.

After openly exploring the perceived benefits derived from not taking medication, Bobby was asked to comment on the "downsides." Bobby spoke about the crashing lows that often resulted in a dark depressive state following manic swings that invariably, when he was off his medication, resulted in going to the hospital and experiencing the deep shame and anger of his life being interrupted by a hospitalization again. Bobby was also able to reflect on how his relationships were ultimately unstable as a result of these highs and lows. The clinician fought hard to check the impulse to push down on the side of medication and, rather, sat with and allowed for the tension between the two sides of change to materialize. While Bobby did not leave the session having reconciled his ambivalence, he expressed feeling an increased anxiety and heightened sensitivity to the inner pushes and pulls he experiences around medication.

The third stage of change, preparation, is described as a "window of opportunity, which opens for a period of time" (W. R. Miller & Rollnick, 1991, p. 17). In the preparation stage, "The person is ready to change in the near future" (DiClemente & Velasquez, 2002, p. 210). Some clients progress from this stage to action, while others are not ready to move forward and may go back to the contemplation of their own ambivalence about change (Stage 2). With this in mind, DiClemente and Velasquez argue that

> The first task for the clinician working with the client in preparation is to assess the strength of the client's commitment to change . . . and to assist the client in making a solid realistic assessment of the difficulties she/he might encounter . . . , a plan for each of these contingencies, and a way to know when he/she might need additional help. (p. 211)

It is easy to overlook the nuances and complexities associated with the preparation stage. The challenge for the clinician is to not overcollude with the client's decision to change. We have found it helpful to engage clients in the preparation stage around their expectations of the change process. Sometimes when clients decide to change they believe that they will begin feeling better, when in fact the opposite is often true. For example, clients who are pulling away from alcohol use may begin experiencing feelings they would otherwise not have felt. If clients are not sensitized to this, they can easily become frustrated and slip back into a precontemplative state.

Sophia, a 37-year-old White female survivor of sexual abuse with PTSD symptoms, coped with her symptoms by isolating herself from family and friends. She arrived to her session one day stating that she was ready to attend a sexual abuse survivor's group. The therapist struck an empathic balance between commending Sophia for her decision to participate in this group and supporting her forward movement with a careful appreciation and exploration of the potential barriers, challenges, and feeling states Sophia might encounter in such a group. Sophia was able to anticipate that she might encounter an initial sense of awkwardness, shame, and vulnerability in revealing her sexual abuse to people who she did not know. This exploration yielded a stronger commitment to push through these feelings in service of her moving forward and feeling less isolated.

It is the action stage, the fourth stage of change, which most closely resembles traditional therapy in that the client is now ready to work actively with the therapist to produce change. DiClemente and Velasquez (2002) caution us to remember, however, that

> the danger is that many people, including professional therapists, can erroneously equate action with change, overlooking not only the critical work that prepares people for successful action, but equally important (and often more challenging) efforts to maintain the changes following action. (p. 212)

The challenge for the clinician in this stage is to continue the dialogue cultivated in the preparation stage by reflecting on the current change process, identifying barriers and obstacles, troubleshooting and problem solving around these barriers, and highlighting a commitment to the values and goals underlying change that the client has articulated.

The maintenance stage (Stage 5) is marked by an internalization and crystallization of the change process by the client. It is frequently a challenging stage for the client as he or she works to "sustain the change accomplished by previous action" (W. R. Miller & Rollnick, 1991, p. 17; W. R. Miller & Rollnick, 2002). DiClemente and Velasquez (2002) caution us that "Often change is not completely established even after 6 months or so of action. This is particularly true if the environment is filled with cues that can trigger the problem behavior" (p. 213).

During this time a person is vulnerable to "minor ('slips') or major ('relapses')" (W. R. Miller & Rollnick, 1991, p. 17). We often equate the maintenance stage as being in cruise control while driving on a major highway where one runs the risk of becoming complacent and losing focus. Often in this stage, a romanticization of past behaviors may occur, for example, "That relationship wasn't so bad," or "I can have one Heineken," or "It was lots of fun to meet up with those guys on the corner, I really miss that." Additionally, persons in the maintenance stage may be susceptible to disillusionment, as they may have expected the change process to result in an elevation of mood and feelings that might not happen (W. R. Miller & Rollnick, 2002).

DiClemente and Velasquez (2002) argue that "Throughout this process, relapse is possible (even likely) when moving through the stages of change" (p. 213). Therefore, relapse or recurrence constitutes its own stage of change. DiClemente and Velasquez have noted that clients experiencing a relapse often "seek reassurance and some way to make sense of the relapse crisis. It is important to help these clients see the crisis as an opportunity to learn rather than a failure" (DiClemente & Velasquez, 2002, p. 213). Likewise, as a fluctuation in readiness or motivation to change is common, therapists should not blame themselves or their clients when relapses into old behaviors occur. For more on the relapse stage, relapse prevention, and trigger management, see Chapter 9.

The stages-of-change model can be transformative for therapists because the clinician's tasks change depending on the client's readiness for change. For example, when a client is in the precontemplation stage, the therapist's role is to "raise doubt and increase the client's perception of the risks and problems with the current behavior" (W. R. Miller & Rollnick, 1991, p. 18). Once the client has moved on to the contemplation stage, the clinician's task is to "tip the balance—evoke reasons to change, risks of not changing; strengthen the client's self-efficacy for the change of the current behavior" (p. 18). As the client enters the preparation stage, the therapist's role is to "help the client determine the best course of action to take in seeking change" (p. 18). In the action stage the therapist "helps the client to take steps toward change" (p. 18). In the maintenance stage, the role of the clinician is "to identify and use strategies to prevent relapse" (p. 18). If a relapse occurs, the therapist's task is to then "help the client to renew the processes of contemplation, determination, and action, without becoming stuck or demoralized because of a relapse" (p. 18). These strategies, ironically, also prevent demoralization in therapists committed to helping clients, as the dynamic process of MI provides the therapist with strategies for assessing, addressing, and increasing a client's motivation for change at all stages of this process (W. R. Miller & Rollnick, 2002).

Underlying Principles and Treatment Interventions in Motivational Interviewing: The Initial Model

MI in its initial form has five main principles underlying its therapeutic approach: "(1) express empathy, (2) develop discrepancy, (3) avoid argumentation, (4) roll with the resistance, and (5) support self-efficacy" (W. R. Miller & Rollnick, 1991, p. 55). *Expressing empathy* involves the therapist viewing the world from the client's perspective (W. R. Miller

& Rollnick, 2002). *Developing discrepancy* occurs when clients begin to recognize that their values and goals conflict with their current behaviors. *Avoiding argumentation* is an important component of MI, in that it is counterproductive to the treatment and therapy relationship for clinicians to enter into confrontations with their clients. W. R. Miller and Rollnick (1991, 2002) view "resistance" as occurring when clients view the therapist as imposing the therapist's own perspective on the problem and taking away the clients' autonomy.

Rolling with the resistance is one strategy for avoiding this type of conflict or confrontation. Therapists invite clients to explore alternative points of view without imposing their viewpoints. Finally, there is an emphasis throughout MI on *supporting self-efficacy*, that is, the belief of clients that they have the power to change within themselves. This is important because clients may have tried to change in the past and relapsed. W. R. Miller and Rollnick (2002) encourage therapists to explore past successes and to emphasize the internal strengths that the client already possesses. Examples of these strategies are given throughout this chapter.

MI has been used clinically with clients who have presented with serious conditions, such as substance abuse (W. R. Miller & Rollnick, 1991, 2002), anxiety, posttraumatic stress disorder (PTSD), obsessive–compulsive disorder, depression, suicidality, eating disorders, and other psychological problems (Arkowitz et al., 2008). Many of these clients had traditionally felt misunderstood and pressured to make changes that were difficult and slow going. This often resulted in a cycle composed of alienation and frustration on the part of the client and repeated disappointment on the part of natural supports and treatment providers. By first understanding and empathizing with the client's reality, this cycle can be interrupted. This process of engagement also encourages the therapist to establish therapeutic rapport with the client.

W. R. Miller and Rollnick (2002) have developed the acronym OARS as an aid to therapists to remember the strategies of their approach: Open-ended questions, Affirmations, Reflections, and Summaries. Open-ended questions are worded in such a way as to avoid simple yes or no answers. They invite the client to describe his or her experience in more detail. Affirmations build on the client's strengths, reframe his or her experiences in a more positive way, and communicate that what a client says is important and matters. Reflections involve the process of reflective listening, which is described in more detail below. Summaries are important parts of the reflective listening process. They can be used to sum up key issues that the client has presented or to develop discrepancy between both sides of a client's ambivalence.

As indicated above, MI is built upon the underlying principles of empathy on the part of the therapist toward the client, which include interpersonal warmth, reflective listening, and acceptance (Miller & Rollnick, 1991, 2002). The following excerpt captures the role of empathy in treatment:

> Through skillful reflective listening, the therapist seeks to understand the client's feelings and perspectives without judging, criticizing, or blaming. It is important to note that acceptance is not the same thing as agreement or approval. It is possible to accept and understand a client's perspective but not to agree with it. . . . The crucial attitude is a respectful listening to the client with a desire to understand his or her perspectives. Paradoxically, this kind of acceptance of people as they are seems to free them to change, whereas insistent non-acceptance ("You're not OK; you have to change") can have the effect of keeping people as they are. This attitude of acceptance and respect also builds a working therapeutic alliance, and supports the client's self-esteem— an important condition for change (Miller, 1983). . . . (W. R. Miller & Rollnick, 1991, pp. 55–56)

Reflective listening is an important part of the process of expressing empathy and is one of the most important clinical skills that a therapist can possess. Therapists can become trapped in the process of continually asking questions of their clients because, at times, this may seem easier than true reflective listening. W. R. Miller and Rollnick (1991) point out that such repetitive questioning about meaning can actually "distance clients from experiencing it" (p. 74) and result in a therapist being more active than the client. It can also distance the therapist from the client.

W. R. Miller and Rollnick (1991, 2002) indicate that reflective listening involves making a statement that is guessing about the client's underlying meaning. It does not involve simply parroting back the client's words. The therapist seeks to form a hypothesis about the client's meaning and then gives voice to that hypothesis. Reflective listening requires a great deal of skill in which tone of voice, body language, and eye contact are crucial elements. When it is done well, the client feels heard and understood. It is not just the words but also a warm, accepting, nonjudgmental tone that is important.

For many clients, the process of having someone genuinely interested enough to be concerned about them and their thoughts and feelings can be a new experience. The therapist's reflection of his or her understanding of their message can be validating and help clients, particularly those caught in long-term patterns of shame and isolation, to feel connected to another human being in a new and meaningful way. For example, a client begins the session by angrily stating that "I am sick and tired of treatment. I am fed up." A therapist who applies reflective listening would be more likely to respond, "What I am hearing you say is that you are really upset and angry and you are fed up with therapy because change does not seem to be happening quickly enough. Did I understand you correctly?" This approach is utilized instead of becoming defensive and following the normal human urge to justify the therapy process. Rather than shutting down dialogue, which a defensive response may be likely to accomplish, the reflective listening response indicates the therapist's willingness to tolerate the client's anger and to understand the reasons for it.

The process of reflective listening can also be used in family and couple therapy sessions. Here, the therapist must be conscious of balancing and using reflective listening to convey an understanding of the position of all parties. The following case example illustrates this point.

Justin, a 15-year-old African American male, was seen in therapy with his mother, who was very concerned about his cutting school and "running the streets." He and his mother, 38-year-old Martha, had developed an extreme continuous pattern of interacting in which one would yell and accuse the other, who would then defend his or her position and offer a return accusation. There was no interchange because neither of them heard the other person. In one session, both the mother and the son became especially angry. The mother yelled, "I am worried about you because I just read about a kid being caught in the crossfire of gang-related violence and dying." The son angrily responded, "I went to school twice this week but instead of giving me any credit you'd rather yell at me because of some kid neither of us even know."

The therapist used reflective listening with both parties and was careful to balance his comments. To the mother, he said, "I hear you saying that you feel really worried about Justin and afraid that he is locked in a pattern that could really put him in harm's way. You are scared that you may lose him and have him die like the boy in the newspaper. You both made some progress this week, and then seemed to go backward. You are really worried and frustrated."

To Justin, the therapist said, "You feel that you made some strides this week in going to school two days, but you feel that all you are hearing is negativity and pessimism from your mother. You feel your efforts are not being acknowledged, and it makes you feel angry and disappointed. I hear you saying that you need your mom to understand that you are trying really hard. Can you talk to each other about this, and when you do, mom, can you listen for your son's attempts to make a change, and Justin, can you try to hear the love and concern in your mother's words rather than the anger and criticism?"

This reflective listening intervention by the therapist was said in a warm, caring way and conveyed his empathy, understanding, and acceptance to both parties. It interrupted the angry exchange between them. This led to a tearful discussion between this mother and son in which they began to hear each other in a different way.

―――――――――

Many clients with serious mental health or substance abuse issues have felt shamed by others because of their behavior. MI is valuable in that it avoids a shaming approach. The process of developing discrepancy recognizes that within each human being there are parts that want change and parts that do not. MI honors both sides of this ambivalence by encouraging clients to talk openly about how their stated desire to change is contradicted by their continued involvement in the problem behavior. The case below demonstrates this process.

―――――――――

Ricky, a 58-year-old Jamaican American man with schizophrenia who lived in a supported housing apartment, was speaking to his case manager about wanting to get more consistent with taking his medication after being evaluated in an emergency room the previous day because of his erratic behavior. He requested information about mental health recovery groups he might attend to gain support and acceptance around medication use.

Later in the week, the case manager made a visit and discovered that Ricky had not taken his medication for the last three days. The case manager empathically reflected back to Ricky an appreciation for the internal struggle that he is facing in trying to make this change. On the one hand, Ricky struggles with the stigma of his diagnosis and side effects associated with his medication. Not taking medication makes him feel "normal." On the other hand, he reminded Ricky how passionately he spoke of making changes and how upset he was about having to go to the emergency room. The case manager emphasized that it is ultimately up to Ricky to grapple with these two sides and communicated a belief in Ricky's ability to change.

―――――――――

Many clinicians (like Ricky's case manager) find themselves engaged with clients in a process of resistance. As noted above, it is important that clinicians avoid arguing with their clients when disagreements are expressed. Argumentation is counterproductive and can lead to more resistance from clients (W. R. Miller & Rollnick, 1991, 2002) and further entrenchment in the problematic behavior. As in this case, expressing empathy, reflective listening, rolling with the resistance, developing discrepancy, and supporting self-efficacy allow clinicians to avoid these arguments with their clients and help them to move toward change.

W. R. Miller and Rollnick (2002) state that change is not able to occur unless a client has an element of belief and confidence in his or her ability to do so. Supporting self-efficacy is the vehicle through which therapists communicate a belief in the client's ability to make changes, emphasize strengths, and ultimately cultivate the client's connection to his or her inner capacities. Ultimately, it is important that these messages are conveyed with an appreciation for the client's self-determination and responsibility to make changes for him- or herself. These messages should always be conveyed in an empathic, nonjudgmental way. The following case example illustrates these principles.

Mary, a 30-year-old Irish-American woman, was referred to the therapist because she had been drinking on a daily basis and it had begun to interfere with her functioning. At home, her constant arguments with her partner about her drinking had made their once-loving relationship increasingly distant. At work, "hangovers" made her irritable with her supervisors and coworkers. In fact, she was recently passed over for a much-desired promotion. She was referred for treatment by her partner who was often critical of her behavior. She reported that when she felt depressed or anxious she drank and this initially relieved the tension that she felt and allowed her to feel "happy for the first time all day." However, every morning she woke up feeling terrible about her drinking. The tension with her partner intensified and she reported that she was "sick and tired of her and everyone else telling her to stop."

She acknowledged to the therapist that her drinking was one of the ways in which she rebelled against her partner, maintained a sense of her own independence, and resisted this pressure to change. The clinician responded empathically to her situation. He recognized that this had been difficult for her. He understood her belief that the drinking "took the edge off" of the anxiety and depression that she often felt.

Initially, Mary reported that she expected the clinician to also put pressure on her to stop. Instead, he asked her to tell him what she liked about drinking. She reported that her first drink initially relieved the tension that she was feeling. It took the edge off of her depression and made her feel normal. In addition, she felt some satisfaction and a sense of control in that no one could tell her what to do. The therapist used reflective listening skills to convey his understanding of the benefit she felt she gained from tension relief and her increased sense of control. Next, the therapist explored the things about the drinking that concerned her. She stated that she would really have liked to have gotten that promotion and dreamed of going to graduate school in order to further her career. She realized that embarking on this journey would require sustained sobriety.

The therapist explored further her desire to go to school and her concerns about the ways in which her drinking might interfere with this goal. He then worked toward developing the discrepancy by acknowledging empathically that there seemed to be two conflicting trends within her that were at odds with each other. On the one hand, she liked the relief that she initially felt from drinking and the sense of rebellion and control she felt in her relationship with her partner. At the same time, she felt some ambivalence about it because she often felt awful in the morning and she desperately wanted to progress at work but she knew she would have to stop drinking to do this. The therapist acknowledged her dilemma and the fact that this was tearing her up inside. He said, "Let's talk about where you want to go with this dilemma."

At the end of the session, it was clear that Mary was not ready to stop drinking. She became angry and stated that she was tired of the pressure from everyone to stop. The therapist avoided an argument and rolled with the resistance by stating: "Right now, you are not feeling like you want to deal with this and you're sick of the pressure." In addition, the therapist acknowledged that Mary was the only one who could ultimately make the decision. He also added that he believed that if she made her mind up to stop she could do so.

Over time, the therapist continued to honor her ambivalence and to create a climate in which she no longer needed to rebel against others. The battle was redefined from an external one with her partner and others who were pushing her to change to an internal process in which she was conflicted about both sides of her own ambivalence. Gradually, as she explored the personal benefits of changing—most importantly, her desire to advance in her career and go to graduate school—she began to stop drinking and to attend regular AA (Alcoholics Anonymous) meetings.

Well-meaning therapists can sometimes find themselves working on change before the client is ready, a situation especially prevalent when working with clients engaging in serious and potentially harmful behaviors such as substance abuse. This can lead to a battle for control. The metaphor of a seesaw is helpful in understanding this process. When you press down on a seesaw, the other side goes up. Similarly, if a therapist puts pressure on the client to change before the client is motivated to do so, the part of the client that does not want to change inevitably grows in intensity. We have often said to our supervisees: "If you get into a tug of war with a client, drop the rope." MI gives therapists a process through which to build motivation in resistant clients. MI does not seek to extinguish ambivalence, but gives the therapist the tools to honor and help clients to reconcile it. MI can provide a great measure of relief to therapists working with clients who describe engaging in destructive, harmful, and dangerous behaviors. Therapists then often find themselves feeling overly responsible for changing this behavior. By adapting the principles of MI to this situation, therapists are enabled to abandon their initial impulse to say, "Oh no! You've got to stop it!" and try to assert control when they recognize the power to change lies totally with the client. By reminding us that the client ultimately has the final choice in terms of his or her own behavior, we can overcome our feelings of frustration, powerlessness and, in some cases, burnout.

Change Talk

W. R. Miller and Rollnick (2011) define change talk as "statements by the client revealing consideration of, motivation for, or commitment to change" (p. 5). The therapist's role is to help to gently guide the client to statements involving change talk. As these statements increase, the likelihood of a more positive outcome increases. W. R. Miller and Rollnick have identified the following 10 strategies for eliciting and supporting change talk. These strategies are highlighted in Box 6.1.

The Evolution of Motivational Interviewing: Latest Developments

In the third edition of their book, W. R. Miller and Rollnick (2013) describe the evolution of MI, and incorporate many new ideas and new language. For example, as discussed above, the initial model used the term *rolling with the resistance* (W. R. Miller & Rollnick, 1991, 2002). Resistance was characterized as "any apparent client movement away from change" and usually referred to "signs of discord in the counseling relationship" (W. R. Miller & Rollnick, 2013, p. viii). Concerned that the term *resistance* might denote client blame, W. R. Miller and Rollnick (2013) reconceptualized this process and changed the term to *sustain talk*, which is composed of verbalizations that favor the status quo. They are the opposite of change talk.

Rolling with sustain talk gives therapists an effective strategy for avoiding a power struggle with their clients. It allows them to respond to a client by saying, "Okay, you are not ready to deal with this right now" (W. R. Miller & Rollnick, 2013). This helps to keep the client involved in the process and does not alienate him or her from the therapist, and leaves the door open for further discussion when the time is appropriate.

W. R. Miller and Rollnick (2013) describe four processes that MI comprises: engaging, focusing, evoking, and planning (p. vii). The first process, *engaging*, establishes "a helpful connection and a working relationship" (p. 36). This is consistent with the processes of joining and establishing the therapeutic relationship (our first core mediational process) discussed in Chapter 4. Within engagement, W. R. Miller and

BOX 6.1. Eliciting Change Talk

1. **Ask Evocative Questions:** Ask an open question, the answer to which is likely to be change talk.

2. **Explore Decisional Balance:** Ask for the pros and cons of both changing and staying the same.

3. **Good Things/Not-So-Good Things:** Ask about the positives and negatives of the target behavior.

4. **Ask for Elaboration/Examples:** When a change talk theme emerges, ask for more details. "In what ways?" "Tell me more?" "What does that look like?" "When was the last time that happened?"

5. **Look Back:** Ask about a time before the target behavior emerged. How were things better, different?

6. **Look Forward:** Ask what may happen if things continue as they are (status quo). Try the miracle question: If you were 100% successful in making the changes you want, what would be different? How would you like your life to be five years from now?

7. **Query Extremes:** What are the worst things that might happen if you don't make this change? What are the best things that might happen if you do make this change?

8. **Use Change Rulers:** Ask: "On a scale from 1 to 10, how important is it to you to change [the specific target behavior] where 1 is not at all important, and a 10 is extremely important? *Follow up:* "And why are you at ____ and not ____ [a lower number than stated]?" "What might happen that could move you from ____ to ____ [a higher number]?" Alternatively, you could ask "How confident are you that you could make the change if you decided to do it?"

9. **Explore Goals and Values:** Ask what the person's guiding values are. What do they want in life? Using a values card activity can be helpful here. Ask how the continuation of target behavior fits in with the person's goals or values. Does it help realize an important goal or value, interfere with it, or is it irrelevant?

10. **Come Alongside:** Explicitly side with the negative (status quo) side of ambivalence. "Perhaps _____ is so important to you that you won't give it up, no matter what the cost."

From W. R. Miller and Rollnick (2011, p. 6).

Rollnick emphasize listening and understanding the person's dilemma, incorporating the core interviewing skills and OARS (discussed above), and exploring the client's values and goals.

Once engagement has occurred, the second process of *focusing* involves working collaboratively with the client to establish the strategic direction for the discussion about change. Rather than using traditional styles of directing or following the client, W. R. Miller and Rollnick (2013) describe a guiding style that is a "collaborative search for direction, a meeting of expertise in which the focus of treatment is negotiated" (p. 99) between the therapist and the client. They describe clear strategies for circumstances in which the goals of the client and the therapist may differ. They provide ethical guidelines and caution therapists that when coercive power is combined with a therapist's personal investment in the client's behavior and outcomes, the use of MI may be inappropriate. In their discussion of exchanging information, W. R. Miller and Rollnick advocate a two-way exchange of ideas that shows respect for the client's perspective and his or her own needs, rather than having therapists asking a number of expert questions and then giving advice to the client.

These first two processes are consistent with many other forms of therapy discussed in this book. It is the third process, *evoking*, that is most particular to MI. Evoking involves recognizing, eliciting, and responding to change talk in treatment. W. R. Miller and Rollnick (2013) have expanded on the concept of ambivalence and described strategies for evoking the client's motivation for change. The major shift that happens in the course of MI is the increase in change talk and the decrease in sustain talk as sessions progress.

Planning is the final process in which the therapist must assess the client's readiness to change and begin to develop a collaborative plan to make it happen. W. R. Miller and Rollnick (2013) caution therapists that ambivalence may resurface in any part of this process. They encourage clinicians to be alert to changes in a client's motivation during the planning stage. When this occurs, therapists may have to use their clinical judgment and go back to an earlier process, such as engaging or evoking. They recommend testing the waters regarding the client's current readiness for change and listening carefully to the quality of the change talk before proceeding to develop a plan. Clinicians should be alert to change talk in this process that contains mobilizing statements such as "I am willing [ready, prepared] to . . . " (p. 286). The therapist's job at this stage is to help to strengthen the client's commitment to change. Finally, the therapist supports the client's change by encouraging persistence, replanning, and refocusing. W. R. Miller and Rollnick (2013) advocate for a two-way exchange of ideas that shows respect for the client's perspective and his or her own needs.

Combining Motivational Interviewing with Other Therapeutic Approaches

Research has shown that MI can be used effectively as a "stand-alone" treatment (Arkowitz et al., 2008; Hettema, Miller, & Steele, 2005). Arkowitz et al. also point out that MI "has been used successfully as a pretreatment to enhance motivation in subsequent treatment" (p. 10). "Meta-analyses of MI have found larger effect sizes (Burke, Arkowitz, & Menchola, 2003) and longer-lasting results (Hettema et al., 2005) for MI as a pretreatment than when used as a stand alone" (Arkowitz et al., 2008, p. 10). For example, it has been combined successfully with cognitive-behavioral therapy for alcoholism (Arkowitz et al., 2008; Connors, Walitzer, & Dermen, 2002). Arkowitz and Westra (2004) have also employed MI during the course of using another treatment, as a means of helping a clinician work with client resistance, lack of motivation, or ambivalence.

In our own work, we have found this approach to be helpful as we support clients in the real world who, although at times are committed to change and working hard to take action in their lives, often express ambivalence or recycle through earlier stages of change during the course of treatment. We find it helpful to consider MI as the foothills to treatment, where techniques to support the resolution of ambivalence are utilized more strongly and frequently in the beginning of treatment, then used again when the desire to change wavers.

Administrative Dilemmas for Clinicians

Clinicians and other mental health and substance abuse counselors often feel a great deal of pressure from their supervisors, administrators, and funding sources to produce change in clients. If administrators continue to pressure clinicians to push their clients to agree to change behaviors, they are likely to increase client resistance and frustrate their staff. It is important, therefore, that agencies, clinics, and hospitals support the use of MI.

MI is not a "one-shot" approach or merely a series of steps but instead comprises an ongoing dialogue with a client that can gradually lead to the client's decision to pursue change. This gradual process must be understood and interwoven in an ongoing treatment approach. The following case example demonstrates the gradual nature of this process.

Alberta, a 40-year-old African American woman, had been living in a residential facility for clients with mental illness since her discharge from a psychiatric hospital. She had been diagnosed with major depression and she had diabetes and hypertension. She was a compulsive overeater whose excessive intake of sweets threatened her health. Over the course of a few months, she had a number of diabetic crises and had been rushed to the emergency room. The doctor put her on a strict diet, but she often snuck out to the corner store in the middle of the night to purchase large amounts of her favorite snack foods.

Karla, her therapist, had the responsibility, in tandem with her case manager at the residence, to monitor Alberta's food intake. Initially, Alberta showed no interest in changing her eating habits. In the first session, she refused to acknowledge the therapist's concern that she might die if she did not change her pattern of eating. Alberta said, "I have been eating this way all of my life and I'm not dead yet. If it ain't broke why fix it? Besides, my eating is not as bad as some of the other residents." The therapist used reflective listening and said, "So what I hear you saying is that you honestly don't think that your eating is that big a deal. You've been eating this way for a long time and you've seen a lot of other people here who eat more than you. It sounds like you feel frustrated and that you're being picked on and singled out." Alberta agreed and added that she hated "this whole diabetes thing . . . the insulin shots . . . and the always having to prick my finger."

Her therapist felt frustrated with this response but discussed food with Alberta and helped her to develop a food plan. Two days later, the therapist learned that a member of the night staff found Alberta in the kitchen of the residence, gorging on jelly donuts. The night staff member reported that Alberta "cursed her out and defiantly ate the whole box of jelly donuts." The therapist's first thought was "What are you doing? I just told you that you might die if you keep eating like this." The therapist restrained herself, however, and did not voice that thought. Instead, she used the MI techniques that she had been learning through a training in her agency. She said empathically to Alberta, "Boy you really love snack foods. Tell me about it." Alberta responded that she had a sweet tooth, and especially loved to eat pastries.

The therapist decided to explore the eating and asked Alberta to tell her more about what made her want to eat and what she liked best. Alberta gave a long list of foods, most of which were forbidden for diabetics and not on the food plan Karla and Alberta developed together, and again stated that she particularly loved sweets. The therapist said, "I see what you mean. You really get a lot of enjoyment out of eating, especially from eating sweets. How do they make you feel?" Alberta responded that it "really makes me feel good and calm, especially if I am feeling kind of down." The therapist responded, "I hear what you're saying. Besides tasting good, sweets make you feel better." Alberta perked up as she began to feel understood and not judged by her therapist.

The therapist then said, "Okay, so I see that there are some real plus-ses to eating sweets, is there a downside to eating them?" Alberta at first couldn't think of anything. Later, she responded, "I guess I could get sick and have to go back to that stupid hospital." She also added that her children and her mother got really worried when she got sick. The case manager developed the discrepancy by saying, "So, to be honest, you have a sweet tooth and it makes you feel good to eat sugary sweets. Not only do they taste good but they also make you feel good and calmer. On the other hand, you really hate having to go to the hospital when your diabetes acts up and you would like to be healthier so that your children and your mom wouldn't worry about you so much. This is a really tough dilemma. What would help you figure it out?" The therapist also emphasized Alberta's personal responsibility by saying, "The choice is yours. No one can force you to change your eating habits unless you want to."

This process continued over many months. One week, the therapist learned that Alberta "cursed out" another member of the night staff (who had discovered her eating donuts) but that this time she left the kitchen after eating only a few donuts rather than all of them. The therapist affirmed her gain. She focused on the positive and said, "I know how much eating those donuts means to you and it must have been really hard to walk away without eating the whole box while being so upset." Alberta talked more about this experience and also about how angry she was that everyone kept "bugging" her about what she eats. The therapist reflected that she was "really angry and fed up that people keep getting into her business."

Gradually, however, Alberta's eating pattern began to change. The therapist validated and affirmed her for eating less. Alberta reported that she only ate three sugary snacks one night. A week later she reported one snack. The therapist reflected how really difficult this must be for her but praised her for her continuous gains.

Conclusion

MI is a highly effective, widely adaptable set of principles, strategies, and clinical interventions. It is continually evolving and expanding its treatment model (W. R. Miller & Rollnick, 1991, 2002, 2013). At its core, MI seeks to accomplish three overarching goals. First, it inspires an increase in intrinsic motivation for change. This is significant because if people are going to take on the difficult challenge of overcoming pro-tracted difficulties in the areas of mental illness, substance abuse, and physical health, the change effort has to be connected to deeply held internal needs and values. In the case of Alberta, her change effort was stimulated by her desire not to let down her family members and to avoid being bogged down by frequent hospitalizations.

Secondly, MI's goal is to inspire hope and optimism that one can embark on sustained change over time. As noted above, in order for people to push into unfamiliar territory, one must first have confidence that he or she has the capacity to make these changes. Lastly, MI seeks to honor ambivalence and support the client in identifying and reconciling it. This is best accomplished through rolling with resistance, empathic reflection, decisional balancing, and a continuous development of discrepancy (W. R. Miller & Rollnick, 1991, 2002). Ultimately, the emphasis on the client's responsibility for change frees the therapist from an overidentification and attachment to his or her own change agenda and allows for the client's inner change argument to manifest (W. R. Miller & Rollnick, 1991, 2002, 2013).

This chapter has discussed the evolution of MI over time and has illustrated the parts of the model that we have found most useful in our clinical work and in the training of other therapists. One of the most important aspects of this model has been its emphasis on the spirit of MI, which encourages clinicians to form partnerships with their clients, accept them as human beings, show compassion for them, and work collaboratively to evoke the motivation for change (W. R. Miller & Rollnick, 2013).

CHAPTER 7

Cognitive–Behavioral Therapy

2 different frames
a numerical ^

Introduction

Cognitive-behavioral therapy (CBT) is an evidence-based treatment model that helps clients become more aware of the relationship among their thoughts, feelings, and behaviors (J. S. Beck, 2011; Padesky, Kuyken, & Dudley, 2011; Persons, 2008). It teaches clients to reflectively identify automatic thoughts and to appreciate how these thoughts contribute to negative emotional responses and keep them entrenched in self-defeating behaviors (J. S. Beck, 1995, 2011). Cognitive-behavioral therapy is our fourth core mediational process and is an evidence-based approach that has been found to be helpful in treating a range of presenting problems and diagnoses including mood and anxiety disorders, personality disorders, psychosis, addiction, and sexual dysfunction (Barlow, 2008).

As a treatment, CBT is goal oriented, problem focused, and time limited. The therapist's primary goal includes symptom relief leading to the remission of psychological disorder(s). Establishing a therapeutic relationship, client–therapist collaboration, and the active participation of clients in their own treatment, are central to the CBT framework (J. S. Beck, 2011; Padesky et al., 2011; Persons, 2008).

In the initial stages, CBT is concerned with treating symptoms as they occur in the present. Through treatment, the therapist works to teach clients the necessary skills to address current problems and prevent relapse in the future (J. S. Beck, 2011, Meichenbaum, 2008; Persons, 2008). In this way, CBT teaches clients how to address issues themselves and avoid dependency on the therapist (J. S. Beck, 2011; Meichenbaum, 2008). Because a wide variety of CBT techniques addressing clients' unhealthy thoughts, feelings, and behaviors may be incorporated into the treatment process in general (Barlow, 2008; J. S. Beck, 2011), we have identified CBT as a core mediational process and a skill that is important for therapists practicing in the real world.

In this chapter we discuss engagement and collaboration within the CBT framework, and then review the basic tenets of this model including core beliefs, schemas, automatic thoughts, and cognitive distortions. We then focus on the use of common CBT interventions such as behavioral activation, homework, behavioral experiments, exposure therapy, role playing, and relaxation techniques, and explore the importance of their integration into the treatment process.

The Therapeutic Relationship and Collaboration with the Client

As we noted in Chapter 4, research has consistently demonstrated that the therapeutic relationship is one of the most important predictors of treatment outcome (Norcross, 2002, 2011a). With this in mind, CBT theorists and researchers have emphasized the importance of establishing a strong therapeutic relationship (J. S. Beck, 2011; Meichenbaum, 2008; Persons, 2008). CBT, like many other forms of therapy, emphasizes the importance of conveying to our clients that we care about and value them and advocates checking in with clients regularly to see how they are experiencing the treatment process (J. S. Beck, 2011; Meichenbaum, 2008).

As discussed in our introduction to the core mediational processes (see Chapter 1), Meichenbaum (2008) emphasizes the importance of instilling hope in the client. Instilling hope also includes a message that the therapist is confident that treatment can work for the client, and that other patients with similar problems have been helped by treatment in the past. Similarly, conveying that the therapist will not be overwhelmed by the client's problems, even though the client may feel overwhelmed, is also important to giving a client hope and confidence in the treatment process (J. S. Beck, 2011).

Collaboration between the client and the therapist is another important concept within CBT (J. S. Beck, 1995, 2011; Meichenbaum, 2008; Padesky et al., 2011; Persons, 2008). Creating the idea of a team working together is central to effective treatment. Within this context, it is important to seek feedback from clients about how they are experiencing the treatment process. For example, at the end of a session, a therapist might say, "This was a heavy session. You worked very hard. How was this session for you?" Similarly, if a client appears uncomfortable or distressed by something in the session, the therapist might say, "You look upset. What was just going through your mind?" (J. S. Beck, 2011,

p. 20). This gives the client the opportunity to share his or her experience with the therapist, which can help to deepen the therapeutic alliance and enhance the relationship.

Core Beliefs, Schemas, and Automatic Thoughts

Another key component in CBT is the concept of core beliefs. Core beliefs are ideas that people begin to develop in childhood that influence the ways in which they view themselves, their families, other individuals, and their world (J. S. Beck 2011; Meichenbaum, 2008; Padesky et al., 2011; Persons, 2008). A. T. Beck (1964) referred to these core beliefs as schemas. Three main categories of negative core beliefs have been identified: those related to helplessness, those related to unlovability, and those related to worthlessness (A. T. Beck, 1999; J. S. Beck, 2005). Some clients may experience these negative core beliefs only when they are in stressful situations. Other clients may have negative core beliefs that are constantly activated. Core beliefs often lie beneath the surface of automatic thoughts, and the reactive coping or compensatory strategies are used to counteract these thoughts (J. S. Beck, 1995, 2011). Often these compensatory strategies are used by the client to prevent coming into contact with anxiety-provoking stimuli that are either internal or external. For example, a client who is extremely anxious about driving on major highways may have an automatic thought that he or she will be in a car accident and die. This fear may lead the client to avoid this type of driving as a way of preventing anxiety in the short term. Unfortunately, however, this avoidance (the client's compensatory strategy) may seriously limit this person's life and work opportunities, further reinforcing his or her core belief of helplessness in the long term. *avoidance maintains*

The CBT model indicates that it is not necessarily the situation itself that causes negative emotion, rather it is the client's interpretation of the situation that is the issue (J. S. Beck, 1995, 2011; Meichenbaum, 2008; Padesky et al., 2011; Persons, 2008). For example, a client walking down the street sees a close acquaintance walking toward him or her. Rather than stop and talk, the acquaintance abruptly crosses the street without saying hello. The client may automatically interpret this event as the acquaintance purposely avoiding him or her. As a result, the client feels depressed and rejected and, in turn, becomes preoccupied at work, unable to focus and get through his or her day productively (Cohen, Mannarino, & Deblinger, 2006). In working with this client, a therapist using a CBT approach might seek to help the client expand his or her automatic interpretation of that event. The therapist may challenge the client's certainty that the acquaintance was purposely avoiding him or her and may help the client to explore other interpretations that would explain the acquaintance's behavior, for example, the acquaintance didn't see the client, he or she was preoccupied, and so on. The clinician might help the client to think through these alternate interpretations of the event and the resulting effect that his or her new automatic thoughts would have on his or her subsequent feelings and behaviors.

Because automatic thoughts are often brief, clients may be less in touch with them than they are with the emotions that they feel. Within the CBT model, the therapist first explains these automatic thoughts to clients and explores what they were thinking in order to help them determine how their thoughts may affect their emotions (J. S. Beck, 1995, 2011; Persons, 2008). The therapist helps clients to learn to access their actual thoughts and not their interpretations of those thoughts (J. S. Beck, 2011). For example, a man who was avoidant of social interactions with women and afraid of rejection was asked by his therapist what he thought when he was introduced to an attractive woman at a party. Initially, he responded that he had started to worry about what she thought of him. When the therapist discussed this with him further, they were able to clarify his actual automatic thought as "She won't like me" (J. S. Beck, 2011). It is this actual automatic thought that produces the negative emotional reaction that a client experiences.

The search engine Google represents a particularly useful metaphor for challenging initial interpretations and exploring alternative explanations (Collis, 2010). For example, if you were to search "lamps" in Google, the first few listings are colored differently than the subsequent 1,000+ listings. These initial links are colored differently because they are sponsored links (e.g., companies such as Lamps Plus paid Google money to have their website emerge as a first hit whenever someone searches for lamps). These initial listings are compelling and seductive, and designed to lure people into their websites rather than exploring the other 1,000+ listings. Similarly, a person struggling with generalized anxiety disorder (GAD) will experience several automatic thoughts when triggered. These thoughts that are "sponsored" by generalized anxiety, too, can be seductive and alluring and cause one to be blinded to alternative possibilities and information. It is not until one can appreciate the compelling nature of these "sponsored" or typical automatic thought cycles of GAD that the content of these thoughts can be challenged (Collis, 2010).

Cognitive Distortions

The CBT model recognizes that clients may have errors in their thinking that lead them to distort their experiences. The therapist labels these cognitive distortions and teaches clients to learn to label them also (J. S. Beck, 2011). The following are a few of the examples of cognitive distortions:

- *All-or-nothing thinking* (also called black-and-white, polarized, or dichotomous thinking): Example: "If I am not a total success, I'm a failure."
- *Catastrophizing* (also called fortune-telling): You predict the future negatively. Example: "I'll be so upset; I won't be able to function at all."
- *Disqualifying or discounting the positive:* You unreasonably tell yourself that positive experiences, deeds, or qualities do not count. Example: "I did that project well, but that doesn't mean I'm competent; I just got lucky."
- *Labeling:* You put a fixed, global label on yourself or others without considering that the evidence might more reasonably lead to a less disastrous conclusion. Examples: "I'm a loser"; "He's no good."
- *Mind reading:* You believe you know what others are thinking, failing to consider other, more likely possibilities. Example: "He thinks that I don't know the first thing about this project" (J. S. Beck, 2011, p. 181).

The therapist who uses CBT teaches clients to recognize these and other cognitive distortions and to learn to evaluate their thinking in different circumstances when their automatic thoughts might be overly negative or might distort the situation. J. S. Beck (2011) gives many illustrations from sessions that help therapists to explore these issues with their clients. She also indicates certain situations where a therapist might use selective self-disclosure to illustrate a point for a client and to normalize his or her experience. For example, a therapist may use his or her own experience of challenging the thoughts that contribute to his or her own people-pleasing tendencies with a client who struggles to make everyone in his or her life happy. By using selective self-disclosure, the therapist may normalize the client's experience and model how to challenge one's maladaptive automatic thoughts.

One useful strategy is to help clients to develop thought records of the cognitive distortions they may experience (J. S. Beck, 2011; Padesky et al., 2011). Therapists can then help clients develop a list of possible things that they can do when they have these automatic thoughts or when they are feeling anxious or depressed. Clients are encouraged to write these strategies down in a journal or a notebook so that they are available to them between therapy sessions or even after they have completed therapy. For example, J. S. Beck (2011) gives the following examples of entries that therapists helped clients to make in their notebooks that discuss ways to address these dysfunctional thoughts and upsetting feelings:

> When I think "I'd rather stay in bed," tell myself that I always feel a little better when I get something done and worse when I do nothing. (p. 189)

> Strategies for when I'm anxious
>
> 1. Do a Thought Record.
> 2. Read coping cards.
> 3. Call [friend].
> 4. Go for a walk or run.
> 5. Tolerate the anxiety. It is an unpleasant feeling but it's not life threatening, and it will decrease once I turn my attention to something else. (p. 191)

Behavioral Activation

Depressed clients have often withdrawn from interactions with others and may avoid activities that were once positive parts of their lives. Through behavioral activation, which can help clients look at factors that impact their moods in daily life, therapists support clients in improving their mood and sense of self-efficacy by becoming more active and involved in how they respond to daily stressors. Behavioral activation was identified as equivalent to medication and more effective than cognitive therapy in a randomized placebo-controlled trial (Dimidjian, Martell, Addis, & Herman-Dunn, 2008; Dimidjian et al., 2006). CBT therapists may help their clients to make lists of the activities that make them feel better and those that make them feel worse throughout the course of their day. Below is an example of a list of activities for someone struggling with depression:

Activities That Make Me Feel Better	Activities That Make Me Feel Worse
• Going for a walk	• Staying home all day
• Playing with my dog	• Watching too much TV
• Dancing	• Withdrawing from family and friends
• Calling my sister	• Eating high-fat foods
• Going to church	• Comparing myself to others on Facebook

At the beginning of each session, the therapist would do a brief mood check in order to establish how the client is feeling on a particular day and review the activities in which he or she participated. Clients can then be helped to see the connection between behavioral activation and positive mood by examining activities such as those in the first column. They can then explore the relationship between more passive activities (such as those described in the second column) and feelings of depression.

Homework

Homework is a central part of CBT. Researchers have found that clients who do homework assignments have better outcomes (Kazantzis, Whittington, & Datillio, 2010; Neimeyer & Feixas, 1990). J. S. Beck (2011) indicates that from the first session, therapists should prepare clients to do homework and to understand its importance. For example, for clients who are depressed, activity scheduling may increase behavioral activation. Monitoring and recording automatic thoughts can also be helpful homework assignments, which later allow the client to evaluate and respond to these thoughts in and outside of therapy. In addition, lists that are constructed during sessions may be helpful to clients. For example, a homework assignment might ask a client to consult a list when considering ways to modify automatic thoughts. In working with a depressed client, a therapist may have the client set an alarm twice a day to remind him or her to read a coping card. This card can include reminding oneself that when one's mood decreases: (1) that depression is an illness that will get better with treatment; (2) to write down all automatic thoughts and to remember that these thoughts aren't necessarily true; and (3) to make plans with friends and remember that if they say no, it's most likely because they are busy, not because they don't want to spend time with the client (J. S. Beck, 2011). In using homework, it is important to tailor assignments to the individual and to develop each one collaboratively with the client (J. S. Beck, 2011). In order to reinforce the importance of these assignments, therapists should review them in each session and discuss the client's responses and experiences to each task.

In the real world, many clinicians can become frustrated when clients do not follow through on designated homework and behavior activation assignments. It is our experience that even when clients do not engage in outside-of-session assignments, that the process of discussing the assignments in session creates a platform for dialoguing on values, expectations, and barriers to be further explored. This dialogue alone can serve as a catalyst for change.

Behavioral Experiments

Meichenbaum (2008) and J. S. Beck (2011) discuss the importance of developing personal behavioral experiments in which clients can test out new behaviors. These may begin as role plays in session with the clinician and the client. They may continue as homework assignments that can then be experienced in the real world. When a behavioral experiment is first attempted, it is important to help the client to set up an experience that might actually be successful.

For example, J. S. Beck (2011) describes a therapy session with a client who was in college and afraid to speak up and assert herself in communicating with her professors. For the first behavioral experiment, the therapist asked the client to describe a professor who she thought would be receptive to her. They role-played an interaction with this professor in session. For her homework assignment, the client was then encouraged to speak to that professor after class. The client came to the next session reporting that she had successfully approached her professor and was proud of her efforts.

Because in the real world clients often encounter situations where others may not respond as positively as we might like, the therapist could then help the client prepare for a possible negative outcome. In a therapy session, the therapist might help the client to discuss and list the possible automatic thoughts or beliefs that would be aroused if she received a negative response from one of her professors. The therapist could then ask the client to construct responses to challenge these negative automatic thoughts, and write them in her journal, as a means of coping with negative experiences and reactions she might encounter in the future.

Modifying Core Beliefs

Once the therapist has helped the client to identify the core beliefs underlying his or her cognitive distortions, there are a number of strategies that can help the client to modify these beliefs (J. S. Beck, 1995, 2011; Padesky et al., 2011). For instance, the therapist might give an example of someone who presents an extreme of the core belief that the client holds. This can be a real person or an imaginary one. Therapists might also use stories, metaphors, or movies that they ask a client to view (J. S. Beck, 2011). For example, a client who struggles with guilt and self-blame was asked to view the film *Ordinary People,* in which the central character, Conrad, struggles with survivor guilt following the death of his brother. The following week, the client expressed how misguided Conrad's behavior was as a result of his distorted self-perception. The client was then more open to taking a look at how negative core beliefs influenced his own behaviors and self-concept.

Exposure

As noted above, anxious and depressed clients often use avoidance as a way to cope with their negative emotions. They may feel that something terrible will occur if they engage in certain activities, and so they do all they can not to engage in them. While such avoidance may be reinforcing for clients, because it brings immediate relief from distress, as a coping strategy, it may perpetuate the clients' problems. With avoidant clients, therapists often explain to clients that they need to gain some exposure to the circumstances they fear (Abramowitz, Deacon, & Whiteside, 2011). The client and therapist develop a hierarchy of the most- and least-feared situations, and discuss coping strategies.

Working together, the therapist and the client identify an activity in this hierarchy that would cause the client low discomfort (J. S. Beck, 2011). The therapist has the client engage in this activity daily, until his or her anxiety about it has decreased significantly. The therapist often asks clients to record these experiences and their reactions to them on an activity chart so that they can be discussed in session. The following is a case example that illustrates many of these concepts.

Cindy, a college freshman, walked into an introductory calculus class, and experienced the automatic thought that she was going to fail the class, appear dumb, and be laughed at by her classmates. Upon entry into the room, she froze and experienced heart palpitations and shortness of breath, which did not resolve until she left the class and returned to her dorm room. Cindy feared both the situation that brought on the anxiety reaction (i.e., the calculus class, as well as the symptoms she associated with the reaction, i.e., heart palpitations, shortness of breath, self-judgment, and recrimination). As a result, she worried that she might withdraw from the class, or fall into a pattern of cutting the class, both of which would reinforce her underlying belief that she was inadequate.

Instead, she began working with a CBT therapist. A critical component of CBT is to help the client to develop an increased awareness of the process in which thoughts, feelings, and behaviors work together to produce the avoidant reaction. Cindy's therapist worked with her to help her to appreciate the power of these automatic thoughts, and to identify, challenge, and interrupt this process.

The therapist then introduced the concept of exposure (J. S. Beck, 1995, 2011) as a practice that could ultimately lead to extinguishing or greatly reducing her symptoms. The therapist explained to Cindy the nature and importance of exposure and began to collaboratively construct a hierarchy of feared stimuli. In moving through this hierarchy of activities, it was hoped that Cindy would develop skills she could use to manage the fear and the avoidant impulse in the moment. The theory was that, as she was able to master these experiences, her anxiety would lessen and the phobia would cease to be a significant life barrier.

The therapist then applied these concepts to Cindy's specific experience. The external stimulus Cindy sought to avoid was the calculus class, while the internal stimuli were the negative thoughts about being subpar and not intelligent, fears of failing the class and being ridiculed by her peers, and the subsequent panic attacks triggered by these thoughts and feelings. Cindy and the therapist co-constructed a hierarchical list of exposure exercises that could be discussed in session, specifically having Cindy focus on and challenge her predictions of failure. This was done by having Cindy explore the evidence that she was inadequate, and look for evidence in past accomplishments that she actually had the ability to succeed. Next, the therapist and Cindy collaboratively constructed a plan for her to attend class and utilize relaxation techniques to enter and remain seated in the class despite the discomforting feelings of inadequacy and the resulting anxiety. The therapist encouraged Cindy to write down her automatic thoughts in a journal and bring them to their next session so that they might collaboratively relabel and restructure her core beliefs. The ultimate goal for Cindy in treatment was to help her be able to regularly attend her calculus class.

Role Playing

Role playing is a technique that is common to many different schools of therapy and that can be utilized for many different purposes (J. S. Beck, 2011). It can be helpful for clients who struggle with learning new social skills, and may help these clients to feel less anxious if they rehearse these skills first with their therapist in a session. Techniques such as assertiveness training (J. S. Beck, 2011; McKay & Fanning, 2005; Wolpe, 1990) are often helpful with clients who feel unable to express their own opinions in certain situations or with certain individuals. Similarly, some forms of exposure can be role-played with the therapist before the client attempts to do them in real situations. This process of practicing a new behavior can be empowering for clients and may increase their feelings of self-efficacy. An example of a role play for Cindy would entail her practicing raising her hand and answering questions while describing and challenging the associated thoughts and feelings she experiences in doing so.

Relaxation Techniques

Relaxation techniques can be helpful to clients, particularly those coping with anxiety (Davis, Eshelman, & McKay, 2008). These techniques include progressive muscle relaxation, imagery, and controlled breathing as relaxation exercises that many clients may find helpful. Although clients may wish to purchase relaxation tapes that they can listen to at home, Beck (2011) encourages therapists to teach relaxation techniques in session so that the therapist and client can observe and process the client's reactions. As with all CBT interventions, it is important that you encourage clients to view this as an experiment that may work for them and that they can discuss in session (J. S. Beck, 2011).

Conclusion

This chapter has presented many of the principles of CBT. CBT is more than just a set of interventions and strategies; it is the fourth core mediational process that sensitizes one to the complexity and power of the relationship between thoughts, feelings, and behaviors. Once one is able to recognize and observe the intricacies of this relationship, he or she gains an increased ability to challenge cognitive distortions and interrupt long-held negative core beliefs.

The next chapter explores the "third wave" of CBT approaches that have incorporated mindfulness and acceptance-based principles (Hayes et al., 2004). Mindfulness principles aid clients in viewing and accepting their own internal experiences nonjudgmentally (Bien, 2010; Kabat-Zinn, 1990; M. G. Williams et al., 2007). Acceptance principles help clients to accept the reality of their conditions and life circumstances, while working with them to identify their values and commit to living a meaningful life (Hayes, Strosahl, & Wilson, 1999, 2011; Hayes et al., 2004). These principles are particularly helpful with clients who have serious mental illnesses, repeated experiences of relapse, and/or substance abuse disorders. ✦

CHAPTER 8

Mindfulness- and Acceptance–Based Principles and Practices

Introduction

One of the developments in the field expanding the tradition of cognitive behavioral therapy (Hayes et al., 2004) is the inclusion and incorporation of mindfulness- (Bien, 2010; Hick & Bien, 2010; Kabat-Zinn, 1990; M. G. Williams et al., 2007) and acceptance-based principles and practices (Hayes et al., 2004). Taken together, mindfulness- and acceptance-based principles constitute the fifth core mediational process. These principles have led to the development of a number of therapies including, but not limited to, acceptance and commitment therapy (ACT; Eifert & Forsyth, 2005; Hayes, Strosahl, & Wilson, 1999, 2011), dialectical behavior therapy (DBT; Linehan, 1993; Robins, Schmidt, & Linehan, 2004), mindfulness-based cognitive therapy (MBCT; Segal, Teasdale, & Williams, 2004), and mindfulness-based relapse prevention (MBRP; Bowen et al., 2011; Marlatt et al., 2008; Witkiewitz, Marlatt, & Walker, 2005). We have found these approaches to be profoundly helpful in real-world practice, particularly with clients with serious mental illness and dual diagnoses (i.e., mental illness and substance abuse). Because many of these clients may experience the reemergence of symptoms at various points in their lives, unrealistic expectations of a complete "cure" of their illness often lead to frustration, shame, relapse, and a sense of hopelessness. Mindfulness- and acceptance-based principles help clients to accept the reality of their illness, and to recognize that while they may have periods when symptoms reappear or relapse occurs, they can still live a meaningful and value-filled life pursuing their core values and goals (Bowen et al., 2011; Eifert & Forsyth, 2005; Hayes, Strosahl, & Wilson, 1999, 2011; Marlatt et al., 2008; Witkiewitz et al., 2005).

Mindfulness- and acceptance-based principles move treatment away from an agenda focused solely on the elimination and control of symptoms, to a more nuanced appreciation for and the incorporation of natural painful experiences in a client's life. In other words, pain is a part of life, and suffering occurs when one overidentifies with, fights against, and/or actively avoids pain (Hayes, Strosahl, & Wilson, 1999, 2011; Hayes et al., 2004; Linehan, 1993). From this perspective, clinical work is not about trying to remove feelings; it is about helping a person develop a healthier and more flexible relationship to the totality of his or her thoughts, feelings, and internal evaluations. Rather than modifying automatic thoughts and core beliefs as in traditional CBT (J. S. Beck, 2011), mindfulness- (Hick & Bien, 2010) and acceptance-based practices focus on modifying one's relationship to these thoughts (Eifert & Forsyth, 2005; Hayes, Strosahl, & Wilson, 1999, 2011). In the real world, clients often present with myriad psychosocial stressors and complex mental health diagnoses. Mindfulness- and acceptance-based principles create a context for the client and therapist to collaboratively let go of the cure agenda, and develop an acceptance of pain while teaching the skills necessary to alleviate suffering.

The first part of this chapter discusses the use of mindfulness as a conceptual framework and a practice that can inform the work of therapists and help them in the development of therapeutic relationships with their clients. There have been many applications of mindfulness to different psychiatric disorders and substance abuse recovery (Bowen et al., 2011; Marlatt et al., 2008; Witkiewitz et al., 2005). (See Chapter 9 for a discussion of mindfulness-based relapse prevention [MBRP].) This chapter illustrates the use of mindfulness in the treatment of two specific disorders: (1) treatment of depression using mindfulness-based cognitive therapy (MBCT; Segal et al., 2004), and (2) the treatment of obsessive–compulsive disorder (J. M. Schwartz & Beyette, 1996). Next, we examine the combination of mindfulness- and acceptance-based principles in acceptance and commitment therapy (ACT) through the work of Hayes, Strosahl, and Wilson (1999, 2011) and Eifert and Forsyth (2005). Finally, we give a brief discussion of the incorporation of mindfulness and "radical acceptance" in the practice of dialectical behavior therapy (DBT) (Robins et al., 2004).

Mindfulness-Based Principles

Hick and Bien (2010) describe mindfulness as "focusing attention, being aware, intentionality, being nonjudgmental, acceptance, and compassion" (p. 5). It is a present-focused state of being in which a person acknowledges and accepts without judgment, each thought, feeling, and bodily sensation that arises in his or her experience (Hick & Bien, 2010).

Human beings often live in the past or future, and have a hard time staying with their feelings and experiences in the present, particularly when they are upsetting. Mindfulness, grounded in Eastern philosophy, encourages clients to live in the present. Eifert and Forsyth (2005) define mindfulness as "fundamentally an acceptance-oriented psychological process derived largely from 2,500 years of Buddhist philosophy and meditation practice" (p. 74). Based on the work of Kabat-Zinn (1990, 2005) and Robins (2002), these concepts have been incorporated into the theory underlying many mindfulness- and acceptance-based treatments (Hayes et al., 2004). Eifert and Forsyth (2005) have indicated that many clients spend an incredible amount of time fighting against their distress in an effort to alleviate it. They assert, however, that once a client learns through mindfulness to observe and endure their pain without evaluating, fighting, or acting against it, they can achieve a sense of pain without suffering and experience peace.

Kabat-Zinn (1990) is credited with developing the first mindfulness-based intervention, mindfulness-based stress reduction (MBSR). It combines an emphasis on being present with and aware of sensations within the body. Classes are taught in mindfulness-based meditation, and mindfulness-based body movements are taught through yoga and other movement techniques (Hick & Bien, 2010). Segal, Williams, and Teasdale (2002) have developed another mindfulness-based intervention called mindfulness-based cognitive therapy (MBCT) that has been shown to reduce the potential of relapse in clients with depression. In recent years, mindfulness-based research has documented its effectiveness with a wide range of presenting symptoms and conditions including chronic pain (Kabat-Zinn,, 1990), suicidal behavior (Linehan, Armstrong, Suarez, Allmon, & Heard, 1991), depressive relapse (Segal et al., 2002), eating disorders (Kristeller & Hallett, 1999), and stress (Shapiro, Schwartz, & Bonner, 1998).

Mindfulness and the Therapeutic Relationship

As indicated in Chapter 4, research has consistently shown that the therapeutic relationship is more important to therapy outcome than the specific techniques or theoretical orientation used (Duncan et al., 2009; Norcross, 2011a). Mindfulness can provide an important theoretical understanding of the therapeutic relationship. Hick and Bien (2010) have described it in this way: "Within the client–therapist relationship, mindfulness is a way of paying attention with empathy, presence, and deep listening that can be cultivated, sustained, and integrated into our work as therapists. . . . " (Hick & Bien, 2010, p. 5).

Some approaches to mindfulness have incorporated meditative techniques, which are utilized by the therapist and client in order to focus and connect (Hick & Bien, 2010). Other approaches, such as acceptance and commitment therapy (ACT) (Eifert & Forsyth, 2005; Hayes, Strosahl, & Wilson, 1999, 2011) and dialectical behavioral therapy (DBT) (Linehan, 1993), incorporate nonmeditative mindfulness-based concepts and techniques into the treatment process as a way of building and strengthening the therapeutic alliance.

Hick and Bien (2010) point out that many therapists, particularly in their early years, are focused on the "doing" of therapy. This is consistent with the modern pressures of the 21st-century world that often lead us to focus on "doing" rather than "being." The therapist's own use of mindfulness can help him or her to avoid being distracted in the therapeutic encounter with a client, and to experience the "here and now" of the therapy relationship (Hick & Bien, 2010).

This process becomes particularly important for clinicians who are working on tight schedules, whether in public agencies or in private practice. These demands are often challenging for therapists, who feel pushed by productivity requirements to go immediately from one session into another with little opportunity to refresh and focus on the here and now encounter with the next client. This seemingly never-ending cycle can make it difficult to remain present in each session and to have the empathy and compassion necessary to build a meaningful therapeutic relationship (Hick & Bien, 2010; Wilson & Dufrene, 2010). Hick (2010) indicates that the practice of mindfulness can help a therapist to be better attuned to "the ebb and flow of emotions, thoughts and perceptions within all human beings" (p. 13), thereby helping him or her to become less of a detached expert or observer and more of an attentive participant in the therapy relationship. With this in mind, a number of researchers and theorists have gone beyond using mindfulness as simply an intervention or a technique that can be taught to clients in therapy, and instead have begun to see it as a basic attitude or way of being with clients that a therapist can bring to each therapeutic encounter (Hick & Bien 2010; Wilson & Dufrene, 2010).

The Therapist's Use of Mindfulness

As discussed above, many evidence-based treatments incorporate mindfulness-based practice for clients (Hayes et al., 2004). In recent years, however, a number of authors have been investigating the ways in which mindfulness can benefit therapists both in terms of their practice and in their training (Hick & Bien, 2010; Wilson & Dufrene, 2010). There has been an ongoing debate as to whether therapists need to use mindfulness-based meditation and other techniques in their own lives in order to be effective with clients. Clearly, there are a number of evidence-based treatments that do not have this requirement (ACT; Eifert & Forsythe, 2005; Hayes, Strosahl, & Wilson, 1999, 2011; DBT; Linehan, 1993).

Bien (2010), on the other hand, has argued that the philosophies on which mindfulness is based can help to train clinicians to cultivate the type of attitude that can enhance the therapeutic relationship and influence treatment outcome. Drawing on an element of Buddhist philosophy known as the Four Immeasurable Minds, Bien has identified the following components of good therapy—love, compassion, joy, and equanimity. Love in this context is different from romantic love. It is described as "the capacity to offer joy and happiness (Nhat Hanh, 1998)" (Bien, 2010, p. 43). He defines compassion as "the capacity to offer relief from suffering (Nhat Hanh, 1998)" (p. 43). In this context, joy also takes on a broader meaning:

> In the therapy context, joy is an important element, though perhaps not one that is explicitly described in many books about therapy. Joy here means first of all that at times, there can be a lightness in the therapy encounter. While care obviously needs to be taken that one is not out of harmony with the internal state of the client, there can be jokes, stories, and laughter in psychotherapy even when talking about serious and sad things. Joy is also about finding a way to enjoy the company of our clients. (p. 44)

Equanimity is also an extremely important component in the process of establishing a therapeutic relationship. As we discuss in Chapter 4, it allows the therapist to be connected to his or her clients without overidentifying with them. Overidentification can lead to compassion fatigue and burnout. Bien (2010) describes equanimity as "evenness, the capacity to accept whatever comes undisturbed. It is not indifference. It doesn't entail being unfeeling, but means not getting lost in the feeling" (p. 45). This sense of equanimity is an important concept for therapists. It allows us to work with our clients with compassion and caring, but it forces us to remember that we cannot make our clients' choices for them (Bien, 2010). We can hear about their painful experiences and empathize with them without taking on the pain. This concept is revisited in Chapter 15.

Hick and Bien (2010) and Bien (2010) give a number of examples of mindfulness-based exercises that can allow therapists to cultivate these positive values in themselves and in their therapeutic relationships with clients. For example, Bien offers the following mindfulness-based exercise that therapists can utilize in their own lives and in building positive therapeutic relationships:

1. Before seeing clients, sit for a few moments and allow your attention to settle gently on your breath.
2. Imagine yourself as being surrounded and filled with absolute love, cradled in total acceptance, kindness, and benevolence. To make this concrete, think of a time when you felt deeply loved and accepted, or imagine yourself in the presence of an all-loving being, a Buddha or a Christ or whatever image might help elicit these feelings.
3. As you continue feeling loved and accepted, gently hold the following intentions for yourself:

   May I be happy.
   May I be peaceful.
   May I have abundance.
   May I be safe.
   May I have ease of well-being.
   May I be free of negative emotions.

4. Envision yourself as capable not only of receiving but also of spreading this feeling of love and acceptance. Feel the presence of each person you are scheduled to see that day, evoking a global felt sense of them. You might begin with those it is easy for you to feel kindly toward, and gradually expand to include those who are more difficult. Imagine yourself sitting with them, relaxed, open, and at ease, intent on understanding, letting what you say and do flow naturally from this awareness.
5. Gently hold the intentions above for your clients: "May he be happy. May she be peaceful," and so on.
6. End by enjoying a few mindful breaths.

The exact nature and wording of the intentions can vary, and one can freely invent new ones, perhaps ones that grow out of a particular life context. In fact, inventing one's own phrases may at times be especially helpful in that the words which come out of one's own consciousness and experience may be more vivid and help one stay in touch with their meaning without having them degenerate into empty sounds. (pp. 50–51)

The above exercise can be helpful to therapists as they prepare to see clients at the beginning of a busy, hectic day that is so typical of practicing therapy in today's demanding climate. In the course of the day, if a therapist becomes overwhelmed with the demands of nonstop sessions and begins to find that his or her focus seems to drift during sessions, this type of mindfulness-based exercise, coupled with meditative deep-breathing exercises, can be used to calm the therapist and allow him or her to be more present with a client. Bien's (2010) discussion of personalizing the words is also important for therapists. As he indicates, therapists who have a different spiritual or religious practice may incorporate their own words into this process. Similarly, those who consider themselves atheist or agnostic may gain the benefits of deep breathing and positive thoughts without placing any spiritual connotation on the process.

As we indicate in Chapter 15, all therapists face times in their lives when they are preoccupied by their own physical or emotional pain; the illness, death, or loss of a loved one; or job or family stress. Because we are all human, these feelings can come right into the therapy room with us and can distract us from our ability to be present with clients. Mindfulness-based exercises such as the one described above can allow us to address our own feelings and refocus on the needs of our clients. A mindfulness-based process can also be helpful in a session if we feel distracted, sense our concentration shift, or become overidentified with a client or a particular outcome for therapy. Bien (2010) notes that in these situations therapists can return to an awareness of their breath, mindfulness of the moment, or a word or intention (such as love, peace, etc.) that can be used to refocus attention to the present moment. It is important to remember that these exercises are internal within the therapist and need not be shared with the client. They are a part of the process by which therapists can use mindfulness to "let go" when they feel that they are more invested in the client's behavior change than the client.

As noted above, these processes can also be used by therapists to refresh themselves between sessions. In the current real world of agency productivity requirements and the financial demands of private practice, therapists often find that they are scheduled back to back in the course of a day. Bien (2010) describes ways in which brief mindfulness-based processes can be useful between sessions, especially those that have been emotionally taxing, in order to help therapists to clear their mind and be more available to their next client. Specifically, he recommends taking time between each session to return to our breath and awareness, noticing and ultimately letting go of any negative effects that a session has had on our body or mind (Bien, 2010).

Mindful Listening

Mindfulness has also made a contribution to the way in which therapists listen to clients. Bien (2010) has demonstrated that one of the essential components of therapy is the clinician's "capacity to listen in a skillful way that avoids a lot of judgment, that is accepting and receptive—a way that demonstrates to the client that one is more intent on understanding than on evaluating, diagnosing or fixing" (p. 38). Many therapists are familiar with the process of reflective listening as it is represented and taught in many different schools of therapy including motivational interviewing (W. R. Miller & Rollnick, 2002; see Chapter 6 in this book). Those who have worked to train new clinicians, however, have often found that the process can become rote and rigid if therapists focus too heavily on getting the words right. They may be so absorbed in their own process that they lose sight of the client. With this in mind, researchers and trainers in the field have searched for new ways to teach the process of developing empathy for their clients. One of the most promising strategies for therapists in building therapeutic rapport, establishing empathy, listening deeply, and conveying compassion is mindful listening (Hick, 2010; Shafir, 2010). Shafir has indicated that mindful listening involves clinicians partnering with clients by establishing trust within the therapeutic relationship. This is accomplished by being present in the moment with clients and being accepting of them.

Many therapists who are new to the field focus on learning the techniques of psychotherapy. Shafir (2010) has indicated that mindful listening should not be conceptualized as a skill but rather as an attitude or a state of mind that allows the therapist to focus on the needs and concerns of the client in a caring way. This process also benefits therapists in that it keeps them from taking on the burdens of their clients and serves to refresh them despite back-to-back hours of clinical work. This concept is extremely important for therapists in terms of their own self-care and is a central part of the process of avoiding vicarious traumatization, compassion fatigue, and burnout (Dass-Brailsford, 2007; see Chapter 15 in this book). To accomplish this, a number of authors have recommended that therapists incorporate meditative processes into their regular clinical practice as well as their lives outside of their offices (Bien, 2010; Shafir, 2010; Shapiro & Izett, 2010).

Others, such as Wilson and Dufrene (2008), advocate a nonmeditative approach. In their book *Mindfulness for Two: An Acceptance and Commitment Therapy Approach to Mindfulness in Psychotherapy*, they provide a "collection of attitudes, sensitivities, and practices, the goal of which is to increase conscious attention on the part of both the therapist and the client in a psychotherapeutic situation" (p. xii).

Mindfulness and the Treatment of Depression

One of the ongoing challenges in the treatment of major depression has been the potential for relapse in these clients (Segal et al., 2004).

ı mind, mindfulness based cognitive therapy (MBCT) has
ıe need to reduce depressive symptoms and provide ongoing
this treatment, cognitive therapy techniques are utilized to
address depressive symptoms while mindfulness principles are utilized
to prevent relapse and the recurrence of depression (Segal et al., 2004).
Utilizing Kabat-Zinn's (1990) mindfulness concept that "your thoughts
are just thoughts and they are not 'you' or 'reality'" (p. 69), MBCT seeks
to establish an alternative way of processing depressive feelings. Clients
are trained in mindful awareness of their bodily sensations, feelings,
and thoughts, and the ability to respond to them with openness and
acceptance. This allows them to be aware of the early signs of depressive
symptoms and to avoid a relapse (Segal et al., 2004).

Unlike traditional CBT, MBCT places less emphasis on changing
the "content of thoughts; rather the emphasis is on changing awareness
of and relationship to thoughts, feelings and bodily sensations" (Segal et
al., 2004, p. 54). This approach is a characteristic of all of the treatments
discussed in this chapter.

Mindfulness and the Treatment
of Obsessive–Compulsive Disorder

Today, many psychological disorders are understood as having a neuropsychiatric component. Highlighting the biological underpinnings of a
client's problem provides an excellent way of reframing psychological
disorders such as obsessive–compulsive disorder, bipolar, psychosis,
schizophrenia, and so on (J. M. Schwartz & Beyette, 1996). In his
discussion of the use of mindfulness in the treatment of obsessive–
compulsive disorder (OCD), J. Schwartz recognizes that the symptoms
of this disorder can be difficult for clients but that the combined use
of medication and mindfulness can profoundly affect the quality of their
lives. He first reframes OCD for his clients as a "brain related medical
problem" (J. Schwartz, 2011). He then uses mindfulness to convey to his
clients that they can learn to use their minds to influence their brains. For
example, he recommends that clients first learn to attend to their inner
experience and note any discomfort that arises without worrying that
it will overwhelm them. J. Schwartz states that even the simple act of
attending to one's experience and emotions can begin to convey to clients
that they have the power to change the way in which they react to their
thoughts and feelings.

J. M. Schwartz and Beyette (1996) and J. Schwartz (2011) describe a
four-step approach to their mindfulness-based treatment of OCD. First,
they help clients to put their disorder into perspective by "relabeling"
and recognizing the intrusive thoughts they experience as a symptom of

OCD. This may seem deceptively simple, but it is extremely powerful in that it reminds the client that OCD is a treatable medical condition that impacts the brain. In this way, clients learn to "mindfully observe" their feelings related to their OCD and relabel them as a symptom of their disorder, thereby beginning to change their response to it. J. Schwartz contends that this process of mindfulness and understanding is so powerful that it can even impact the brain chemistry underlying OCD.

"Reattribute" is the second step in this process. Once a client becomes familiar with the aspects of OCD, the therapist is able to attribute the client's obsessive thoughts and feelings of being bombarded by them to a "biochemical imbalance in the brain" (J. Schwartz, 2011). This conveys to clients that they are not their disorder or to blame for it, and allows them to reattribute any negative feelings to their disorder. Thus clients learn to say, "It's not me it's the OCD" (J. Schwartz, 2011, p. 3). This is an extremely important realization for many clients with OCD and forms of serious mental illness, as it allows them to release the blame and shame they associate with their condition. In some cases clients can be helped to distance themselves from their illness and call it "the OCD," or "the anxiety disorder," or "the bipolar disorder" and to recognize the role of their neuropsychiatric condition and its effect on the brain. In this way, clients learn that while they still may experience symptoms from time to time, they do not have to become immersed in trying to fix or change these symptoms. They can instead decide to control the things that they can, by focusing on living a meaningful life.

"Refocus" helps the client to "work around the OCD symptoms by focusing attention on something else" that the client feels invested in. The client is encouraged to "not wait for the feeling to go away [but to]—work around it by doing another behavior, even though the feeling is still bothering you" (J. Schwartz, 2011, p. 3). Clients are told to mindfully accept that their symptoms are present, but to not let these symptoms control them. They are asked to do this by redirecting their attention away from their emotional response and toward values that are important to them, such as doing "good things."

The fourth and last step in the process leads the client to "revalue," or put a different value on their symptoms and disorder. In this step, clients learn to look at and interpret their feelings in new ways with a different meaning. For example, in the midst of feeling anxiety, a client would learn to mindfully state, "that's just the medical symptom. I don't need to listen to that. I'm going to refocus and do an adaptive behavior" (J. Schwartz, 2011, p. 3). Clients who have integrated the fourth step may still experience the once-paralyzing feelings, but then after acknowledging them, go on to do something positive, such as engaging in a fun activity with a friend or their significant other.

It is important for clinicians and clients alike to recognize that this process is not easy and can often take several weeks or months. Schwartz is also careful to acknowledge that medications may be a helpful part of the treatment process for many of these clients. As an example of the synthesis of CBT and mindfulness, J. Schwartz's (2011) work helps clients choose not to expend energy trying to avoid or extinguish a distressing experience but rather to nonjudgmentally integrate these experiences into a more flexible and value-based behavioral path.

Acceptance-Based Principles

Acceptance is another core concept within many of these models (e.g., DBT [Linehan, 1993; Robins, Schmidt, & Linehan, 2004], ACT [Eifert & Forsyth, 2005; Hayes, Strosahl, & Wilson, 1999, 2011], and MBCT [Segal et al., 2002]). As we indicated above, this is a particularly useful concept when working with clients with serious mental illnesses and/or substance abuse (Bowen et al., 2011; Marlatt et al., 2008; Witkiewitz et al., 2005; see Chapter 9 of this book). Instead of focusing on a cure, clients are encouraged to accept that they may have a particular condition (e.g., depression, bipolar disorder, obsessive–compulsive disorder, substance abuse disorder) that may be a part of their lives. Clients are encouraged to accept their feelings and thoughts (e.g., anxiety, depression) without the need to struggle against or change them. This can then lead to a freedom or liberation from the constant struggle and battle to change these experiences (Eifert & Forsyth, 2005; Hayes, Strosahl, & Wilson, 1999, 2011).

One crucial point in describing acceptance-based principles is that the concept used here is not a giving up or a passive form of acceptance, it is an active acceptance. Clients are encouraged to actively accept and mindfully experience the thoughts and feelings that they have avoided in the past (Hayes et al., 2004; Hayes, Strosahl, & Wilson, 1999, 2011). According to this model, upsetting feelings are natural and normal, embedded in our nervous system and a part of our human experience (Hayes et al., 2011). The problem is not the anxiety itself but all of the difficulties brought on by trying to banish it, such as the tendency to negatively judge, evaluate, fuse, avoid, dread, or deny these feelings. It is here that the concept of acceptance becomes so important: once individuals can actively accept and be willing to have internal discomfort and upsetting feelings, they can learn to step out of their internal struggle to be rid of these inevitable experiences and direct their energies to pursuing meaningful goals and values. Acceptance- and mindfulness-based clinical work is therefore critical in that it helps a person to identify and make room for what he or she cannot control (e.g., anxiety, panic, depression) and to more effectively work with that which is in his or her control (e.g., transforming his or her relationship to these feelings and experiences and moving toward valued goals).

Similarly, dialectical behavior therapy (DBT) (Linehan, 1993; Robins et al., 2004) has introduced the concept of "radical acceptance," which combines mindfulness and the ability to focus on the current moment and to accept difficult and often painful feelings. This approach has proven particularly effective with clients with borderline personality disorder who often struggle with painful and dangerous experiences of suicidality.

Far too often, we have encountered people in our clinical work who are criticizing and blaming themselves for experiencing symptoms of anxiety, obsessive–compulsive disorder, depression, addictions, psychosis, borderline personality disorder, bipolar disorder, and other problems. In addition to blaming themselves for having these experiences, they are also caught up in an endless struggle to figure out why it is that they feel this way or what specific life experiences have caused these feelings. In our experience, this mental struggle can make the situation worse as it perpetuates further entanglement with distressing feelings that often have multiple determinants. It is when we work with clients to accept these feelings and no longer expend so much psychic energy trying to control them that they begin to relax their internal judgments, make room for these experiences, and free themselves to move forward in a valued direction.

Once clients are able to accept their feelings and thoughts in the present moment, they can address the process of committing to the values and goals that they would like to achieve in their lives (Hayes et al., 2011). The ACT model presented below is one of many treatments that illustrate the combination of mindfulness- and acceptance-based principles and the process of helping clients to make a commitment toward living a more meaningful life.

Acceptance and Commitment Therapy

As noted above, there are a number of treatment approaches that incorporate mindfulness- and acceptance-based principles and practices (Hayes et al., 2004). In order to further illustrate the use of these concepts, we describe acceptance and commitment therapy (ACT) in more detail. ACT is an evidence-based treatment developed by Hayes, Strosahl, and Wilson (1999, 2011). These authors argue that pain (i.e., anxiety, depression, grief, loss, etc.) is a normal human condition that most people experience in the course of their lives. It is not the experience of pain that is the problem but our reactions or relationship to it, which can include judging and blaming ourselves for experiencing it. ACT promotes the development of greater psychological flexibility and seeks to assist the client with developing alternatives to strategies such as avoidance of uncomfortable feelings or an overidentification with these feelings (Hayes, Strosahl, & Wilson, 1999, 2011). Unlike earlier treatment models that focused on understanding the root causes of depression, anxiety, and fear, acceptance and commitment therapy is unique in that it encourages individuals to accept the continued presence of such upsetting emotions without allowing them to prevent pursuit of a meaningful, committed, productive life.

In order to accomplish this, a primary goal of ACT is to help clients accept distressing thoughts or feelings whose presence cannot be controlled (Eifert & Forsyth, 2005). One empowering aspect of this model is that it shifts the focus away from trying to discover an unconscious meaning, conflict, or early experience that explains one's symptoms to developing an overall acceptance and tolerance of what it means to be human. It is similar in intent to the serenity creed that forms the basis of 12-step programs: "Accept with serenity what you cannot change, have the courage to change what you can and develop the wisdom to know the difference" (pp. 7–8).

ACT incorporates six core processes: acceptance, cognitive defusion, being present, self as context, values, and committed action (Eifert & Forsyth, 2005; Hayes, Strosahl, & Wilson, 1999, 2011). Acceptance is an alternative to experiential avoidance. Cognitive defusion is the process by which ACT changes the way a client relates to his or her thoughts "by creating contexts in which their unhelpful functions are diminished" (Hayes, 2006, p. 2). For example, a person who has the thought "I am no good," would relabel that as "I am having the thought that I am no good." This distances the individual from the negative consequences of the original thought (Hayes, 2006; Hayes, Strosahl, & Wilson, 1999, 2011). Being present is one of the most important ACT concepts. It encourages conscious attention to the present without drifting into defeating thoughts, which are often based on past experiences or anxieties about the future.

Self as context is a stance in which the "self is not the experience but simply provides the context for the experience" (Eifert & Forsyth, 2005, p. 180). This process helps clients to learn to observe the self without judging or labeling it as "good" or "bad" (Eifert & Forsyth, 2005). Values are the goals, directions, and things that are important in a person's life. Some clients might value family, career, education, service, or spirituality. These values give a person a purpose in life that can transcend painful experiences. Committed action is another important concept within ACT. Once clients have clarified their values, they begin to develop patterns of effective action linked to those values. For example, a client with a serious mental illness may have a value of education and may have dreamed of going to college and graduate school, but allowed the experience of his or her illness to stop him or her. Once his or her values have been clarified, the client can begin to work toward committed action to obtain the education that has been so important to him or her (Eifert & Forsyth, 2005; Hayes, Strosahl, & Wilson, 1999, 2011).

The following case example illustrates how a client with anxiety and depression was helped through acceptance.

John, a 50-year-old White man, entered treatment to address issues of trauma from experiences early in his life. He reported feelings of anxiety and depression whenever he remembered the physical abuse he suffered as a child at the hands of his father. Six months earlier, his father had died and John reported that he had been sad and angry since then. He burst into tears in the session and reported that he was crying all the time. Repeatedly, in the first session, he asked the therapist in a pleading tone, "Can you make these feelings go away?" The therapist reflected that John was sick of these feelings and wanted desperately to get rid of them. He then asked John, "In your experience, do you feel that you can really make them go away completely?" John responded that this had not been his experience. The therapist replied that "The abuse that you suffered from your father as a child was really terrible. You still feel sad and angry at your father even though he has died. It is a part of your history and it may cause you pain at different times. Maybe it is not about getting rid of the feelings but sitting with them and allowing yourself to have them. You can learn to relate to them in a different way. If you can learn to accept these feelings as a part of your life, you can choose to go on with your life and do meaningful things that you value."

John responded angrily that it was not fair that these things had happened to him. The therapist reflected that he could hear that John was angry and that it was not fair that he had to go through so much pain. Over a series of sessions, the therapist began to help John to understand that his painful and upsetting feelings were an outcome of his early traumatic experiences and he might not always be able to control those experiences or those feelings. But he could decide to accept those feelings and learn to control his response to the memories of those traumatic experiences with his father and thus the way in which he responded to his feelings of anxiety and depression.

They began to explore John's dreams and goals in life that he felt his early experiences and feelings of anxiety and depression were keeping him from pursuing. Over a number of sessions, John struggled as the therapist tried to help him to clarify the things that would make him feel that he was living a valued life. After so much difficulty on John's part, the therapist finally asked him, if he were to die tomorrow, what would he like his epitaph or his eulogy to read? John responded that he would not want it to read that he was paralyzed by feelings of anxiety and depression.

This session seemed to release something for John as he acknowledged how his feelings had caused him to distance himself from his wife and children. He then spent a number of sessions talking about the fact that his children were growing up and he felt less and less a part of their lives. He loved his wife but they did almost nothing pleasurable, particularly since his father's death. Gradually, he and the therapist began to work on John's goal of continuing to have a meaningful relationship with his wife and children despite his sadness and anger. Once John was able to accept the feelings, he was able to turn his attention to the important relationships in his life and to commit to something that added a great deal of value to his life.

As this case illustrates, one way of addressing the issue of adding value to a person's life is to raise the question of how they would like their epitaph or eulogy to read. Hayes and Smith (2005) describe an exercise in which a person is helped to imagine attending his or her own funeral. The person is asked to first write down what might be said at his or her funeral "if the struggle you are currently engaged in continues to dominate your life or even grows" (p. 167). Later the client is asked to imagine that someone is giving a eulogy about him or her that reflects a life lived true to the client's most important values. The following case illustrates how a client can learn to choose how she responds to her feelings, while pursuing goals and values that are meaningful to her.

Jane, a 30-year-old White woman, entered treatment because her marriage of five years was ending. She and her husband had been different in temperament and life goals. His decision to leave the marriage and file for a divorce was experienced by her as abrupt and arbitrary. She had attempted to convince him to go into couples therapy, but he had refused. She reported feeling devastated and experiencing emotional pain so intense that she could not escape it even in sleep. Each night she lay awake for hours feeling terrible. This loss had reopened earlier painful experiences and brought back memories of her abandonment by her father and an abusive relationship in her 20s. She reported that she desperately wanted to escape from these upsetting emotions and memories and to start feeling better.

The therapist first reflected her pain and stated, "I know that this breakup is causing a lot of pain and is stirring up a lot of upsetting memories. You wish that you could make all of these feelings go away." Jane nodded, but did not say anything. The therapist then added that Jane was feeling a lot of pain because she had never allowed herself to feel the pain of these earlier experiences and now this loss of her husband was pulling up all of the old feelings. He introduced the concept that it was not the feelings that were the most difficult, but the constant fight to make the feelings go away (experiential avoidance) that caused the problem. He told her that this was a human response and that feelings were a part of making us human.

This treatment was difficult and Jane alternated between feeling angry and depressed. The therapist began to explore her values and dreams. She talked about her dream of going to law school and her value of offering some of her services pro bono to clients who could not afford legal representation. She had abandoned her values and dreams when she got married because her husband was threatened by her plans. The therapist began to introduce the importance of accepting the feelings that she had and going on with her life in spite of them. Jane was initially confused and said that she had always thought that she had to make these upsetting feelings and memories go away in order to focus on the contribution that she wanted to make. With the therapist's help, she was able to begin the process of applying to law school and accept that she would sometimes have upsetting feelings related to her divorce and earlier losses. She recognized that she had a choice about how she responded to these feelings and she was able to pursue a commitment to meaningful work.

Acceptance- and Mindfulness-Based Exercises for Clients

As indicated above, acceptance means "letting go of fighting the reality of having fear and anxiety" (Eifert & Forsyth, 2005, p. 162). Mindfulness is an important part of this "letting go" process. Eifert and Forsyth assert that mindfulness can help clients to observe their thoughts, feelings, and experiences without judging, evaluating, fighting against, or suppressing them. Mindfulness then, ultimately facilitates acceptance, as acceptance involves a willingness to experience (rather than fight against) distressing thoughts and feelings so that one can ultimately choose to spend one's time and energy participating in activities that are meaningful and important to him or her (Eifert & Forsyth, 2005).

One contribution of mindfulness principles to our work with clients has been the notion that everyone experiences pain in life. As human beings, we do not wish to feel pain so we attempt to push it away; it is this process of attempting to avoid the pain—labeled "experiential avoidance" (Hayes, Strosahl, & Wilson, 1999, 2011)—that can lead to suffering. Eifert and Forsyth (2005) draw upon the work of Marsha Linehan (1993), the founder of dialectical behavior therapy (DBT), another evidence-based approach that incorporates mindfulness, to underscore the ways in which mindfulness can help clients to understand the differences between pain and suffering. They note that mindfulness facilitates freedom from suffering by helping clients to accept pain as it is, without adding the struggle of nonacceptance (Eifert & Forsyth, 2005).

Mindfulness-based acceptance exercises often involve components that are found in different forms of meditation and in some other forms of CBT. These might include deep breathing and relaxation exercises. The purpose of these exercises is to help clients experience anxiety-related thoughts and feelings without attempting to eliminate or change them (Eifert & Forsyth, 2005; Hayes, Strosahl, & Wilson, 1999, 2011; Segal et al., 2002). An example of a mindfulness-based acceptance exercise that offers clients new ways of responding to or relating to anxiety symptoms can be seen in Box 8.1.

Follow-Up with Clients

Hayes, Strosahl, and Wilson (1999, 2011) and Eifert and Forsyth (2005) also caution clinicians to check in regularly with clients to explore how they are processing and experiencing these exercises. Some clients may begin to use these mindfulness- and acceptance-based processes as just another technique to fix or control their anxiety (Eifert & Forsyth, 2005). Even when clients report positive changes, they may still be viewing these exercises simply as a way to manage their anxiety. In these cases, therapists may need to gently review the principles of mindful acceptance in order to move the client away from the allure of utilizing these techniques as another way to distance him- or herself from directly experiencing internal affect. Therapists should be assessing whether the techniques are being used by the client to promote true, nonjudgmental openness to all experiences. For example, if a client says, "I've been doing these mindfulness exercises and I'm still feeling awful," this presents another opportunity to work with the client on reexamining the potential power of present-moment awareness and acceptance.

Mindfulness- and Acceptance-Based Approaches with Clients Who Have Experienced Trauma

One useful technique with clients who have experienced trauma involves a process of "peeling back the layers." Often, clients with symptoms related to trauma engage in continuous cycles of avoidance of these feelings. This avoidance, a control strategy, is seen as a symptom itself that contributes to long-term consequences such as substance abuse and chronic anxiety (Follette, Palm, & Hall, 2004; Follette & Pistorello,

BOX 8.1. Mindfulness-Based Acceptance Exercise

1. Go ahead and get in a comfortable position in your chair. Sit upright with your feet flat on the floor, your arms and legs uncrossed, and your hands resting in your lap (palms up or down, whichever is more comfortable). Allow your eyes to close gently [pause 10 seconds].

2. Take a few moments to get in touch with the physical sensations in your body, especially the sensations of touch or pressure where your body makes contact with the chair or floor. Notice the gentle rising and falling of your breath in your chest and belly. There is no need to control your breathing in any way—simply let the breath breathe itself [pause 10 seconds]. As best you can, also bring this attitude of allowing and gentle acceptance to the rest of your experience. There is nothing to be fixed. Simply allow your experience to be your experience, without needing to be other than what it is [pause 10 seconds].

3. It is natural for your mind to wander away to thoughts, worries, images, bodily sensations, or feelings. Notice these thoughts and feelings, acknowledge their presence, and stay with them [pause 10 seconds]. There is no need to think of something else, make them go away, or resolve anything. As best you can, allow them to be . . . giving yourself space to have whatever you have . . . bringing a quality of kindness and compassion to your experience [pause 10 seconds].

4. Allow yourself to be present to what you are afraid of. Notice any doubts, reservations, fears, and worries. Just notice them and acknowledge their presence, and do not work on them [pause 10 seconds]. Now see if you can be present with your values and commitments. Ask yourself, "Why am I here?" "Where do I want to go?" "What do I want to do?" [pause 15 seconds].

5. Now focus on a thought or situation that has been difficult for you. It could be a particular troubling thought, worry, image, or intense bodily sensations [pause 10 seconds]. Gently, directly, and firmly shift your attention on and into the discomfort, no matter how bad it seems [pause 10 seconds]. Notice any strong feelings that may arise in your body, allowing them to be as they are rather than what you think they are, simply holding them in awareness [pause 10 seconds]. Stay with your discomfort and breathe with it [pause 10 seconds]. See if you can gently open up to it and make space for it, accepting and allowing it to be [pause], while bringing compassionate and focused attention to the sensations of discomfort [pause 15 seconds].

(continued)

BOX 8.1. (*continued*)

6. If you notice yourself tensing up and resisting what you have, pushing away from the experience, acknowledge that and see if you can make some space for whatever you're experiencing [pause 10 seconds]. Must this feeling or thought be your enemy? [pause 10 seconds]. Or can you have it, notice it, own it, and let it be? [pause 10 seconds]. Can you make room for the discomfort, for the tension, for the anxiety? [pause 10 seconds]. What does it really feel like moment to moment to have them? [pause 10 seconds]. Is this something you must struggle with or can you invite the discomfort in, saying to yourself with willingness, "Let me have it; let me feel what there is to be felt because it is my experience right now"? [pause 15 seconds].

7. If the sensations or discomfort grow stronger, acknowledge their presence, stay with them [pause 10 seconds], breathing with them, accepting them [pause 10 seconds]. Is this discomfort something you must not have, you cannot have? [pause 10 seconds]. Even if your mind tells you that you cannot, can you open up a space for it in your heart? [pause 10 seconds]. Is there room inside you to feel that with compassion and kindness toward yourself and your experience? [pause 15 seconds].

8. Apart from physical sensations in the body, you may also notice thoughts coming along with the sensations, and thoughts about the thoughts. When you notice any such thoughts, also invite them in . . . softening and opening up to them [pause 10 seconds]. You may also notice your mind coming up with evaluative labels such as "dangerous" or "getting worse." If that happens, you can simply thank your mind for the label [pause 10 seconds] and return to the present experience as it is, not as your mind says it is, noticing thoughts as thoughts, physical sensations as physical sensations, feelings as feelings—nothing more, nothing less [pause 15 seconds].

9. Stay with your discomfort for as long as it pulls on your attention [pause 10 seconds]. If and when you sense that the anxiety and other discomfort are no longer pulling for your attention, let them go [pause 15 seconds].

10. Then, when you are ready, gradually widen your attention to take in the sounds around you in the room [pause 10 seconds]. Take a moment to make the intention to bring the sense of gentle allowing and self-acceptance into the present moment [pause 5 seconds], and when you are ready slowly open your eyes.

From Eifert and Forsyth (2005, pp. 163–166). Copyright 2005 by New Harbinger Publications. Reprinted by permission.

2007). When a client describes obsessive, controlling, or anxious thoughts and feelings, the therapist asks the client to "peel back the layers and to look and see what is underneath those feelings." This mechanism supports clients in breaking cycles of avoidance that lead to greater suffering and thus develop greater psychological flexibility (Follette & Pistorello, 2007). The following case illustrates this process.

Malinda, a 25-year-old Latina, was in a relationship with Manuel, age 26. They had been together for about a year and were experiencing a great deal of arguing and fighting due to Malinda's need to obsessively schedule every part of their lives. She was constantly mapping out plans for everything and was aware that this was alienating her from her boyfriend, but she could not stop. She described this urge to plan as an "itch that you constantly scratch."

The therapist explored with her, "Suppose you did not scratch this itch to plan?" Malinda replied that she had never been able to refrain from this activity. The therapist then asked her, "Suppose you were to peel back this urge to plan and control, what would we find underneath it?" Malinda was silent for a few minutes and then her face distorted and she reported, "I was a victim of a date rape . . . the one time I did not plan. . . . " She reported that friends had encouraged her to "loosen up" and go on a blind date with a man who then raped her. It became clear that she had always been a "planner" but that she became obsessive about it after the date rape. The therapist responded, "So you came to believe that not having plans led to that trauma of the date rape. Planning is your way of protecting yourself from something bad happening. It gives you a sense of control. Planning may also be your way of avoiding those upsetting feelings. But, look at the price you pay for controlling and avoiding these feelings—your relationship is in jeopardy."

The therapist then discussed with Malinda the fact that the fear, anxiety, and feelings of helplessness that the date rape stirred up for her were normal human emotions in response to a painful event. In her effort to avoid and control them by trying to plan every aspect of her life, she was cutting off a major part of her life and destroying her relationships. When he explored Malinda's values, it was clear that she wanted to have a good, meaningful relationship and hoped to get married and have children one day. The therapist validated that she had a number of meaningful goals in her life. He also talked with her about pursuing her dreams in spite of her stressful feelings and letting go of trying to control them by planning every aspect of her life. He helped her to accept that she might continue to have these feelings and obsessive thoughts, but rather than allowing them to control her she could accept and disentangle herself from her painful experiences and thus develop the flexibility to move on to pursue the life, relationship, and family that she so desired.

The above vignette is also illustrative of many core mindfulness- and acceptance-based principles. First, the therapist was able to introduce the concept of workability (Harris, 2009; Luoma, Hayes, & Walser, 2007) by getting Malinda to reexamine her efforts to eliminate and control otherwise uncontrollable painful memories and experiences. The concept of workability asks the question "Is what you're doing working to make your life rich, full, and meaningful?" (Harris, 2009, p. 22). If the answer is yes then the strategies are workable; if the answer is no, they are unworkable. Workability is consistent with acceptance-based principles because from this perspective it is not the existence of painful private experiences that is the problem, rather it is our overidentification with and repeated attempts to get rid of painful feelings that result in suffering (Hayes, 2006; Linehan, 1993). Second, the therapist was able to introduce the concept of acceptance and disentanglement as an alternative to avoidance and control. A principal aim of acceptance-based therapies is to assist a person in developing the skills necessary to detach from painful symptoms and to willingly accept that which one cannot control. As a person develops this capacity, he or she experiences the increased flexibility to have painful private thoughts and feelings and expose oneself to previously avoided internal and external experiences (Eifert & Forsyth, 2005). Finally, the therapist was able to engage Malinda in a discussion about values. This is critical in acceptance-based therapies because helping individuals to clarify their values as well as to develop the commitment to pursue valued directions in the face of painful private experiences anchors the change process and allows the person to live a meaningful life (Hayes et al., 2004; Luoma et al., 2007).

Conclusion

While CBT focuses on the interrelationship among thoughts, feelings, and behaviors, mindfulness- and acceptance-based principles comprise a fifth core mediational process that addresses a person's responses to those thoughts, feelings, and behaviors. Mindfulness, the practice of present-moment awareness, is a skill that can assist clients with being fully present in the here and now of symptomatic experiences without overidentifying with or avoiding them. The utilization of mindful awareness lowers reactivity to painful thoughts and feelings and broadens a person's ability to choose how to respond to them in a less reactive and more value-driven way. When this approach is coupled with acceptance, which is the fundamental belief that pain is unavoidable and does not have to be extinguished, clients can experience increased flexibility to move on with their life goals in the face of difficult experiences.

CHAPTER 9

Relapse Prevention, Trigger Management, and the Completion of Treatment

Introduction

Relapse prevention and trigger management are part of the ongoing lexicon of cognitive-behavioral therapy (J. S. Beck, 1995, 2011), motivational interviewing (W. R. Miller & Rollnick, 2002), substance abuse therapy (Bowen et al., 2011), and mental health treatment and recovery in general (Ralph & Corrigan, 2005). Its proven value as a best practice justifies setting it apart as the sixth core mediational process. From this perspective, treatment is not about a cure but rather the nurturing of skills necessary to pursue life goals in the face of recurring challenges. Inherent in this perspective is the notion that people with mental illness can live a value-filled life as they learn to harness and activate personal strengths and competencies in the service of ongoing change and recovery (Hayes, Strosahl, & Wilson, 1999, 2011).

As a core mediational process, relapse prevention and trigger management help clients to develop the flexibility necessary to navigate the inevitable twists, turns, and detours often associated with the recovery process. Inherent in this mediational process is the belief that persons in recovery from mental illness and/or substance abuse can learn to manage and sustain change long after the conclusion of formal treatment. Therefore, discussing client goals and the criteria necessary for ending or reducing treatment at the first session is critical (J. S. Beck, 2011). Relapse prevention as an intervention facilitates from the first day of treatment the establishment of self-directed processes that empower a client to become his or her own therapist in the long term. In other words, the emphasis of treatment lies in developing a client's internal, self-directed capacity for change that can be taken out of the therapy room and into his or her life (J. S. Beck, 2011).

The first part of this chapter provides an overview of the history of relapse prevention interventions in the fields of addiction and mental health. It explores relapse prevention and trigger management as they relate to cognitive-behavioral approaches to addiction (Marlatt & Donovan, 2005), stages of change (DiClemente & Velasquez, 2002; Prochaska & DiClemente, 1982), MI (W. R. Miller & Rollnick, 1991, 2002), and mindfulness (Bowen et al., 2011; Marlatt et al., 2008). The role of relapse prevention in CBT for mental illnesses is also discussed (J. S. Beck, 2011; Meichenbaum, 2008).

The second part of this chapter expands on these contributions and discusses our work on relapse prevention and trigger management as core mediational processes that should be included as a part of effective treatment. The final part of this chapter explores the completion of therapy and the role of relapse prevention in this phase of treatment.

Relapse Prevention in the Addictions Field

Relapse prevention has a long history in the addictions field. Chaney, O'Leary, and Marlatt (1978) first explored relapse prevention in the treatment of alcohol disorders using a CBT approach. Marlatt and Gordon (1985) subsequently introduced one of the earliest relapse prevention approaches and in 1986, Brownell, Marlatt, Lichtenstein, and Wilson published an extensive review of early approaches to relapse prevention in the field of addictions. Marlatt and Donovan (2005) have developed evidence-based strategies that describe relapse prevention as

> a self-management program designed to enhance the maintenance stage of the habit-change process. The goal of RP [relapse prevention] is to teach individuals who are trying to change their behavior how to anticipate and cope with the problem of relapse. . . . RP is a cognitive-behavioral treatment (CBT) with a focus on the maintenance stage of addictive behavior change that has two main goals: to prevent the occurrence of initial lapses after a commitment to change has been made, and to prevent any lapse that does occur from escalating into a full-blown relapse (relapse management). (p. ix)

Another advance in the field has been the recognition that clients with dual diagnoses, and co-occurring disorders (e.g., depression and substance abuse) are at high risk for relapse. As a result, a number of authors have recognized the necessity of addressing both mental health and substance abuse problems as part of a comprehensive relapse prevention strategy (Drake, Wallach, & McGovern, 2005; Marlatt & Donovan, 2005; Mueser et al., 2002).

Relapse prevention teaches clients to identify high-risk situations or triggers that may lead to a relapse. In the field of substance abuse treatment and research, the main goals of this approach are to prevent a relapse, maintain abstinence from drugs and alcohol, and utilize a harm reduction approach (Marlatt & Witkiewitz, 2005). Harm reduction is a public health philosophy and set of strategies that aims to reach people "where they are," and assist them in reducing the negative consequences associated with high-risk behavior, with the ultimate goal of reducing or eliminating the behavior such that it no longer acts as a barrier to valued living (Wofsy & Mundy, 2010a).

Within the field of CBT, it is recognized that whenever someone attempts to change a problematic behavior, it is highly likely that a lapse or experience of the prior behavior may occur (Marlatt & Witkiewitz, 2005). These authors emphasize, however, that a lapse does not have to lead to a full-blown return to the problematic behavior (i.e., a relapse). As Marlatt and Witkiewitz have shown, "Another possible outcome [of a lapse] is the individual getting "back on track" in the direction of positive change (prolapse)" (p. 2).

Marlatt and Witkiewitz (2005) also discuss the self-blame, guilt, and loss of perceived control that individuals often experience after violating their commitment to abstinence (Curry, Marlatt, & Gordon, 1987). This reaction to breaking one's self-imposed change rules often contains both an affective and a cognitive component:

> The affective component is related to feelings of guilt, shame, and hopelessness (Marlatt, 1985), often triggered by the discrepancy between one's prior identity as an abstainer and one's present lapse behavior. The cognitive component, based on attributional theory (Weiner, 1974) assumes that if the individual attributes a lapse to . . . an irreparable failure or due to chronic disease determinants, then the lapse is more likely to progress to a relapse (Miller, Westerberg, Harris & Tonigan, 1996). . . . The individual who views a lapse as a learning experience is more likely to experiment with alternative coping strategies in the future, which may lead to more effective responses in high risk situations. (Marlatt & Witkiewitz, 2005, p. 3)

Thus, Marlatt and Witkiewitz (2005) emphasize the importance of helping clients to see current and future lapses not as failures but as opportunities for learning and skill building around maintaining change.

Trigger Identification and Management

Marlatt (1996) and Marlatt and Donovan (2005) have developed assessments to identify the various risk factors or triggers that may precipitate a lapse or relapse. These include interpersonal, intrapersonal, environmental, social (including familial), and physiological factors that can serve as risks or triggers (Marlatt, 1996). Once triggers are identified, CBT approaches are helpful to assist the client in developing self-management strategies to cope with them (Marlatt & Donovan, 2005). These interventions operate on the premise that identifying triggers, preparing clients for lapses, normalizing lapse/relapse experiences, and teaching effective cognitive-behavioral techniques to cope with and plan for triggers can lead to effective self-management and prevent a full relapse in the future. Self-management strategies may also include classic cognitive-behavioral techniques such as relaxation training or stress management (Marlatt & Donovan, 2005).

Identification of these triggers or risk situations can help the therapist and the client to construct "relapse road maps" that examine the possible outcomes associated with the different choices that can be made when a client is in the midst of a high-risk situation (Marlatt & Donovan, 2005). This process of developing, mapping out, and role-playing different high-risk scenarios can help prepare the client to develop effective coping strategies when faced with one of these triggers. This strategy of planning ahead for and thinking through possible triggers can prevent a lapse or can stop a minor lapse from becoming a major relapse.

Different Kinds of Triggers

Orlin and Davis (1993) and Straussner (1993) reviewed a broad range of triggers for clients with dual diagnoses of mental illness and drug and alcohol abuse, who were treated in psychiatric settings. Triggers may include feelings, thoughts, persons, places, and things that set the context for high-risk situations leading to relapse (Marlatt & Gordon, 1985; Marlatt & Donovan, 2005). For example, in treating dual-diagnosis clients in a group format, Orlin and Davis (1993, p. 117) asked clients to list those triggers that they believed were related to emotional illness and those that were related to addiction. Not surprisingly, these authors found that many of the triggers listed by clients fell under both headings:

Emotional Illness	Addiction
Anxiety	Anxiety
Denial (forgetting)	Denial (forgetting)
Depression	Depression
Family and peer pressures	Family and peer pressures
Feeling paranoid	Feeling paranoid
Loneliness	Loneliness
Anger	Anger
Holidays and anniversaries	Holidays and anniversaries
Stopping medication	Physical craving for substance
	Too much money

For persons with dual diagnoses of mental illness and drug and alcohol abuse, Orlin and Davis (1993) recommend the use of group therapy, as it can address issues of "denial, isolation, lack of social skills, and [the] absence of pleasurable activities," which can in and of themselves be risk factors or triggers for relapse. It is important for clinicians to remember that more lapses and relapses may occur, and treatment may take longer, for clients who have dual versus single diagnoses (Orlin & Davis, 1993). Unlike some earlier drug abuse treatments that called for the elimination of all medications, psychotropic medications are also essential for clients with serious mental illness, as stopping these medications can be a major trigger for relapse. In treating dually diagnosed clients, Orlin and Davis emphasize the importance of psychiatric availability and an interdisciplinary treatment team (Orlin & Davis, 1993).

Mindfulness–Based Relapse Prevention

More recently, a number of research studies have demonstrated that mindfulness-based meditation can contribute a great deal to the treatment of substance abuse (Marlatt, 1996; Witkiewitz et al., 2005). Mindfulness-based interventions have presented a different approach to addressing the challenges faced by individuals with addictions (Bowen et al., 2011; Marlatt et al., 2008) and/or mental health issues (Eifert & Forsyth, 2005; Hick & Bien, 2010). As discussed above, mindfulness is the cultivation of present-moment self-awareness as a capacity to engage in the nonjudgmental reflection of moment-to-moment experiences, no matter how painful or pleasurable. Mindfulness-based relapse prevention (MBRP) (Witkiewitz et al., 2005) is an evidence-based program that combines cognitive-behavioral relapse prevention principles with mindfulness-based meditation practice (Bowen et al., 2011). It is based in part on the MBSR (mindfulness-based stress reduction) technique developed for chronic pain (Kabat-Zinn, 1990) and mindfulness-based cognitive therapy (MBCT) developed by Segal et al. (2001) as a treatment for depression. Bowen et al. (2011) have conceptualized MBRP as an aftercare program for clients who have completed inpatient or outpatient treatment programs and are now ready for an approach that can address lifestyle changes and long-term recovery. This model requires clinicians who become group facilitators to develop their own personal mindfulness-based meditative practice as an essential part of their training (Bowen et al., 2011; Marlatt et al., 2008).

Similar to other mindfulness-based meditative approaches, MBRP helps therapists and clients to develop a nonjudgmental and compassionate approach to the cravings, triggers, and discomfort that are part of the recovery process for so many individuals (Marlatt et al., 2008). Unlike earlier approaches that attempted to fix, suppress, or stop these cravings, this mindfulness-based meditation approach "may disrupt habitual craving responses by providing heightened awareness and even acceptance of the initial craving response without judgment or reactance" (Marlatt et al., 2008, p. 109). These authors have stated:

> The goal of MBRP is to develop awareness and acceptance of thoughts, feelings, and sensations through practicing mindfulness, to observe both pleasant and unpleasant experience, and to accept whatever is present without judgment. . . . The focus is not on "doing what's right" or making a "good decision," but rather on a state of "just being" (Segal et al., 2002). Identification of one's individual high-risk situations for relapse remains a central component of the treatment. Clients are trained to recognize early warning signs for relapse and to increase awareness of substance-related cues, such as people and places that have previously been associated with substance use. Mindfulness practice provides clients with a new way of processing situational cues and monitoring reactions to environmental contingencies. (p. 110)

The MBRP approach includes eight 2-hour group sessions that occur over 8 weeks (Bowen et al., 2011; Marlatt et al., 2008). This approach uses many different mindfulness-based techniques. For example, Marlatt et al. describe a technique called "urge surfing":

> Urge surfing uses the imagery of a wave to help a client gain control over impulses to use drugs or alcohol. The client is first taught to label internal sensations and cognitive preoccupations as urges, and then to foster an attitude of unattached, curious observation of the experience. The technique focuses on identifying and accepting the urge, rather than acting on or attempting to fight it using suppression

or avoidance strategies. The curious and accepting attitude taken by facilitators and trainers toward the experiences of participants models this stance. The thoughts, feelings, and sensations experienced by participants are identified simply as arising events, without judgment, evaluation, or attempts to alter and control them. . . . In a recent study of vipassana meditation in reducing substance use (see Bowen et al., 2006; Marlatt et al., 2004), clients reported that "staying in the moment" and being mindful of urges were the most helpful coping strategies. (pp. 110–111)

Stages-of-Change and Motivational Interviewing Approaches to Relapse Prevention

Prochaska and DiClemente (1982) identified the six stages of change in clients struggling with addictive behaviors—precontemplation, contemplation, determination, action, maintenance, and relapse. (See Chapter 6 for a more detailed description of each stage.) In their research, they conceptualized this process as a wheel, with clients often needing to go through these stages three to seven times before they become stable in their recovery process (W. R. Miller & Rollnick, 1991, 2002; Prochaska & DiClemente, 1982). This model emphasizes that the experience of relapse may be a normal part of the cycle and may occur at any point in the stages of change.

MI is another set of principles that has contributed to the thinking on relapse prevention. While we acknowledge and agree with W. R. Miller and Rollnick (2009) that the stages-of-change model (Prochaska & DiClemente, 1982) and MI (W. R. Miller & Rollnick, 1991, 2002) are different approaches, we have found it helpful to conceptualize them together as we apply MI to our work with clients. W. R. Miller and Rollnick (1991, 2002) have emphasized that taking action to make changes definitely does not guarantee that the road to recovery will be a smooth one.

The MI approach normalizes the recovery process by indicating that "human experience is filled with good intentions and initial changes, followed by minor ('slips') or major ('relapses') steps backward" (W. R. Miller & Rollnick, 1991, p. 17). Thus, a relapse prevention perspective pervades all stages of change and becomes a major emphasis of the maintenance stage (W. R. Miller & Rollnick, 1991, 2002). If a relapse does occur, the counselor's role is to normalize the process and help the client to avoid discouragement and becoming stuck in the relapse process (W. R. Miller & Rollnick, 1991, 2002).

A natural tendency in the maintenance stage is to romanticize past behaviors and minimize the stress, pain, and consequences associated with those precipitating behaviors. W. R. Miller and Rollnick (1991), in their description of the process of relapse in their book on MI, indicate that they sometimes tell their clients, "Each slip or relapse brings you one step closer to recovery." They also state that "This is not, of course, meant to be an encouragement to relapse; rather, it is a realistic perspective to keep them [clients] from becoming disheartened, demoralized, or bogged down when a relapse occurs" (W. R. Miller & Rollnick, 1991, p. 39).

MI can make explicit this natural pull to reengage in self-defeating behaviors and support clients in staying connected to the values that have driven the change process thus far (W. R. Miller & Rollnick, 2002). When a client begins feeling pulled toward past behaviors, ambivalence may be heightened and the client may subsequently feel torn between reverting back to familiar patterns and maintaining his or her recovery (DiClemente, 1991; W. R. Miller & Rollnick, 1991, 2002). The case example below illustrates this process.

Chuck, a 52-year-old White man in recovery from alcohol and depression, worked with his therapist on managing triggers that he might encounter if he should attend a family barbecue. He had not attended this barbecue in several years, but had recently had successful reconnections with family members and had identified several value-based reasons to attend. However, he knew there would be alcohol there, and he knew that he would experience shame and guilt, among other painful feelings, especially when interacting with family members he had not been in contact with for many years. He and his therapist reviewed the skills that he had developed on his recovery path. Together they explored barriers and triggers that Chuck might encounter at the barbecue and discussed how to apply his recovery philosophy and skills base to manage these encounters while focusing on his main value—enjoying a long-held family tradition. The potential pain and discomfort were normalized and established as the necessary flipside to enjoying his family once again.

Once at the barbecue, Chuck adeptly managed his cousins' invitations to drink and clearly stated to them his recovery efforts in a way that was comfortable to him and limit setting to his cousins. He felt shaken when some of these cousins invalidated his recovery efforts and told him to "be a man." Additionally, the scouring looks and hurtful asides thrown his way by his great aunt, who had never let him forget his brief incarceration many years ago, stung in a way that Chuck had not anticipated. Old feelings related to guilt of his past actions and hurt from familial rejection he experienced surfaced in a way that was overwhelming for him, and he ended up drinking that night.

He called the therapist the next day and requested a session. He presented in session full of remorse and expressed feelings of failure and hopelessness. He expressed awareness that these things happen, that recovery requires steps backward in order to make two steps forward, yet he expressed feeling demoralized. He questioned what the point of doing all this work was if he ended up slipping anyway. Chuck expressed that it felt easier at this point to keep drinking. The therapist reflected Chuck's desire to keep drinking and that it felt easier and familiar at that point, a stressful moment in his life. He ultimately reminded Chuck that, at the end of the day, it would be his choice to continue drinking or not, but requested Chuck's willingness to look at this event and the choices before him in a different way. The therapist praised Chuck's progress thus far and spoke to Chuck and the values that drove him to make these difficult and significant changes in his life. The therapist asked Chuck if he would be willing to consider that what happened to him was normal and part of the recovery process, and commented on how tricky, complex, and nuanced the twists and turns of recovery can be. The therapist invited Chuck to see if there was an opportunity here for further learning. The therapist reminded Chuck that this was likely not the only time that Chuck would be blindsided by events that were out of his control and could easily precipitate urges to drink. Every time Chuck could turn a lapse such as this into an opportunity, he could emerge stronger from learning about the existing crevices of vulnerability in his recovery effort. Chuck commented that this dialogue was helpful to him and that there was strength in recognizing and learning from one's own weaknesses. He tentatively expressed optimism and said that, for the time being, he would try and refrain from drinking.

CBT Applications of Relapse Prevention in Mental Health Treatment

As a core mediational process, relapse prevention and trigger management can be applied to both mental health and substance abuse recovery. As indicated above, CBT approaches have influenced the development of relapse prevention techniques in the addictions field (Marlatt & Donovan, 2005). J. S. Beck (1995, 2011), Ludgate (2009), and Meichenbaum (2008) have described the use of these techniques in the field of mental health. Within the CBT model, J. S. Beck (2011) conceptualizes this approach as providing not only symptom remission but also skills that clients can utilize throughout their lives. With this in mind, she argues that therapists should begin relapse prevention even in the first few sessions of treatment. J. S. Beck (2011) actually presents clients with a graph that provides a visual representation of the ups and downs of the process of improvement. This serves to normalize the change process and the experience of setbacks or difficulties along the way.

Consistent with other principles of CBT, J. S. Beck (2011) emphasizes the process of using the techniques and skills learned in treatment when old feelings or issues reemerge. A part of the process throughout therapy is helping clients to address and prepare for potential setbacks. Beck recommends addressing this directly with clients early in treatment. In discussing this with a client, a therapist might ask, "Since it's possible you could have a setback, I'd like to discuss in advance how you would handle it" (p. 321). Beck then normalizes this process by encouraging clients to view thoughts and feelings such as depression as "only a setback, which is normal and temporary" (p. 321).

J. S. Beck (2011) also cautions therapists about the problem of fostering dependence in therapy. Using relapse prevention techniques and normalizing the ups and downs of the process of change and recovery helps to validate clients' sense of self-efficacy.

Core Mediational Processes of Relapse Prevention and Trigger Management

As illustrated above, relapse prevention and trigger management are well established in both substance abuse and mental health treatment. In relapse prevention, the focus is on helping the client to understand that his or her struggles may be a recurring presence in his or her life, but that a commitment to change, coupled with a skills-based, practical way to approach lapses, relapses, and struggles, can facilitate long-term change. While the philosophical framework that mental illness may be a recurring experience in their lives is difficult and painful to accept, when clients internalize these principles, they put themselves in the position of developing parts of themselves they would not have otherwise nurtured. Thus, in this sixth core mediational process, the management of triggers is shifted away from being framed as a barrier. Rather, it becomes viewed as an opportunity for learning, growth, and increased fortitude that would otherwise not exist. The next section will discuss two components of this core mediational process of relapse prevention and trigger management.

Component 1: The Therapist Introduces the Client to the Idea of Ongoing Relapse Prevention and Trigger Management Work

As noted above, criteria for discharge should be raised in the first session and maintained as a discussion point throughout treatment. The therapeutic process is presented as an opportunity for the client to develop ongoing skills that he or she will begin to acquire in treatment and further strengthen and hone throughout his or her entire life. Th only shifts focus away from a dependency on the therapist–client _, ___ but also establishes the client's responsibility to experience and view him- or herself as a proactive participant in his or her own life. Whether one is in therapy or not, recurrent exposure to triggers and painful experiences is inevitable, thus it is important for clients to view skills development and utilization as a necessary part of the ongoing recovery process. The following case example illustrates this component.

Sam, a 45-year-old White man, entered therapy because of ongoing feelings of depression and anxiety. He had been to a lot of different therapists and had recently relocated to the East Coast. He stressed that he wanted to find a therapist right away. In the first session, the therapist explored Sam's goals and asked him what he expected to get out of therapy. Sam replied that he had been in therapy for a long time, he liked coming to sessions, and saw them as an opportunity to vent. In exploring Sam's challenges and difficulties, it was revealed that Sam suffered frequent panic attacks. These panic attacks continued and in some cases worsened despite years of therapy. Sam was able to say that even though he had a lot of insight as to why he might be anxious, he stated that he never developed the tools to deal with his panic symptoms in the moment.

The therapist explored with Sam what he would be doing if he were not so affected by these panic attacks. Sam discussed going back to school to get his degree in the culinary arts, but immediately dismissed it as an impossibility because he could never imagine himself engaging with the public in that way. The therapist explored this dismissal and began to open up the possibility for Sam to obtain a new set of skills that would help him to develop a new relationship to his panic symptoms. These skills could be utilized in his outside life, regardless of the role of treatment in it. The therapist discussed an orientation to treatment that emphasized that he could take these skills with him wherever he went, and that the utilization of these skills would uncover strengths and capacities not otherwise recognized and developed.

The therapist noted that Sam became notably uneasy when the end of treatment was raised. Sam expressed that he never contemplated life without therapy, that a weekly appointment made him feel connected and provided an opportunity to vent and be heard. The therapist responded by reflecting Sam's concerns empathically and talked about recent changes in the mental health field, emphasizing that the work had become less about uncovering and doing away with symptoms and more about developing new ways of being with difficult feelings and symptoms. The therapist expressed the importance of the treatment focusing on taking what is learned and developed in therapy and applying it increasingly more and more in his natural life. The therapist emphasized that the therapy would be about helping him get in touch with a set of skills that he would always have with him in the face of adversity and discomfort. The therapist expressed a firm belief in Sam's ability to pursue school, and that there was no reason why Sam should not be able to move forward in the direction of his choosing.

Component 2: Therapist Sets the Stage That Lapses Are Going to Happen and Are Opportunities to Develop These Tools and Skills

Inherent in the framework of relapse prevention is the realization that no recovery will occur in a straight line but that true recovery is marked by detours and unexpected lapses that set the stage for further refinement of the recovery process. It is necessary to emphasize this from the beginning of treatment (J. S. Beck, 2011) because such lapses can be met with a sense of futility and defeatism. By generating an appreciation of the inevitability of lapses, clients can greet these opportunities as an invitation to learn and grow.

One of the most demoralizing aspects of clinical work is that clients come in wanting to feel better, and to be "cured" in the hope that this will mean no pain and no symptoms. This can be particularly challenging for clients with severe mental illness (e.g., bipolar disorder, schizophrenia, major depression). It can also be problematic for clients who have had recurrent drug-related lapses and relapses. A developing trend in the literature is the belief that collaborating with this desire for "cure" in the client is falling into a control-and-elimination perspective that is ultimately unobtainable (Eifert & Forsyth, 2005; Hayes, Strosahl, & Wilson, 1999, 2011; M. G. Williams et al., 2007). One of the potential traps in treatment is that after 6 or 7 months, if this expectation of a complete cure is not addressed, clients can feel that the work is not resulting in progress or that they aren't working hard enough, and a sense of futility can result. Similarly, therapists might feel overresponsible for making change occur and embroil themselves in this dance of unobtainable results. It is important therefore, for both the client and the therapist to establish realistic expectations in line with the recovery research- and acceptance-based work that is so prominent in the recovery literature. It is important to help clients realize that there may always be ebbs and flows, and that pain and comfort may exist side by side. In the case of Sam discussed above this was evident.

———————

Sam, when asked by the therapist about expectations of treatment, invoked the idea that eventually he would be "fixed" and would be rid of anxiety

and painful feelings. The therapist validated Sam's need to feel l
gently introduced the possibility that these feelings might reappea
ent points in his life, particularly when he might be experiencing s
two discussed how life was not without its joy or without its discomfort.
That for every moment of joy there may be sadness, guilt, and shame. The
therapist pointed out that anytime there is a value, such as going to culinary school, there is a vulnerability, such as fear of making an embarrassing
comment in class or failing to succeed. This statement resonated with Sam,
and the therapist asked Sam to envision himself actually going to culinary
school, and the two began exploring if Sam could do this without feeling, sometimes very intensely, the risks attached to taking such steps, and
that the two—values and vulnerabilities—go hand in hand. The therapist
stressed that these moments of feeling intense anxiety can be, alternatively,
viewed and experienced as opportunities to learn how to manage and push
forward alongside such adversity.

Ultimately this core mediational process addresses the idea that
struggle, pain, and difficulties that arise out of having a mental illness
need to be honored and integrated into the person's whole life rather
than seen as an enemy that needs to be battled with and resolved (Hayes,
Strosahl, & Wilson, 1999, 2011; Linehan, 1993). In this approach the
symptomatic experience is seen as a painful experience, but also as an
opportunity to transform one's relationship to these experiences and
ultimately to transform oneself.

This idea that symptomatic experiences and triggers may be viewed
and experienced as opportunities for learning and growth can be
extended to the notion that symptoms take one to the corners where
exposure is most needed. Willingness-based, internal exposure to symptoms thus becomes an essential part of relapse prevention and trigger
management. It is through these newly developed pathways where value-
based functioning takes hold. If Sam from the case example above can
develop the willingness and capacity to experience his symptoms as
opportunities to move into, rather than avoid, the overwhelming barriers he experiences when considering going to school begin to dissolve,
and the conditions for ongoing relapse prevention and trigger management are established.

Ronald Siegel (2005) similarly states:

> While few people ever say they are glad to have had a psycho-physi-
> ological disorder, it is not unusual for patients to appreciate the les-
> sons they have learned through their recovery. In retrospect, many
> people come to understand their symptoms as wake-up calls, signals
> that their approach to life was in some way out of balance. A surpris-
> ing number of people become drawn to regular mindfulness practice,

and to the philosophical principles with which it has been historically associated. . . . The reality of the impermanence of all things becomes clearer. They may develop an appreciation of the experience in the present moment, realizing that this is where life is actually lived. They also gain confidence that they can learn to bear both emotional and physical pain, and no longer need to rush to resolve it. . . . When adversity becomes an opportunity for learning and growth, life is enriched. (p. 195)

The Completion of Therapy

Discussions of relapse prevention and trigger management are important throughout treatment beginning at the first session. However, they are particularly important as the time for the completion of therapy approaches. Many treatment models in the mental health field use "termination" to describe the ending of therapy (J. S. Beck, 2011). We prefer the word *completion* for a number of reasons. First, for some of our clients, the word *termination* invokes an image of a permanent ending. In our conceptualization, we use the metaphor of life as a book with different chapters. With this in mind, the experience of therapy is framed as one chapter that has been successfully completed. Clients are validated for the work that they have done and are told that life may present new issues in the future and that they always have the option of opening a new chapter of treatment. They may also choose to come in for one or two booster sessions rather than open an entire new chapter (J. S. Beck, 2011). Clients should always be encouraged to attempt to address problems after completing therapy on their own first before contacting the therapist (J. S. Beck, 2011).

In this process, it is important that clinicians recognize the need to avoid promoting dependency on the therapist. Since empowerment of clients is always the goal, it is important that clients be given credit for their own improvement or their gains in therapy (J. S. Beck, 2011; Meichenbaum, 2008). It is also helpful during the process of completion for the therapist to gradually begin tapering sessions from once per week to every other week. J. S. Beck suggests that as clients are able to handle this schedule, the therapist should spread out the sessions to every three or four weeks in preparation for ending treatment. J. S. Beck also reminds therapists that some clients may feel anxious about completion. She recommends that therapists discuss the advantages and disadvantages of tapering sessions with clients. A chart can be made collaboratively with clients to list the advantages and disadvantages. It is then important for the therapist to reframe disadvantages positively.

For example, J. S. Beck indicates that a therapist might reframe a client's stated disadvantage, " I might relapse," to, "If I'm going to relapse, it's better for it to happen while I'm still in therapy so I can learn how to handle it" (p. 322).

Clients can be encouraged throughout treatment to keep notebooks or journals of helpful strategies to use if they should encounter a setback. These can be particularly helpful in the completion process. Therapists can help clients to prepare lists of the steps they would take if they should experience a setback (J. S. Beck, 2011).

In addition, acceptance and commitment therapy (ACT) (Eifert & Forsyth, 2005; Hayes, Strosahl, & Wilson, 1999, 2011) encourages clients to clarify their values and goals and to accept that they may have setbacks but that they can still make a commitment to pursuing their goals and having a fulfilling life (see Chapter 8). It is helpful to review these principles again with a client during the completion process.

Booster Sessions

Another process that is common to CBT approaches and other evidence-based treatments is the use of booster sessions (Barlow, 2008; J. S. Beck, 2011). Typically, during the completion process, clients are encouraged to schedule booster sessions that will occur after they have completed treatment. J. S. Beck reports that this process serves a number of purposes: it can alleviate the anxiety of some of our clients about completing treatment, it provides an opportunity for the therapist to review the client's coping strategies, and it offers an opportunity for the therapist and the client collaboratively to predict possible future difficulties and to develop strategies for addressing them. It is also important that these booster sessions focus on positive experiences as well as the problems that clients may encounter.

Conclusion

Recovery is most often characterized by a two-step-forward, one-step-back process. Inherent to the core mediational process discussed in this chapter is the recognition that people will continue to experience setbacks, challenges, stress, and bumps along the road after treatment. Relapse prevention and trigger management create a framework to anticipate and accept these challenges, as well as to utilize the skills developed in treatment to mediate these experiences. The completion of treatment provides another occasion to empower clients to view setbacks or relapses as opportunities to learn and grow.

PART III

Systems Interventions

Family, Multisystems,
and Group Treatment

CHAPTER 10

Family Therapy

Introduction

Family therapy has evolved considerably since its early days in the 1950s. Nichols (2011), in his comprehensive review of the field, has identified over 14 different models and related approaches. (Readers are referred to his book *The Essentials of Family Therapy* [Nichols, 2011] for an excellent overview.) This chapter addresses a number of the issues faced by therapists in translating family therapy approaches to the real world of clinical work. Topics discussed in this chapter include engagement, strength-based approaches, problem solving, tapping the family's creativity, and reframing. Because many clinicians associate family therapy with the presenting problems of children and adolescents, we also explore how family interventions can be extended to the treatment of adults. As an example, in the last part of this chapter we discuss the use of family therapy and approaches such as family psychoeducation (McFarlane et al., 2003) when identified clients are adults diagnosed with serious and/or chronic mental illness.

As we have indicated throughout this book, one of the first realities facing family therapists in the real world is the fact that many families are not self-referred (Boyd-Franklin, 2003; Boyd-Franklin & Bry, 2000a). Many are sent for treatment by schools, hospitals, courts, child welfare systems, probation departments, etc. As a result, many families, including those that are poor and ethnic minority, may enter treatment initially with a great deal of suspicion (Boyd-Franklin, 2003). Some have had a history of negative experiences with the multisystems mentioned above; others may be responding to "healthy cultural suspicion" related to experiences with discrimination and racism (see Chapter 3). As a

179

result, two extremely important concepts for therapists in the real world to be aware of are the therapist's use of self and the concept of establishing therapeutic rapport or "joining" (Boyd-Franklin & Bry, 2000a; see Chapter 4 of this book).

The Therapist's Use of Self and the Process of Joining

Because so many families are not self-referred, the "therapist's use of self" is essential to the process of joining or establishing therapeutic rapport. One of the most important functions of training and supervision in family therapy should be to help therapists increase their self-knowledge and discover ways in which they can personally connect or join with families. It is also important for therapists to be aware of the ways in which they may be perceived by their clients and families. For example, a young White therapist may be perceived as culturally different and inexperienced by an African American family. Similarly, a middle-class African American therapist may be perceived as different by a poor family of the same racial and cultural background. One of the most important lessons for therapists is to recognize that these judgments may be inaccurate and have nothing to do with who they are personally, but reflect the experiences that the client or family has had with other providers of their race and age. With this in mind, it is important that therapists not take these initial reactions personally, but work to join or connect past them (see Chapter 3). The therapist's use of self often involves basic responses that convey warmth, genuine interest and concern, and a relaxed demeanor that can help put clients and family members at ease.

Identifying the "Real" Family: Cultural Considerations

Throughout this book, we have adopted a broad definition of "family" that includes the social supports and important people involved in a person's life. Cultural definitions of family may vary. For example, some African American families may include "blood" (e.g., mother, father, siblings, grandparents, aunts, uncles) and "nonblood" members (e.g., friends, neighbors, godparents, ministers, church family members). In working with families, therapists should have an awareness of these multiple definitions and structures of family and take this into account when considering whom to include in the treatment process.

Assessment of Families

Joining is not only an engagement process but is also an opportunity to observe and begin an assessment of the family system. As stated above, our first goal must always be to connect with the family and establish therapeutic rapport. The early joining phase also offers the therapist the opportunity to elicit the perspective of each family member, while at the same time observing the interactional patterns that make up the family dance (Nichols, 2011). When you are joining with a family, you are participating in the family's everyday pushes and pulls, which allows you to identify dynamics such as:

- Who talks to whom?
- Hierarchy: Who is in charge?
- What are the alliances and coalitions?
- The permeability and rigidity of boundaries
- Nonverbal communication patterns
- Family roles including scapegoat, caretaker, parentified child, and identified patient (Minuchin, 1974; Nichols, 2011)

Enactments or *interactions* are an important part of the assessment process and the therapist often encourages family members to role play a discussion in the therapy room (S. Minuchin, 1974; Nichols, 2011). These enactments bring "the kitchen table" to the session. The family demonstrates to the therapist the places in which they are "stuck," thus giving the therapist a unique vantage point to target interventions. For example, a mother arrives with four children, who proceed to tear the office apart. What does the mother do? Is she frozen? Does she overreact? How do the children respond? Through these actions, the family is presenting to the therapist the dynamics that occur at home. These enactments and interactions may serve as microcosmic representations of the family's larger difficulties and represent points of entry for intervention.

Another important assessment tool is the process of *mapping* an interactional diagnosis of family relational patterns (S. Minuchin, 1974; Nichols, 2011). Once the therapist has successfully joined with the family and experienced its natural "pushes and pulls," he or she is equipped to formulate a structural hypothesis about the family dynamics. Each family has its own unique map. The map is designed as a guide for therapists to help families get "unstuck" in their interactions and relate to one another in more adaptive ways.

When working with complex families, it is beneficial to remember important family systems concepts in the assessment process.

Two central concepts are the circles of causality and complementarity (Nichols, 2011). These concepts involve multidirectional cycles of co-construction in a family system and can reveal symptomatic cycles within families. The following examples illustrate these circles of causality and complementarity:

- *Example 1:* A child acts out in school, which elicits Mom's activation out of her depression and Dad becoming more involved after being mostly absent.
- *Example 2:* Dad yells at his adolescent daughter, who withdraws. Daughter's withdrawal elicits further yelling on the part of Dad.
- *Example 3:* Partner A pursues a distancer (Partner B). This results in further distancing by Partner B and further pursuit by Partner A.

Understanding the circles of causality and complementarity can help families get "unstuck" from these symptomatic patterns of interaction, of which they might not always be aware.

Stages of Change

As we discussed in Chapter 6, Prochaska and DiClemente (1982) and DiClemente and Velasquez (2002) challenged a long-held belief in the mental health field regarding the readiness of clients for treatment. Many therapists have been trained to assume that the clients and families sitting in front of them are committed to therapy and the process of making changes in their lives. In their work with substance abusing clients, Prochaska and DiClemente challenged this assumption. They introduced the concept of ambivalence with which many clients approach treatment and the process of change. These concepts are also relevant in our evaluation of families.

With this in mind, they identified the following stages of change: precontemplation, contemplation, preparation, action, maintenance, and relapse (see Chapter 6). Prochaska and DiClemente (1982), and many other theorists who have discussed stages of change, have focused primarily on the individual (DiClemente & Velasquez, 2002). There has been little exploration of these concepts in terms of families. In our experience, however, different family members often present for treatment at different stages of change and readiness for family therapy. It would not be unusual, for example, to have a mother in the action stage who is ready to work, an adolescent (the identified patient) in the precontemplation stage who has a great deal of resistance to treatment and change, and a father in the contemplation stage who is still ambivalent about the treatment process.

The therapist's role is to assess where the family members are in this process of change and to engage them in treatment by meeting them where they are in this process. To accomplish this goal, the family therapist may use a number of different strategies including reframing the problem in a way that feels less judgmental to the family members. The case examples below illustrate this process.

The stages-of-change approach encourages clinicians to honor and respect family burnout and ambivalence. It also emphasizes the importance of recognizing all perspectives of different family members. This has the effect of widening the lens with which we view the family and allowing us to positively reframe their responses. For example, instead of viewing a father's initial refusal to become involved in family therapy as final, therapists are encouraged to "roll with the resistance" (W. R. Miller & Rollnick, 2002) and keep the dialogue open with the hope that the father might eventually move through his resistance or ambivalence.

Engagement versus Involvement of Family Members

Given the reality that family members may be at different stages of change, one of the challenges faced by therapists doing family therapy is the fact that some family members may refuse to come into the office for treatment. This is particularly problematic if the family member(s) is powerful in the family system and exerts a great deal of influence over other members. Most family therapists have been trained to reach out in order to involve these family members in the treatment process. By involvement, many therapists expect the family members to meet together in traditional office sessions. This is ideal when it occurs. Unfortunately, however, many experienced family therapists report that this continues to be a challenge even after many years of clinical work.

With this in mind, we would like to propose a reframe of this involvement process. Often the therapist's view of involvement might include some level of commitment or behavior change on the part of different family members. For example, a therapist working with a mother on reunification with her children who are in foster care may have faced a challenge in trying to engage the grandmother, who has been a source of social support for the mother in the past. The grandmother may be "resistant" to becoming involved initially. She explains that she has been through the process of removal of her grandchildren many times because of her daughter's drug use. Each time reunification has occurred, she and the children have felt disappointed when their mother again relapsed into drug use.

Recognizing this concern, the therapist does not insist that the grandmother come in to participate in the family therapy sessions. Instead, she obtains written permission from the mother to reach out to the grandmother. She calls her on the phone, and in their brief conversation it becomes clear that this grandmother is still angry with her daughter, but she loves and cares about the future of her grandchildren. With this in mind, the therapist does not ask her to come in right away, but she says, "You are one of the most important people in your grandchildren's lives. Would you be willing to talk to me occasionally and give me your input as I work with them?" The grandmother responds positively, and the therapist has engaged her in the treatment process.

The above example illustrates an important distinction in the process of family therapy (i.e., the difference between engagement and involvement). It has been our experience that many family members are "burnt out" in their efforts to help other family members over many years. This is particularly apparent in our work with the families of adult clients who are substance abusers or who have serious mental illness. Sometimes these clients have angered family members who have tried to help and intervene with them numerous times. In these cases, well-meaning therapists can sometimes alienate a family member by pushing for involvement prematurely, particularly if that involvement involves providing housing or attending regular treatment sessions. Similarly, therapists on inpatient units or in residential programs can sometimes alienate a family member by pushing prematurely for that family member to take the client into his or her home to live after discharge.

In these situations, engagement may be a more appropriate initial goal. This might involve phone contact of the type described in the case example above. It might involve one session in which a willing family member shares the history with the therapist. Later in the process, the client might be reconnected with one or more family members without undue pressure upon them for more involvement. Similarly, for grandparents, aunts, and uncles of children placed in the child welfare system, little attempt has been made in some cases to maintain contact and regular supervised visits with these family members, particularly if they indicate that they are unable to raise or adopt the child(ren). One sad consequence of our current child welfare laws has been the push for family members or foster parents to adopt a child. Like many child welfare laws, this was grounded in good intentions. Unfortunately, particularly for older kinship relatives or foster parents, they may love the children but feel overwhelmed by the prospect of assuming the full responsibility of an adoptive parent. For many of these individuals, this results in a systemic cutoff from these children, who often lose an individual or family to whom they are attached. This occurs because the system often discourages contact once the child has been removed.

By our definition, many of these individuals may be seen by the child as "family." Even in cases where ongoing involvement is no longer possible, engagement of these individuals, even for periodic supervised visits, would help to address the feelings of loss, abandonment, and emotional cutoff that so many of these children feel. With clients who have been through multiple placements through the child welfare system, or for a prolonged stay in residential treatment, the construction of a "life book" (Backhaus, 1984) offers the opportunity for the therapist to identify family members who may have been involved in the child's life in an earlier period.

Establishing Family Connections

The therapist might work with the family members who are willing to come in for sessions, while gradually reaching out to other key members who are initially reluctant to become involved. The goal here is a more gradual, incremental connection that is established over time; first through the therapist and then involving other family members, including the identified client. This approach often requires therapists to rein in their enthusiasm and modulate the rate of contact with these family members. It requires meeting family members where they are, while building credibility and trust.

For example, as described in the case example involving the engagement with the grandmother above, reaching out through periodic phone contact might be a way to engage these family members. Therapists may also take a more indirect route. This might involve establishing "vicarious dialogue" with the absent family member. Sending home messages or questions can also be helpful, as illustrated in the following example.

Juan, a 12-year-old Latino boy, was referred for treatment for fighting in school. In response to the therapist's request for the whole family to attend the first session, the mother arrived with Juan and his three brothers (ages 10, 6, and 5) and his baby sister (6 months). The father lived with the family and was described as "not able to get off" for the session. It quickly became clear that the mother was feeling overwhelmed with all of the children, especially Juan, and that the father was not home a great deal. The mother reported that he was away from home because he worked long hours.

Although all of the boys spoke English, the mother and the father spoke only Spanish. Since the therapist did not speak Spanish, she invited an intern who was bilingual to become her cotherapist. With the help of their supervisor, they decided to first use a vicarious dialogue to engage this father.

After a discussion with Juan, his mother, and his brothers about the reason why he might fight in school, they asked the mother to go home and ask the father what he thought was causing Juan to fight at school.

In the next session, the mother and Juan were excited to give the therapists the father's response. Mother reported that he said, "so they won't see him as a punk." Another lively discussion ensued in this session in which the therapist encouraged the mother to talk to Juan about this issue. Juan told a number of stories about the expectation of his peer group that he fight to show that he was not a "punk." At the end of the session, the therapists encouraged the mother and Juan to go home and praise the father for his insight. The bilingual therapist then said that she would like to call the father to learn more about his understanding of this issue.

The next evening, she called the father at home, late after work, and explained that she was one of the counselors working with Juan and the family at the clinic. She then praised the father for his understanding of what his son was up against with peers who might view him as a "punk" if he did not fight. She told the father that he was one of the most important people in his son's life and that she needed his input on how best to help his son. She and the father then talked for a half hour about his understanding of the problems that his son faced. The therapist told him that she would like to call him sometimes in order to get his opinion about their attempts to help his son. They spoke a number of times on the phone over the next 2 months.

At the beginning of the spring semester, Juan was involved in an angry fight in school and was suspended for a week. In the family session, Juan was sullen and refused to speak and the mother was again overwhelmed and crying. The therapist discussed with the mother the importance of getting the father's input so that they could work together as a team to help Juan. She called the father that night and told him that this was a serious crisis. Juan had been suspended and was being threatened with expulsion. She told him that they needed his input to help his son. She offered to hold a home-based family session later in the evening so that the father could attend. Because they had by now established a therapeutic relationship, the father was willing to allow the therapist to come to his home for the session.

In the meeting, the therapists greeted the father and the intern explained to him that the other therapist did not speak Spanish so she would translate for her. She praised the father for the insights that he had given over the last few months into Juan's behavior. She asked him to speak to Juan about his fighting. Since it had been a productive line of questioning earlier, she asked the father to explore with Juan his theory that he did not want to be called a "punk" by his friends for not fighting. The father and Juan had a lively conversation about this issue. The father shared that he had to deal with these issues himself as a boy growing up in "el barrio." The therapist emphasized that the father was an "expert" on these issues because he had been through them himself. They discussed a number of ways in which Juan could walk away from a fight and not be considered a "punk."

The therapist encouraged the father and Juan to talk for a few minutes each night to discuss the day's events. The two therapists also encouraged the mother and the father to talk each night before bed to discuss alternatives for Juan.

The therapists were excited about the father's participation in this session. In their eagerness, they invited him to join them for the next session. The father was obviously uncomfortable and responded that he had been forced to leave work early in order to attend. He explained that he worked two jobs in order to pay the family's bills. He was afraid that he would lose his job if he continued to take time off. The therapists realized their error and backed off this request. The bilingual therapist asked the father to connect with Juan and with his wife each night and that she would check in with him in a week.

The night before the next family session, the therapist called the father. He reported that he had spoken to his son on a number of occasions. The therapist asked his advice about interventions that he would suggest to his son to avoid fighting. The father told her a number of experiences that he had had as a young adolescent.

In a future phone session some months later, the father shared that he had been a lightweight boxer as a young man. The therapist discussed this with him and asked if he had ever told Juan or his other sons about this experience. He said no. The therapist encouraged him to do so. She asked if he had any pictures of himself as a boxer. He told her that he did. She encouraged him to share them with Juan, his mother, and his brothers. The therapist told him that she and her cotherapist would also like to see these pictures. He reported that he could not take off but that if they held the session later in his home, he would try to return from work by the end of the session. On the night of the session, everyone in the family was excited about the father's involvement. The therapists came to their home, looked at the pictures and shared the enthusiasm of Juan and the other family members. The therapist asked if the father still boxed. He replied that he still did occasionally at a local gym where he used to work but that it was rare because of his work schedule. The therapist asked the father and the mother if they might be willing to try something in order to help Juan. The therapist asked the father if he might be willing to take Juan and give him some boxing lessons. The father said that he would. She asked if he would be willing to do it only as a reward for Juan. If he had a "good week" in school (i.e., no fights), then his father would take him on the weekend to box.

Juan was thrilled and the mother strongly supported the plan. Juan's behavior improved markedly over the next few months and he was able to increasingly avoid fighting at school.

―――――――――――

This case illustrates a number of issues. First, it was important that a bilingual therapist was able to be a part of this treatment process. This allowed her to reach out directly to the father. Her contribution was more than her ability to speak Spanish. She was able to utilize her cultural sensitivity to join with the father using the cultural values of *personalismo* and *respeto* (personalism and respect) (Garcia-Preto, 2005) to connect with the father in a down-to-earth personal manner and to convey her respect for him and for his input about Juan's problem.

It was important to first establish a "vicarious dialogue" with the father, by sending home messages to him in the form of questions. The therapist then progressed to calling the father and asking his advice about the treatment of his son. Once again, as indicated in the earlier case example involving the engagement of a reluctant grandmother, it was necessary to acknowledge the father's expertise in the raising of his son and to emphasize the importance of his relationship. She conveyed to him that he was "one of the most important people in his son's life" and that his input was critical. Through this process, the therapist established a gradual relationship with the father—one based on mutual respect.

Juan's suspension and threatened expulsion presented a "crisis" that the therapists used to involve the father in a home-based family session. He was reframed as a caring father with a very demanding work schedule. Change began to occur in Juan's behavior when his father took the time to speak with him in the evening and when he was encouraged to discuss Juan's behavior with his wife. Initially, the session went so well that the therapists moved prematurely to try to involve the father in ongoing sessions. He objected, again raising his work schedule. The therapists "rolled with the resistance" (W. R. Miller & Rollnick, 2002) and did not push the issue at that time (see Chapter 6).

In a later phone conversation, the therapist learned about the father's experience as a boxer as a young man and the fact that he sometimes worked out at a nearby gym. The father agreed to tell Juan and his other sons about this and to show them his pictures. The therapist expressed interest in seeing them also. It is noteworthy that it was less of a problem to convince the father to agree to another home-based session when the agenda was a positive one rather than one focused on Juan's fighting. Joining with the family's enthusiasm, the therapist then encouraged the parents to discuss the possibility of using boxing lessons for Juan and his brothers from the father as a reward for a week of good behavior in school (i.e., no fighting).

It was important that boxing be used as a reward for positive behavior only. Too often, parents "give away" these powerful positive reinforcements without tying them to behavior change. The mother and the father agreed on this strategy. In the next few months, Juan had only one incident of fighting and the father, who had been peripheral to the family, was now involved in a positive activity with Juan and his brothers. The strategy of including the brothers was important because if only Juan received this attention from the father, there was a potential that the other boys might begin acting out in order to gain his attention.

Strength-Based Interventions

The case of Juan also illustrates the process of moving from a problem-saturated focus to a strength-based one (Berg, 1994; Boyd-Franklin & Bry, 2000a). The father was resistant to becoming involved in treatment when the emphasis was on Juan's problem behavior. Many parents are concerned that therapists may blame them for their children's misbehavior. As the emphasis shifted to the father's strengths and he was validated for his input, he became more engaged in the process, even though he rarely attended a session. The therapist's response—that of paying attention to the father's strength as a boxer—allowed for the development of a therapeutic relationship. Both therapists also made it clear repeatedly that the father was the expert on his son and that they respected him for it.

Strategic family therapists such as Jay Haley (1976) and Cloe Madanes (1981) describe the technique of using the boxing lessons as a reward for not fighting as "prescribing the symptom." Juan was in trouble for fighting, but the father's strength as a boxer was prescribed as a way to bring father and his sons closer together and to reward Juan for avoiding fights at school.

The Utility of the Structural Family Therapy Approach

The case of Juan also illustrates the value of the structural family therapy approach. In families where there is a child with a problem, one parent is often overinvolved and overwhelmed like Juan's mother in the above case. The other parent is often peripheral to the daily life of the family and less involved with the children (Haley, 1976; S. Minuchin, 1974; Nichols, 2011). The child acts out at least in part to gain the attention of the peripheral parent, and the child's behavior provides a great deal of the contact and conversation between the parents. In the case of Juan, this led to the mother often complaining to the father about how overwhelmed she was by Juan's behavior. The therapists worked to build more of a positive relationship between the parents by asking the mother to ask the father his opinion about why Juan fought at school.

The mother's report of the father's feedback opened the door for the therapist to praise the father to the mother and the children, including Juan, and to reach out to the father directly.

As mentioned above, the therapist's use of self is important in this case as well as her cultural knowledge. She praised the father for his input. Boyd-Franklin and Bry (2000a) remind us to "Never underestimate the power of praise." So often, parents of children who are referred for treatment fear that they will be blamed for their child's misbehavior. They often become more and more critical of their child and more removed from them as the behavior persists and they feel increasingly helpless to change it. This becomes a parallel process because as they are blamed by schools and other agencies for their child's behavior, the parents in turn often blame their children. Validating their opinions and praising them for their appropriate behavior may be a new experience for the parents who we treat.

In keeping with the structural family therapy approach, the peripheral parent is connected with the child in trouble. What is different about the case of Juan from many early examples of this approach is that the therapists worked indirectly and rolled with the father's resistance (W. R. Miller & Rollnick, 2002) to becoming involved. They engaged him first more indirectly through phone calls and then gradually involved him in the treatment process. Respecting his value of working hard to support his family, they did not force the issue of his becoming "involved" by attending all family therapy sessions. Instead, they focused on "engaging" him in the process of connecting with Juan and his other sons. It was also crucial to emphasize the importance of having the parents work together to decide when Juan should be rewarded. The therapists realized their error of prematurely pushing for more involvement in the form of the father's attendance at sessions and worked instead on engaging him in the process at a pace and in a manner with which he was comfortable.

Home–Based Family Therapy

Another important intervention in this case was the use of home-based family therapy sessions. Although many of the sessions took place in the clinic, the therapists found that the father's work schedule made it difficult for him to meet at the clinic. However, he was willing to allow the therapists to come to a meeting in his home at a later time in the evening. This was possible only after the therapist had joined with him on the phone and had begun to establish a therapeutic relationship. This is an important lesson for therapists who are doing primarily office-based family treatment. In our experience, even one well-timed home visit can make an enormous difference in the outcome of the treatment process (Boyd-Franklin & Bry, 2000a).

Home-based family therapy has also been used as a distinct treatment modality with families that are difficult to engage in treatment and with those who may present with multiple problems (Berg, 1994; Boyd-Franklin and Bry, 2000a). The messages given throughout this book on joining are crucial in home-based family therapy. This is particularly necessary in cases of mandated treatment. Boyd-Franklin and Bry encourage therapists to remember their own "home training" as they enter a client's home:

> Family therapists can benefit greatly from the exercise of putting themselves in family members' position and considering how they might feel if a stranger came into their home asking painful, difficult, and sometimes intrusive questions. Imagine further that the person is there without their invitation or permission but at the behest of an outside authority such as the courts, and that they are mandated to comply. Given this complex context, it is not unusual for family members to be guarded and uncomfortable in the first home-based session. Family therapists can do a great deal to put family members at ease during this first contact. Never underestimate the value of a pleasant personality; personal warmth will help put family members at ease. (p. 38)

These guidelines are helpful to family therapists whether they do home- or office-based sessions (or a combination of both). The value of calling first and beginning the joining process on the phone, as the therapists above did with Juan's father, is particularly helpful. Another lesson from Juan's case is that it is important that therapists remember that they are on the client's "home turf" (Boyd-Franklin & Bry, 2000a, p. 39) and that it is important to respect the person's home. This can require some flexibility from therapists who are used to having only office-based sessions. For example, if family members are watching the television when the therapist enters, it may be considered rude to ask the family to turn off the television in their first meeting. Boyd-Franklin and Bry offer the following helpful hints to therapists in the first home-based session:

> One rule for the first session is to learn to "go with the flow" of the family. Do not be in a hurry on a first visit to impose rules or your own sense of order. Try to relax, fit in, and get to know all of those present. An error sometimes made by beginning family therapists is to try to draw too rigid a boundary around the family in a first session. If visitors arrive during your session, greet them, but do not plunge

into an exploration of personal family matters without asking the parents or parental figures whether they are comfortable talking now or whether they would prefer for you to return later. Take your cues from the parents or parental figure. (p. 39)

Ironically, sometimes a visit of a family friend or an extended family member will help to connect the therapist with another resource for the family or for a particular client. In cultures such as African American and Latino families, these close friends may actually be "like family" and may be referred to as if they were relatives (Boyd-Franklin, 2003; Garcia-Preto, 2005; McGoldrick et al., 2005).

Families with Multiple Problems and Many Stressors

In the real world of clinical work, especially in agencies or clinics in urban areas, families often present with multiple problems and stressors. As we discuss in Chapter 11, this can prompt therapists to bring in multiple services, which can lead to a large number of multisystemic agencies involved with a single client or family. Chapter 11 also gives a number of examples of how clinicians can utilize the multisystems model and interdisciplinary case conferences to help to coordinate care (Boyd-Franklin, 2003; Boyd-Franklin & Bry, 2000a; E. N. Cleek, Wofsy, Boyd-Franklin, Mundy, & Howell, 2012).

Berg (1994) gives the following advice to therapists as they work with clients and families that present with many problems:

1. Do not panic! . . . be calm.
2. Ask the client what is the most urgent problem that he [or she] wants to solve first. Follow his [or her] directions, not yours. Be sure the goal is *small,* realistically achievable and simple.
3. Ask yourself who is most bothered by the problem. Make sure it is not you; you do not want to be the "customer" for your own services.
4. Get a good picture of how your client's life would change when that one goal is achieved. . . .
5. Stay focused on solving that one problem first. Do not let the fact that the client is overwhelmed affect you. . . .
6. Find out in detail how the client made things better in the past. . . .
7. Be sure to compliment the client on even the smallest progress and achievements. Always give the client the credit for successes.
8. When one problem is solved, review with the client how he [or she] solved it. What did he [or she] do that worked? (p. 199)

There are many words of wisdom in Berg's (1994) list. One that is particularly important to remember is number 7, "Always give the client the credit for successes." Without an emphasis on the client (or family's) own self-efficacy in producing change, therapy can foster dependency on the clinician. This is the difference between empowerment and helping (see Chapter 4).

Techniques

Therapists who are working with families in the real world have found it helpful to adopt an integrative model (Nichols, 2009) and to incorporate techniques from many different family systems models, depending on the needs of each family. This section discusses the following important techniques and their utility in the treatment process:

- Decreasing blame and negativity and breaking the cycles of mutual reactivity
- Relational processes
- Increasing hope and optimism
- Acceptance
- Highlighting strengths
- Eliciting values
- Interventive enactments
- Rolling with the resistance
- Reframing
- Organizational theme
- Fostering improved problem-solving and communication skills
- Generalizing skills

Decreasing blame and negativity and *breaking the cycles of mutual reactivity* are two of the most central family systems concepts (M. White & Epston, 1990; Nichols, 2011). Family members often enter treatment caught in self-defeating and limiting cycles of relating to each other. The technique of illuminating these cycles has the power of shifting the locus of control from inside the individual to the relational dynamics in the family or couple system, thus externalizing the blame (Freedman & Combs, 1996; M. White & Epston, 1990) and establishing *relational processes*. The following therapist response illustrates these processes.

"Thank you for showing me what is going on. I can now see why you are stuck and how you are experiencing each other. Mom, you are clearly angry and frustrated at your son's disregard for household rules, and son, you are clearly reactive to your mother's criticism and anger. Mom, each time you express your anger, the more shutdown your son becomes. Son, the more defensive and withdrawn you become, the angrier your mom gets. This has been going on for so long now, it has become a part of your reality; at this point, it is not about whose fault it is, it's about both of you participating in changing this pattern."

Increasing hope, optimism, and highlighting strengths is another important part of the family treatment process. Many families come into therapy feeling demoralized and defeated by the problems that they are facing. Often the therapist initially serves as the container for hope and the optimism about the family's potential for change. The clinician's role also includes introducing novelty and discontinuity into the family system, which creates room for an expanded, more flexible experience. For example, in helping the client to see beyond their problematic interactions, therapists can ask questions such as "Who are you outside of these problems?" or "What can we borrow from your past experiences to apply to these current challenges?" Similarly, another technique therapists can use involves having family members engage in a fun mutual activity such as playing a game. This technique is particularly helpful in working with families whose interactional style mostly revolves around fighting as it helps to have these families engage in a neutral or fun activity that requires cooperation and collaboration.

Acceptance (Hayes, Strosahl, & Wilson, 1999, 2011) is also a new concept for many family members. For many people, there is strife in family life. Many are taught to expect and want only the good in life. In order to participate in the human drama, however, there has to be an active acceptance and tolerance of the inevitable pain and disharmony that comprises a full life experience. Providing the client with the following illustration can help them to contemplate the value of the inevitable ups and downs of family and relational life:

> "Choice A is no strife with your wife; yet the cost is that you cannot be in any relationship. Choice B is being in a relationship with the full human range of both harmony and strife."

Many of these ideas are based on concepts incorporated in mindfulness (Hick & Bien, 2010; M. G. Williams et al., 2007) and acceptance and commitment therapy (ACT) (Eifert & Forsyth, 2005; Hayes, Strosahl, & Wilson, 1999, 2011), approaches discussed in Chapter 8 of this book. These approaches can assist family members in recognizing the forces in their lives that they can control versus those that they cannot control. Family members are helped to make the choice to change their relationships to these dynamics.

Throughout this book, we have emphasized the importance of *highlighting strengths*. This is one of the most powerful treatment techniques. Many families have lost sight of their strengths after years of self-defeating patterns and cycles. It is our job to reconnect families to their inherent strengths in order to resuscitate their belief in their capacity to make changes and overcome adversity. Most families present first with their problems and the therapist may have to look beyond their initial angry words to locate their strengths. A wise clinician once commented:

> If you are a vacuum cleaner salesman going door to door, looking for crumbs, you will find crumbs on the cleanest of carpets. Similarly, if you are a clinician looking for strengths, you will find strengths, competencies, and hidden resources in the most problematic of families. (Wofsy & Mundy, 2011b)

Eliciting values is another significant treatment intervention (Hayes, Strosahl, & Wilson, 1999, 2011). People tend to do better and behave better toward one another when their actions are consistent with intrinsic values and meaning. The following response from a family therapist draws upon this premise:

> You all are clearly at odds with one another and have been struggling with these experiences for a long time. At the same time, you are here, which is indicative of the fact that some part of you wants to make changes. In thinking about that, it may be helpful for us to stop and think about what is important to you in terms of your role in this family. On your 80th birthday, if your family was going to talk about you and your character, what would you want them to say about you? And to what degree are you stepping toward these qualities in the here and now? (Wofsy & Mundy, 2011b)

Interventive enactments (S. Minuchin, 1974; Nichols, 2011) are techniques designed to shift and modify the experiential field within the family system. Earlier in this chapter, we have described the utility of enactments during the assessment phase, but these techniques are useful throughout the entire treatment process. Unlike the enactment described in the assessment phase, which encourages the family to show the therapist their normal interactional patterns, interventive enactments encourage family members to experiment with a new way of relating. Drawing on strengths and positive intent, the clinician encourages a here-and-now interaction between family members designed to influence more positive outcomes. The following example illustrates a therapist's use of this technique.

> "Dad, when you talk to your daughter, she seems to be hearing anger and disrespect and not the underlying caring and hurt beneath your statements. Can you turn to your daughter now and speak to her in a way that captures the love and concern that you obviously have for your daughter?"

Rolling with the resistance is a technique drawn from motivational interviewing (MI) (W. R. Miller & Rollnick, 2002; see also Chapter 6 in this book). Although this is often used primarily with individuals, we have found that it is also extremely useful in family and couples treatment. Families automatically look to preserve the familiar, and often come in requesting change, while simultaneously blocking the change effort. If a therapist fights against this drive for homeostasis (Nichols, 2011), this will only increase the resistance and potential sabotage. Recognizing and going with the resistant pockets allows for the family to feel heard and validated, while at the same time remaining in the process that may ultimately serve as a catalyst for change. The following excerpts from a session illustrate this process:

> THERAPIST: Mom, would you be willing to talk with your daughter in a way that she can hear it rather than tune you out and withdraw?
>
> MOM: No, she needs to make the change first; I am the parent.
>
> THERAPIST: Okay, so right now you're feeling like you are the adult in the family. You feel that you need to be respected, and she needs to change first.
>
> MOM: Yeah.
>
> THERAPIST: I hear you. And at the end of the day, the choice is up to each of you as to whether or not you are going to work differently with each other, but we know that in order for patterns to change, it requires more than one person.

The therapist in this case example also utilized a technique known as "stroke and kick" (Nichols, 2011). This is a technique in which you reinforce the person's good intentions, but challenge the behavior. The therapist's remarks below illustrate this process.

"You want to be valued as the parent in the family, and you deserve that. You are a hardworking, dedicated mother. At the same time, the way that you and your daughter are communicating is not working. Is there a way that you can experiment with communicating differently and still be respected in your family?"

Reframing (S. Minuchin, 1974; Nichols, 2011) is the process in which the clinician seeks to shift the perceptual and attitudinal understanding of the problem. It is often used to relabel a behavior or attitude in a more positive way. The following examples illustrate this process:

- *Example 1:* A son who is perpetually viewed as the family problem is cast in a new light in session when the clinician reframes his behaviors as resulting in the family coming together to overcome challenges in ways they have not had the opportunity to do in the past.
- *Example 2:* A mother and daughter who are intensively fighting and emotionally reacting off one another by firing insults can be reframed as two people who care deeply for each other enough to expend this high degree of emotional energy.

An *organizational theme* is a framework that is mutually constructed by the clinician and the family that anchors the process throughout the treatment (Sexton & Alexander, 2004). Once established, it acts as a guiding thread that connects the content of the session with the process of the treatment. For example, the clinician begins each session with a review of the processes and framework that have been previously established. He states:

"This is a family that is very close and emotionally charged and struggling to reconcile past conflicts with present emotional and developmental needs."

Once an organizational theme has been developed and established, reframes put forth, and motivation for change has been affirmed or increased, the family is ready to experiment with and practice relational skill development. This can further *foster improved problem solving, communication skills,* and conflict resolution capacities (Robin & Foster, 2002). Techniques imparted to the family can include active listening, "I statements," finding a middle ground, identifying and working with antecedents of a particular behavior or interaction, and regulating affect to match intent (Robin & Foster, 2002).

All good treatment and clinical interventions should carry over or *generalize* from the session room to the naturally occurring environments of clients. Therefore, there should be an emphasis placed on encouraging family members to root these strategies into the day-to-day interactions at home. This can be accomplished through the work of homework assignments, tapping into support networks, expansion of systems, and booster sessions post discharge (Robin & Foster, 2002).

Families of Adults with Chronic Mental Illness

A great deal of the family therapy literature has emphasized working with families in which a child or an adolescent is the identified patient. In our work with the families of chronically mentally ill adults, we have noted a number of other patterns. Many of these adults have become progressively disengaged from their families of origin, beginning in late adolescence and young adulthood. For some of these individuals, long separations from the family due to residential placements and repeated hospitalizations may have contributed to this process of disengagement. In other cases, a parent or grandparent may have been the primary caregiver or support for this person during his or her childhood and adolescence. As the parents or grandparents age and develop their own medical and other concerns, they often become increasingly "burnt out" and less involved with the client as he or she becomes a young adult. In some cases, other siblings and extended family members have become even more disengaged over time and have relied increasingly on the parent or grandparent to see to the client's care. In some cases, when this primary caregiver(s) dies, or becomes ill, the mentally ill adult is left feeling alone in the world. Some of these individuals become "serially homeless" as a result and live in a cycle of hospitalization, release, referral to a program, temporary housing, loss of housing, homelessness, and rehospitalization.

For those individuals who are both seriously mentally ill and also substance abusers, the process can be even more problematic, sometimes resulting in repeated incarcerations for the possession or dealing of drugs. In both cases, this may lead to alienation from family members who may have been victims of theft in order to support a drug habit.

We share the belief of the National Alliance on Mental Illness (NAMI, 2012) that asserts that people with serious mental illness can learn to manage their symptoms, reduce the impact of their illness, and live satisfying and independent lives, if given the appropriate treatment, medication, and services. Like NAMI, however, we agree that a central part of the treatment process must revolve around helping clients and their families to manage the ups and downs of the illness process.

The Narrative Family Therapy Model
and Externalizing the Blame

Narrative family therapy (M. White & Epston, 1990) with its postmodern emphasis on each person's story or narrative, is particularly helpful when working with these families. Often, families of the chronically mentally ill feel that they are in the position of being pressured by mental health professionals to care for their family members. They often feel blamed for the problems that their family member has developed. They do not fully understand the symptoms of serious mental illnesses such as bipolar disorder, major depression, psychosis, and schizophrenia. In many cases, they begin to blame the family member with mental illness for his or her behavior.

Narrative therapists avoid judgments about what is normal (Nichols, 2009) and view each family as generating a number of story lines that explain the behavior of different family members and their interactions as a family. As Nichols has stated in his summary of the narrative approach, "Stories don't just mirror life; they shape it" (p. 284). One can begin to see how the behavior of a family member with mental illness can contribute to what Michael White (1995) has called problem-saturated stories. Nichols, in his summary of the narrative therapy approach, summarizes the work of narrative therapists Freedman and Combs (1996) and White:

> Narrative theory is put into practice by therapists who (1) take a keen interest in their clients' stories; (2) search for times in their histories when they were strong or resourceful; (3) use questions to take a non-imposing, respectful approach to any new story put forth; (4) never label people but treat them as human beings with unique personal histories; and (5) help people separate from the dominant cultural narratives they have internalized so as to open space for alternative life stories (Freedman & Combs, 1996; M. White, 1995). (p. 287)

The process of *externalizing the blame*, an important concept of the narrative therapy approach (M. White & Epston, 1990), can be helpful in working with mentally ill individuals and their families. Nichols (2009), in his summary of Michael White's (1995) work, argues:

> To counter the ways society convinces people that they are their problems, narrative therapists **externalize** problems. Instead of having a problem or being a problem, clients are encouraged to think of themselves as *struggling against* their problems. Neither the patient nor the family is the problem; *the problem is the problem*. Accordingly, narrative therapists aren't interested in problem-maintaining interactions

or structural flaws. They aren't interested in the family's impact on the problem but rather in the problem's impact on the family. (p. 287)

Externalizing can be used to align the client and the family together to address a problem or the symptoms of an illness. It can be applied to mental illnesses such as bipolar disorder, major depression, schizophrenia, and so on. In other cases, it can be applied to attention-deficit/ hyperactivity disorder (ADHD) and learning disabilities or even serious medical illnesses. It reframes the situation. The client is not the problem; the family is not the problem. The problem is the mental illness or the ADHD and the client and the family can work together to learn to address it and minimize its effects.

Family Psychoeducational Approaches

The family therapy field has a long history of using psychoeducational approaches to help families to understand clients' conditions (McFarlane et al., 2003). These are important in the process of helping family members to avoid blaming the identified patient for his or her mental illness. In our experience, however, it is extremely important to first use the externalizing-the-blame process discussed above with families in order to avoid the inevitable alliance of families and mental health professionals that can perpetuate the definition of the client as the problem.

Families are often unaware of their own feelings and reactions in response to symptoms. They may feel blamed or judged by mental health professionals with whom they interact. They may not fully understand mental illness, substance abuse, ADHD, PTSD, and the associated behaviors. Combining externalizing techniques with psychoeducation gives a new meaning to the process as in the following case.

Martin (age 30) and his parents, Philip (age 51) and Martha (age 50), met with his outpatient therapist following his discharge from the inpatient unit of a psychiatric hospital. Martin, an African American male, had been diagnosed with bipolar disorder 5 years before and had been since hospitalized many times. His parents were confused and his father was also angry because he perceived Martin as "not trying to help himself."

The therapist realized that the family did not fully understand bipolar disorder and were feeling blamed by the doctors on the inpatient unit for the circumstances leading to Martin's latest hospitalization. She decided to use an externalizing-the-blame reframe in order to change the family's perception of Martin as "the problem." To do this, she began with a neurobiological explanation and told them that Martin was not at fault nor were his parents. She presented bipolar disorder in a box and told Martin and his parents that they would need to unite together to manage this illness. She emphasized the belief from NAMI (see above) that Martin could lead a more satisfying life and his parents could also, if they were able to accept and address the bipolar disorder.

Within this context, she was able to use a psychoeducational approach to discuss the diagnosis of bipolar disorder and to describe its symptomatology, behavioral sequelae, medication, and side effects. Most importantly, she spoke with them about working together as a team to learn how to relate adaptively to the symptoms.

Family members typically get caught up in the "drama" of mental illness and addiction rather than partnering with the consumer or client to manage symptoms for the well-being of everyone. The sessions described above allowed the therapist, with the client and family, to *relabel* "Martin is acting crazy" to "Martin is experiencing an intensification of his bipolar disorder." This *relabeling* process can also allow *reattributing* (J. Schwartz, 2011; J. M. Schwartz & Beyette, 1996) behavior as a byproduct of the mental illness rather than as the fault of the individual. This process can empower both clients and families. The therapist could also connect both Martin and his family members to resources and support groups such as those offered by NAMI (National Alliance on Mental Illness).

Involving Other Family Members

The therapist in Martin's case focused primarily on his parents as his "family." While her approach was good and helped to realign this family in their approach to the bipolar disorder, she overlooked the rest of his family. He had two adult siblings who were not involved in his treatment, the externalizing reframe, or the family's psychoeducation. In our experience, this can be problematic in the future if the parents become ill or disabled, or when they die. If the siblings are not included in some form in the treatment process, they may suddenly find themselves involved in his treatment after the loss of their parents. By this time, their life circumstances may have changed—they may have married and may have families of their own and may resent what they perceive as the burden of Martin. If they are involved in some form earlier and are exposed to the externalizing process and the family psychoeducation, they are less likely to blame Martin and see him as the problem, but instead, they can be reframed early as a part of his future team.

Empowerment: The End Result

Throughout this book, we have emphasized the importance of moving from a stance of helping clients and families, to one of empowering them to intervene and take charge of their lives. In this process, "knowledge is power." The reframe described above and the psychoeducation gave Martin and his family a greater knowledge of the bipolar disorder so that they could understand the behaviors that they experienced and witnessed. The mere fact that they could unite together to address the disorder was empowering because it shifted their understanding of the issue. The therapist, at a later point, worked with Martin and his family to support greater independence for him by helping him move first into a residence and then into a more independent apartment setting.

There is a distinct difference between empowerment and helping. Although helping often involves well-meaning mental health providers doing a great deal to help and provide services for their clients, empowerment has as its goal the involvement of clients and families in taking control over their own lives. Empowerment encourages individuals and families to act on their own behalf in order to gain greater control over their lives and futures (Staples, 1990).

Combining Treatment Modalities

Many therapists identify primarily as individual or family therapists and may see these two modalities as separate. As we indicated in the first chapter, this is often an artificial distinction in the real world of clinical practice. In fact, it is not unusual for a therapist who is seeing a client individually to decide to include the family in a number of sessions. For example, in our chapter on risk assessment and suicide prevention (Chapter 13), we describe a number of situations where a therapist was concerned that a client might be suicidal and decided to involve the family as a protective factor in the treatment process. Similarly, there are many times when a therapist may begin meeting with the entire family and decide that a mother needs to be seen individually as well as in family sessions, or that an adolescent would benefit from individual as well as family therapy. In some cases, one or two sessions may be helpful to engage a resistant family member. In other circumstances, the therapist may feel that the client has individual issues to address in addition to family concerns and that both types of interventions may be helpful. Creative therapists have also divided a session to include time for family and individual work, or scheduled individual and family sessions on alternate weeks in order to accommodate family members' schedules and the dictates of managed care companies. Thus in working with individuals and families, we encourage flexibility in the use of these modalities.

Conclusion

This chapter has presented a number of concepts that are central to family systems theory including joining, engagement versus involvement, acknowledging client and family strengths, analyzing and utilizing enactments and interactional patterns, and reframing. We have attempted to blend interventions from a number of different family therapy and other treatment approaches, including narrative family therapy, structural family therapy, motivational interviewing, mindfulness, and acceptance and commitment therapies in an effort to present the many ways in which family treatment can be structured. We have also provided examples of how to best work with and engage resistant or ambivalent family members on the periphery who are often integral to effective treatment. Finally, in working with the multiplicity of family structures and relational patterns, we encourage therapists to be flexible in their willingness to combine treatment modalities and to incorporate a variety of family therapy concepts and approaches into their work with children, adolescents, and adults.

CHAPTER 11

The Multisystems Model and Interdisciplinary Coordination of Care

Introduction

The multisystems model and interdisciplinary coordination of care are essential concepts because mental health care in the real world is often complicated and fragmented for clients and their families. Similarly, many clinicians struggle with the often overwhelming life challenges faced by their clients, particularly those who are poor. Many schools of psychotherapy focus exclusively on the individual. This is unfortunate because most individuals are embedded in multiple systems, including families and communities. For poor clients, there are also life realities such as poverty, racism, discrimination, homelessness, unemployment, substandard housing, failing schools, gangs, violence, dangerous neighborhoods, drug and alcohol abuse, a lack of good health care, and other significant stressors that have an impact on behavior and mental health. Clinicians who are not trained in the multisystems model often find that they do not have a framework to address these issues. The first two sections of this chapter explore the multisystems model and the challenges of coordination of interdisciplinary care within the mental health system. The third section describes a Family Empowerment Program, based on a conceptual framework of the multisystems model that addresses coordination of interdisciplinary care and the process of collaboration with clients from a strength-based perspective (E. N. Cleek et al., 2012).

Our students often ask us whether we identify primarily as individual or family therapists. In our conceptualization of therapy in the real world, this is a false dichotomy (Boyd-Franklin, 2003). As we demonstrate in the second part of this book, a therapist, to be effective, must be well trained in individual, family, group, and multisystems levels and modalities. With this in mind, this chapter presents both individual and family cases conceptualized through the multisystems model with an emphasis on the interdisciplinary coordination of care.

The Multisystems Model

As Boyd-Franklin (2003) has indicated, the multisystems model is a theoretical concept that can help therapists to understand and organize complex information about our clients and their families and to plan interventions at different system levels. Clearly, the therapist will not necessarily intervene at all levels, but it is important for each clinician to be aware of the ecosystemic context that impacts the lives of our clients and their families.

Conceptually, the multisystems model has been influenced by the work of Bronfenbrenner (1977), Aponte (1994a), Falicov (1988), Boyd-Franklin (1989, 2003), Henggeler and Borduin (1990), Henggeler, Schoenwald, Borduin, Rowland, and Cunningham (1998, 2009). Our current framework for this model incorporates nine levels (see Figure 11.1):

- Level I.   Individual
- Level II.   Subsystems
- Level III.   Family household
- Level IV.   Extended family
- Level V.   Nonblood kin and friends
- Level VI.   Churches, schools, and community resources
- Level VII.   Social service agencies and outside systems
               (Boyd-Franklin, 2003, p. 241)
- Level VIII. Work[1]
- Level IX.   External societal forces (e.g., poverty, racism,
               discrimination, sexism)[1]

It is important for therapists to look beyond the client or family in the room and understand the other individuals and systems that might impact their lives. It is not necessary to intervene at each of these levels,

---

[1]These levels represent an expansion of the model.

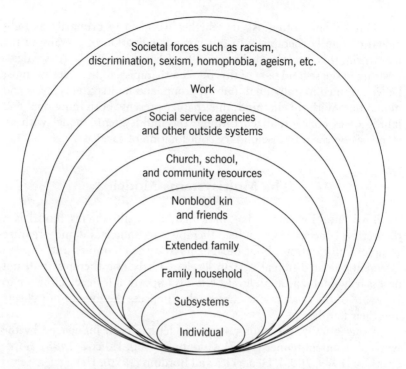

FIGURE 11.1. The multisytems model. Adapted from Boyd-Franklin (2003, p. 242). Copyright 2003 by The Guilford Press. Adapted by permission.

but recognition of these realities can be helpful in understanding the context in which our clients live. Within this framework, for example, a therapist might be working with an individual with serious mental illness and might choose to bring in a spouse or family in times of crisis.

The Multisystems Model in Working with Poor Clients and Families

Another challenge faced by mental health providers is the fragmentation of services that often occurs in the mental health and social service fields. Unlike middle- and upper-class clients and families that may have health insurance and can pay for medical and mental health as well as legal, financial, and other services, poor clients often find themselves at the mercy of multiple systems that may have a tremendous amount of power in their lives. E. N. Cleek et al. (2012) have described the following reality for clients and families that receive treatment at public mental health centers in inner-city communities:

These clients often struggle with multiple psychosocial forces that interfere with their use of inherent capacities and access to effective treatment—all of which challenges providers to go outside the bounds of traditional service delivery. Psychosocial forces often include homelessness, poverty, domestic violence, child abuse, foster care, substance abuse, racism, and other forms of discrimination, which may create a sense of hopelessness. Such families repeatedly interact with multiple outside systems, such as child welfare agencies, foster care agencies, family court, public assistance programs, law enforcement, schools, and shelters. These systems may have contradictory agendas and often fail to coordinate their priorities and services. This impedes each system's effectiveness and creates a sense of confusion, fragmentation, and futility in the family (Micucci, 1998). Insofar as these systems and services focus on individual people and problems, they fail to activate the inherent strengths, competencies, and healing capacities of the family and the community (P. Minuchin, Colapinto, & S. Minuchin, 2006). (p. 208)

Concrete Problems as a Legitimate Part of Therapy

Many schools of therapy focus primarily on internal emotional or psychological problems and symptoms and may ignore the overwhelming life realities presented in treatment, particularly by poor clients. Boyd-Franklin (2003) has indicated that survival issues, such as the lack of money and unemployment, homelessness or poor housing, lack of food, and fears for their safety, are often ever-present concerns for poor clients and families. Beginning therapists may actually ignore these types of survival issues and look instead at feelings, emotions, and psychological concerns. In some of these cases, by not tuning into the concrete issues that are the most pressing priorities for their clients, these clinicians may miss important opportunities to join, establish therapeutic rapport, and build trust. The case below illustrates this process.

Maria, a 40-year-old Latina, was referred for treatment by the social worker in the homeless shelter in which she was living. She presented in treatment as extremely sad and depressed. She also reported constant headaches that a doctor had labeled as stress related. Maria's main concern was that she had been homeless for the last 6 months and that her children had been "taken away" by child protective services because she could not provide for them.

Mary, a psychology intern, was assigned to see Maria in therapy. Recognizing the symptoms of depression, Mary began treatment by doing an assessment of Maria's depression. As the session proceeded, Maria became increasingly agitated. She tried a number of times to communicate to her therapist that it was the fact that she was homeless and that her children had been removed that was contributing to her depressed and sad feelings.

The therapist ignored many opportunities to follow-up on these concerns and to empathize with Maria's sadness about these realities. As a result, Maria left that session feeling that therapy was not helpful to her and she informed her social worker at the homeless shelter that she would not be returning.

This case illustrates the importance of these concrete, real-world issues in a client's life and the disconnect that can occur between the therapist and client if these important issues are ignored.

Utilization of an Eco Map as a Tool in the Multisystems Model

The psychology intern described above was doing her best and following the assessment and treatment strategy that she had learned in her training program. Unfortunately, she had not been exposed to the realities of poverty and the lives of poor clients or to the multisystems model as a conceptual approach. As indicated above, the realities of concrete problems and the intrusion of multisystemic agencies are a part of the lives of many poor, multistressed clients (E. N. Cleek et al., 2012). The multisystems model incorporates the development of an *Eco Map,* a tool that can be extremely useful with clients and families that are struggling with many problems and concerns (Boyd-Franklin, 1989, 2003; A. Hartman & Laird, 1983).

The case below describes a client who was facing many of the same concerns as Maria. In this case, however, the therapist had been trained in the multisystems model and the coordination of interdisciplinary care and was able to explore the many stressors and outside agencies involved in the client's life. This approach played an extremely important part in the building of trust between the therapist and client and in establishing the therapeutic relationship.

Shakeera, a 35-year-old African American woman, was referred for treatment by her child protective services worker. Her three children, Amir (age 8), Mike (age 6), and Ronda (age 3) had been removed last year after she left them alone in the house in order to go shopping at a supermarket. She was gone for a number of hours and a neighbor called child protective services after hearing fighting among the children and crying in the apartment. Shakeera was charged with child neglect and the children were placed in three different foster homes.

Shakeera had become depressed and was referred to a local outpatient mental health clinic by her child welfare worker, who was concerned about her. Prior to the removal of the children, Shakeera had received TANF (Temporary Assistance for Needy Families) funds for her children and food stamps. After their removal, she was informed that she would be required to attend a job training program. In addition, child protective services had mandated that she attend parenting training classes. She was so depressed that she felt unable to meet all of these demands and was feeling completely overwhelmed.

In addition, she was worried about Amir, her oldest son, who had sickle-cell anemia. He was being seen at a local hospital and, although he was now in foster care, she had kept in touch with his doctor. Due to the stress of the last year, Amir had a number of hospitalizations and had been experiencing a great deal of pain.

At the outpatient clinic, Shakeera was referred to Margaret, a White therapist, who had worked at the clinic for 3 years. In the first session, Margaret took the time to join with Shakeera and to understand the challenges that she was facing. She was depressed during the session and reported that she had not been sleeping well at night. She would wake up and begin worrying about her children and was not able to return to sleep. Often she would cry for hours and blamed herself for the removal of her children. Margaret listened carefully and reflected the worry that Shakeera was experiencing as well as her obvious love and concern for her children.

Sensing Margaret's empathy, Shakeera shared the circumstances of the removal of her children. She was angry at herself for leaving the children home alone, but she explained that the children all had colds, there was no food in the house and she didn't know what else to do. There was no supermarket in her neighborhood, so she had to take a bus some distance in order to get the food that they needed. By the end of the first session, Shakeera was feeling more comfortable with Margaret and indicated that she would be willing to return to talk about these issues.

In the fourth month of treatment, Shakeera came into a session anxious and agitated. She reported that she was scheduled to go to court at the end of the month and that she feared that the judge would not return her children to her. She cried and explained that she was so down that she had struggled to attend job training and was inconsistently attending the parenting program. She felt that everyone was making demands of her that she could not possibly satisfy. The therapist began to explore the many challenges that Shakeera faced and the various agencies that were making demands. With her therapist's help, Shakeera constructed an Eco Map (see Figure 11.2) that included all of the agencies and systems that were making demands.

The Eco Map placed Shakeera in the center and drew a line to each of her children. She had only one family member, an elderly aunt who lived in a nursing home whom she rarely saw. The therapist drew a line and a circle to indicate lack of family support. She passed the pen to Shakeera and asked her to help her draw in the various agencies that were pressuring her for

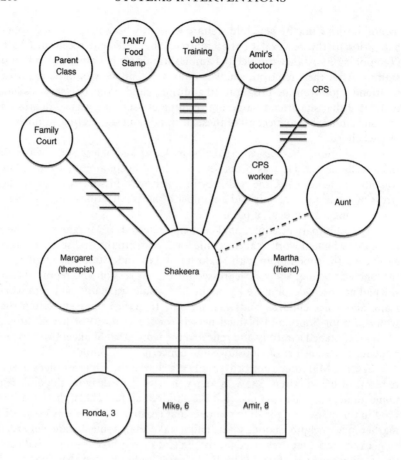

FIGURE 11.2. Eco Map.

changes. Shakeera drew a line to a circle for child protective services, one for the court, another for the parenting training program, one for welfare services, one for job training, and one for the doctor and hospital where her son Amir received his treatment for sickle-cell anemia.

When the therapist asked Shakeera to draw circles for the persons whom she felt were supportive of her, she paused for a long time. Finally, she drew a circle for Margaret, her therapist, and although she experienced child protective services as punitive, she was grateful for the support of her child welfare worker, who had referred her for treatment. She also drew a circle for her one friend, Martha, who had been helpful with child care and general support until she moved away. Shakeera had not been in touch with her in the last year.

Her therapist discussed with her all of these pressures as well as her fear that her children would not be returned to her. Over the next few sessions, the therapist explored Shakeera's dreams for the future and her values in terms of her children and her mothering. She had a tremendous desire to reunite her family and to be a good mother. The therapist validated all of her efforts.

Gradually, the therapist began to explore with Shakeera what she would say to each of these multisystemic agencies if she had the chance. The therapist encouraged Shakeera to write these ideas down and to keep them in a small notebook. She also encouraged her to consider having a multisystems case conference with all of the key agencies in order to address her concerns.

The Multisystemic Case Conference

Shakeera and Margaret collaborated closely and Shakeera contacted each of the agencies that were placing demands on her and requested their attendance at a case conference to be held in the conference room at the outpatient clinic. Prior to the meeting, Shakeera and her therapist had collaborated to prioritize her concerns. The therapist used role playing to empower Shakeera to present these issues herself in the meeting. At first, Shakeera was anxious about speaking in the meeting but the role playing helped to empower her to "speak her mind." On the day of the case conference, the worker from child protective services attended, as well as the social worker from the parenting program, a staff member from the job training program, and a nurse practitioner from the hospital who worked closely with Amir's doctor.

In the case conference, Shakeera was able to prioritize her concerns. She made it clear that she was a good mother and desperately wanted to regain custody of her children. She acknowledged that she had not used good judgment in leaving them alone in the house but that she was desperate and had no one to leave them with.

She stated that she had been depressed earlier in the year but that her therapy was helping and that she had been able to focus more on her parenting class and her job training program, which she was scheduled to complete in 2 months. Shakeera also explained that she was worried about her son Amir, who had sickle-cell anemia and who had been hospitalized due to the stress of this year's separation. The nurse practitioner reported that she and Amir's doctor had been impressed with Shakeera's dedication to her son and her willingness to be involved in his treatment even though he was still in foster care.

The representatives from the job training program and the parenting program both reported that they had seen a clear change in Shakeera in the last few months. She had seemed less depressed, more hopeful, and more focused on completing these programs and working toward the return of her children. With her therapist's support, Shakeera was able to present a timeline for the completion of her programs and her goals regarding the return of her children.

Her worker from child protective services stated that she hoped to put preventive services in the home in order to support Shakeera when the children were returned. She also discussed some respite services that would be available to Shakeera, for example, a babysitter if she needed to leave the children unattended for any reason. She validated Shakeera's efforts and suggested that all of those present at the meeting write notes to the judge documenting Shakeera's attendance at programs and her determination to reunite with her children. Margaret, the therapist, also suggested that Shakeera prepare her own letter in collaboration with her therapist that would document her proposed timeline and the efforts that she had made.

Shakeera's final request was that she be allowed to have "supervised visitations" each week with all of her children together at the therapist's office so that they could stay connected as a family and begin the process of reconnecting before their reunification. The child protective service worker agreed to arrange transportation for all of the children.

The court session was postponed. All of the different service providers prepared letters to the judge. Shakeera and her therapist worked together on her letter and she felt very positive and hopeful about her timeline. When the court date occurred, the therapist accompanied Shakeera to court. The judge extended the timeline, but agreed to begin the process of reunification for Shakeera and her children. He approved the ongoing family therapy sessions with the children. Although it took 6 months longer than she had originally hoped, her children were successfully returned to her. She continued to see her therapist individually and in family sessions with her children during the first year of their reunification as a family. Once all of the children were placed in daycare, schools, and after-school programs, Shakeera began to look for job possibilities.

This case illustrates the value of a multisystems model and of bringing together the key systems involved to address the challenges in a client's life. Shakeera's therapist recognized the multisystemic challenges that she was facing and the sense of being overwhelmed that was contributing to her depression. By addressing the real-world survival challenges that Shakeera was facing, her therapist was able to establish a therapeutic relationship that empowered her to advocate for herself and her children.

Through the multisystems case conference, a process of interdisciplinary coordination of care occurred and Shakeera was able to see these various programs and agencies as aligned with her and collaborating with her in her goal of reunification with her children.

Coordination of Care
and Interdisciplinary Involvement

The fragmentation discussed above can often lead to a duplication or overlap of services provided to a client or family. In addition, many poor clients are not self-referred to any of the agencies assigned to provide care. Past negative experiences with other health, mental health, or social services can lead some poor clients to enter treatment with a healthy suspicion of the process (Boyd-Franklin, 2003). In addition, different agencies may have different philosophies and goals for the client. This can lead to confusion and mixed messages. With this in mind, it is important for therapists to be aware of the different agencies that are working with the client or family and the ways in which these may be contributing to the solution or exacerbating the problems.

Different disciplines may have different perspectives on care. This may be true in the mental health system and even in the same agency, hospital, or clinic. For example, a psychiatrist, who may be providing medication, may not be aware of recent psychological testing that has shed light on diagnostic implications, and the psychologist, who is providing individual treatment to the mother, may not be in touch with the social worker who is providing family treatment. This type of lack of communication is quite common even within the same clinic or agency and can be much more serious when it occurs among agencies, clinics, or hospitals. It can become even more complicated when other disciplines are involved, such as the police, lawyers, judges, child protective services, foster care, schools, and entitlement programs, such as welfare and housing.

With these realities in mind, therapists must recognize the importance of multiple perspectives and the merit of drawing upon these diverse points of view. Clinicians are often trained to conduct therapy in a vacuum, largely ignoring these other perspectives and the external realities of their clients' lives. The case examples presented below illustrate the importance of integrating different philosophies and eliminating divergent agendas. Staying focused on the goals or values of the client or family and remaining client centered can help to provide clear treatment plans.

Coordination of care through bringing together different members of a treatment team can help to eliminate these competing agendas. This is even more important when practitioners are spread out throughout different clinics or agencies. As indicated in the case above, multisystemic case conferences can in fact be an antidote to competing agendas that lead to fragmentation of care. As our case below illustrates, however, it is important that these multisystemic decisions be made with the participation of, and collaboration with, our clients and families.

The case below demonstrates the value of incorporating the multisystems model, identifying the concerns and personal, as well as cultural strengths, and working to coordinate care in close collaboration with the client.

Angela, a 45-year-old African American woman, had a long history of serious mental illness. She had been diagnosed with major depression and had experienced many hospitalizations due to suicidal ideation. Three months prior, she had been evicted from her apartment in Brooklyn, New York. She had lived on the streets for a month before becoming profoundly depressed and suicidal. The police picked her up and she was taken to a psychiatric hospital in Manhattan in New York City. During this hospitalization, she was assigned to Jerome, an African American social worker, for treatment and for case management.

In his sessions with Angela, Jerome had been careful to establish therapeutic rapport with her before bombarding her with many intrusive questions. He learned that Angela had been the only child of her mother, who had been a single parent. They had lived an isolated life due to her mother's drug abuse and subsequent cutoff from the mother's family. When her mother died 6 months earlier, Angela was left all alone. Jerome and Angela spent a number of sessions helping her to explore her relationship with her mother and to mourn her loss. Although she had been suicidal at the beginning of her hospitalization, Angela began to feel less so.

Gradually, as the therapeutic relationship developed, Angela shared with her therapist that the happiest time in her life had been when she had attended a small storefront Pentecostal church in Brooklyn, where the pastor and the congregation had been supportive. She reported that she had not been back in over 3 months and that she had begun to isolate and drift away after her mother's death.

As her therapist began to learn more about her involvement in this church, he began to see this as a personal and cultural strength, which had helped her to cope in the past. During the process of discussing her involvement in the church, Angela's affect often changed and she became more positive. With this in mind, Jerome explored with Angela whether she would be interested in reconnecting with this church after her discharge from the hospital. Angela was excited about this idea, but expressed doubts that they would even remember her. Jerome encouraged her to call the pastor but she was afraid to do so. He explored options with her and discovered that she would be willing to talk with the pastor but was afraid to make the initial call. Jerome obtained a written release form from Angela and arranged to call the pastor during one of their sessions together. She agreed to talk with the pastor once Jerome had reached him and explained her situation. They made the call together. Jerome spoke to the pastor who clearly remembered Angela and who agreed to speak with her. He told Angela that he and the members of the congregation would welcome her return. He also encouraged her to contact one of the deaconesses and a member of the missionary society who she had been close to. Angela followed up and spoke with each of these women. They also visited her at the hospital.

In a session, Jerome discussed with Angela the possibility of discharge to a residential program for adults with mental health issues located in the same area of Brooklyn as the church. She was pleased. As a part of discharge planning, a session was scheduled with the intake worker from the residence. Jerome asked Angela if she would like to invite any members of her church family to attend that meeting. She reached out to her two friends and both agreed to attend.

During the meeting, the intake worker described the program at the residence. Angela asked if she would be able to have visitors from her church family and if she would be able to attend church. The intake worker indicated that she would be encouraged to have visitors and that, after the first month, she would be allowed to leave to attend church services if someone was willing to pick her up and return her to the residence. Both members of her church family indicated that they would be willing to pick her up for church as soon as she was permitted to attend.

After 1 month, by the time of her discharge from the hospital, Angela's therapist had developed a therapeutic relationship and had helped to connect her to systems in her community that would support her recovery after her release from the hospital.

This case is an excellent example of the application of the multisystems model. The therapist used a culturally sensitive, strength-based approach and took the time to develop a therapeutic relationship before taking an extensive history. He learned a great deal about Angela and her strengths. Although she had no close family members and was mourning the loss of her mother, he discovered that she had been involved in a small storefront Pentecostal church and that she felt connected to the pastor and the congregation. Her therapist recognized this as a cultural strength and pursued it.

In the course of these discussions, it became clear that the church was a major support system in Angela's life and that she had become disconnected and isolated during her intense depression after her mother's death. Although Angela was initially reluctant to call her pastor, her therapist encouraged her to call with him. This was important because he did not take over the process for her but empowered her to make that connection again through his facilitation and encouragement. The therapist also recognized that in Angela's African American culture, her church members were her "family" (Boyd-Franklin, 2003), and he encouraged her to include them in a family session for discharge planning.

Also, consistent with the multisystems model, the therapist searched for a residence for clients with serious mental illness in Brooklyn that would address the issue of her homelessness, would provide her with therapeutic support after discharge, and would be near her "church home" (Boyd-Franklin, 2003). All of these interventions were done in close collaboration with Angela and the discharge planning session was also a good example of interdisciplinary coordination of care. Too often, clients like Angela "fall between the cracks" in the mental health system if there is not careful coordination of care between outpatient services, as well as family and community multisystemic support systems.

Collaboration with Our Clients

Angela's case above is also an excellent example of the process of collaboration with our clients. As we have indicated throughout this book, our role as clinicians is to empower our clients. This is best accomplished through collaboration with them. In order to collaborate, clinicians must be able to recognize the strengths in their clients, including cultural strengths, and to work closely with them to explore options that are consistent with their belief systems and values. Despite the discharge pressures inherent in inpatient treatment units, Angela's therapist took the time to develop a collaborative therapeutic relationship with her by joining slowly and exploring the things and values that were most important to her. It was in this context that he learned about her church and recognized the potential of this "church family" to be a multisystemic community-based support for her upon her discharge.

He collaborated with her to explore ways in which this might occur and to empower her to reconnect with that network. Madsen (2007) discusses the importance of this collaborative stance as a major part of successful therapy. Too often therapy has focused on problems. Madsen encourages an emphasis on "the usefulness of organizing therapeutic efforts around an investigation of possibilities in life and beginning our efforts by helping clients envision preferred directions in life" (Madsen, 2007, p. 126). By incorporating this strategy as a part of the multisystems model, Angela's therapist collaborated with her to uncover and explore a positive system (i.e., her church family) and to restore her involvement with these church members.

The last section of this chapter presents the Family Empowerment Program, a multisystemic, interdisciplinary approach to working with multistressed urban families.

The Family Empowerment Program:
A Multisystemic Interdisciplinary Approach to Working with Multistressed Urban Families

The Family Empowerment Program (FEP) is a multisystemic family therapy program that partners multistressed families with an interdisciplinary resource team while remaining attached to a "traditional" mental health clinic.[2] The rationale for this model is that far too often, families presenting at community mental health centers struggle with multiple psychosocial forces (e.g., problems with housing, domestic violence, child care, entitlements, racism, substance abuse, and foster care, as well as chronic medical and psychiatric illnesses) that exacerbate symptoms and impact traditional service delivery and access to effective treatment. Thus, families often experience fragmented care and are involved with multiple systems with contradictory and competing agendas. As a result, services frequently fail to harness the family's inherent strengths. The Family Empowerment Program (FEP) partners the family with a unified team that includes representatives from Entitlements Services, Family Support and Parent Advocacy, and clinical staff from the agency's outpatient mental health clinic practicing from a strength-based family therapy perspective. The goal of the FEP is to support the family in achieving its goals. This is accomplished through co-construction of a service plan that addresses the family's needs in an efficient and coherent manner—emphasizing family strengths and competencies and supporting family self-sufficiency.

Local and National Context

Initiatives in national and local mental health policy have moved the agenda forward for an integrated systems-of-care approach. In July 2003, the President's New Freedom Commission on Mental Health set a new standard for the delivery of evidence-based and best practices in the public mental health service arena. Enumerated in the commission's report (2003) were a series of *Goals for a Transformed Mental Health System*. Among these were the elimination of disparities in access to excellent mental health care, and the establishment of care that was consumer and family driven. Consistent with this report is a trend emerging at the

---

[2]The remaining sections of this chapter were originally published as Cleek, E. N., Wofsy, M., Boyd-Franklin, N., Mundy, B., & Howell, T. (2012). The Family Empowerment Program: An interdisciplinary approach to working with multistressed urban families. *Family Process, 51*(2), 207–217. The text has been edited in part and reprinted with the permission of *Family Process* and Wiley-Blackwell.

state level, wherein state funding across the country has become increasingly contingent upon a system's capacity to deliver evidence-based and best-practice programming with documented outcomes (e.g., Carpinello et al., 2002; New York State Office of Mental Health, 2001; Oregon Senate Bill 267, 2005). The accountable care model (U.S. Department of Health and Human Services, 2011), which highlights integrative partnerships among medical and behavioral health providers, and which will transform payment mechanisms (Jarvis & Alexander, 2011), is emerging in health care policy and highlights another application of coordinated care interventions.

Consistent with the trends noted above, the Institute for Community Living (ICL) designed and implemented FEP. ICL, a New York City-based not-for-profit, meets the specialized needs of over 9,000 adults, children, and families annually through a broad array of programs and services including supportive housing, outpatient mental health clinics, community support and outreach services, and health care services. The FEP is located in East New York, Brooklyn, in a building that houses many ICL resources, including an outpatient mental health clinic, an entitlements counselor, and the Brooklyn Family Resource Center. It engages representatives from each of these programs to better support families in responding to the myriad psychosocial forces that the individuals living in this inner-city neighborhood often experience. The FEP was developed in accordance with Kazdin's (1997) recommendation that blueprints for effective treatments meet the needs of the population served, follow strong theoretical underpinnings, and incorporate best practices within a flexible service structure, enabling the FEP to deliver theoretically sound interventions in a manner that is sensitive to the cultural context of families served (Waldegrave, 2005).

A Proactive Response to Fragmentation of Care

The FEP comprises an interdisciplinary team that partners with multistressed urban families to address the needs most essential to the family being served. The team consists of the family along with staff from collaborative programs, including parent advocates, family therapists, an entitlements specialist, and agency administrators. Additionally, other involved parties such as specialist consultants, outside providers, and family-identified support personnel regularly attend meetings in support of family goals (see Figure 11.3).

The FEP model is driven by a threefold focus on engaging the entire family in treatment, implementing strength-based family therapy interventions, and linking with a multidisciplinary resource team that assists the family in transferring the principles, insights, and skills developed

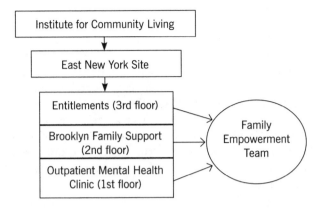

FIGURE 11.3. Composition of the Family Empowerment Program team in East New York, Brooklyn.

in the family session to their experiences within the naturally occurring community environment (Boyd-Franklin & Bry, 2000a; Imber-Black, 1988). As a result, rather than being pulled in many directions, families experience the maximal benefit of the array of services offered.

Through the multiple perspectives represented on the team, the family is better able to address a broad range of mental health and concrete concerns. By balancing family needs and strengths with systemic priorities, the team is better able to prioritize family concerns and thus stabilize family functioning while coordinating services. Three elements lie at the core of this model's success:

- Involvement of parent advocates.
- Response to the concrete service needs of the family through entitlements, counseling, and advocacy.
- Family therapy informed by the evidence-based brief strategic family therapy model (Szapocsnik, Hervis, & Schwartz, 2003).

Central to all of the FEP's interventions is the involvement of the parent advocates from ICL's Brooklyn Family Resource Center. The advocates are parents who have sought mental health services for their children and their families, and serve as flexible resources to families of children with emotional and behavioral challenges (Burns, Hoagwood, & Mrazek, 1999). Advocates offer support and education that stems from their own experience navigating the system on behalf of their own children. Through the Brooklyn Family Resource Center, they provide a wide array of local wisdom and assistance, such as attending school and court meetings along with the family, offering program-funded respite monies in times of crisis, and/or providing after-school parent and child mentoring programs. The local wisdom and lived experience of parent advocates has enhanced the larger service system and provides a new dimension of support to families. Though research is limited, early outcomes suggest that family advocate involvement increases the likelihood that families engage in treatment (McKay et al., 2010). Ireys, Devet, and Sakwa (2002), in their discussion of family support programs, highlight the concept of "weak ties"—"small social groups or networks . . . [which] can themselves be linked by an acquaintance relationship to different social groups" (p. 155):

> The concept of weak ties is integral to understanding the role of experienced peer or support partner. Parents of children with severe emotional or behavioral disorders report many unmet needs when working with traditional service providers. In some instances, a support partner may function as a weak tie by developing only an acquaintance relationship; yet within this relationship, the partner may link a parent to community resources, people, or institutions and thus serve as a relationship or social network bridge-builder. (p. 155)

In keeping with this concept, and in addition to the individual linkage and support work noted above, the Brooklyn Family Resource Center advocates offer an array of workshops and support groups designed to promote an understanding of children's mental health issues, as well as to create a natural support network among parents. Examples of these services include single-parent support groups, workshops on mental health-related topics, and prosocial gatherings such as trips to amusement parks and a monthly family night where dinner and activities are provided. All families involved in the FEP can avail themselves of these offerings. In addition, it provides youth advocacy and mentoring activities that help keep children involved with meaningful activities, and enables them to become part of a larger prosocial peer community. Families attached to the Family Resource Center participate in a community where social support, trust, and connectedness are realized.

An entitlements specialist complements these services by offering expertise in the realms of finance, health care benefits, and housing. For instance, the entitlements specialist can support families by providing information on tenants' rights, supplying the family with an application for needed benefits, and assisting the family with negotiating the complex bureaucratic system that often encumbers access. In agencies where this position does not exist, programs can draw on the expertise of experienced social workers who have worked with accessing entitlements, and/or can cultivate expertise by giving staff the time to attend one of the many free community-based and government trainings that exist around this issue.

The third component of the FEP is family therapy informed by the evidence-based brief strategic family therapy (BSFT) model (Szapocznik et al., 2003). ICL's family therapists were trained in BSFT when the FEP was developed, and BSFT has informed the perspective by which the therapists and families work. Through BSFT, therapists begin treatment by eliciting each family member's point of view on presenting problems, drawing out family strengths, and reframing the presenting problem as one that is rooted in family functioning (Szapocznik et al., 2003). This process is designed to identify symptomatic cycles and to help the family achieve more adaptable patterns of relating by addressing issues with communication, problem solving, and conflict resolution (Szapocznik et al., 2003).

The three core components of the FEP team (family advocacy, entitlements counseling, and family therapy) are implemented and coordinated in collaboration with the family to enhance internal family functioning and resiliency, and to create a more adaptive fit between the family and its naturally occurring environment. At any given time, the FEP team actively works with a caseload of approximately 10 families. Over the last 4 years, 36 families that enrolled in the ICL mental health clinic have enrolled in the FEP, and reflect the diversity of the community.[3]

Families that present as multistressed and multisystem involved during the mental health clinic intake are informed of the FEP and its array of services. Should the family decide to participate in the FEP, they are matched with an advocate from the Brooklyn Family Resource Center, and an FEP team therapist is assigned. The therapist and the advocate meet with the family in order to further orient them to the FEP process, after which a first FEP meeting is scheduled.

The FEP is predicated on the idea that effective treatment must reflect the translation of research to practice. For instance, the FEP's central activities are consistent with the principles of recovery, which include notions of first- and second-order change (Onken, Craig, Ridgway, Ralph, & Cook, 2007). By stabilizing environmental factors and concrete service needs (second-order change), the FEP's integrated approach creates the conditions necessary for successful delivery of evidence-informed treatment targeted to facilitate transformation within the family system (first-order change). The combined effect of the clinical interventions, advocacy work, and concrete specialist services create a synergistic effect that also reflects a multisystemic care coordination framework (Madsen,

---

[3] Of families served by the FEP, 47% have been Latino, 36% African American, 8% Caribbean or of Caribbean American descent, and 5% Caucasian.

1999). The model is influenced by system-of-care (Stroul & Friedman, 1986) theory, which emphasizes that the child and family are central to the initiation and direction of the service process, that service delivery and coordination are localized and community based, and that the development and delivery of services are culturally relevant (Pires, 2002; Stroul & Friedman, 1986).

In order to identify and facilitate the integration of cultural context into the clinical work, clinicians are trained, from the time they are hired, to be sensitive to clients' age, gender, and cultural issues. The process of cultural sensitivity begins during the psychosocial assessment conducted at intake, when all clients are asked to complete a person-centered survey specifically developed to identify cultural needs and background, and individually identified strengths, needs, interests, and goals. Cultural context must be integrated into clinical work, particularly in therapy for individuals and families from racially and ethnically diverse, low-socioeconomic backgrounds (Waldegrave, 2005). Boyd-Franklin (2003) also highlights this need along with the challenges that poor African American families often face in relation to multisystems involvement.

In addition to the integration of cultural context in therapy, parent advocates from the Brooklyn Family Resource Center who are from the same cultural, racial, linguistic, and socioeconomic backgrounds as families participating in the FEP often serve as "cultural bridges," and their involvement fosters a more seamless inclusion of cultural context in the service delivery system. At all times, hope, resiliency, and an emphasis on self-sufficiency within and among family members are the overarching frameworks that guide the FEP.

The manner in which the component parts of the FEP work together in assisting families with stabilizing external systems and internal functioning is illustrated in the following case example.[4]

The Smiths, an African American family, entered the shelter system following their move to New York City. Due to a history of substance abuse, Mr. and Mrs. Smith were referred for specialized counseling. Upon hearing their account of current use, the clinician reported the family to the city's

---

[4]Identifying characteristics have been changed to ensure confidentiality. The FEP team also has preliminary data reflecting symptom improvement from standardized outcome measures such as the Strengths and Difficulties Questionnaire (Goodman, 1999) for children and the Outcomes Questionnaire (Lambert et al., 2003; Wells, Burlingame, Lambert, Hoag, & Hope, 1996) for adults that is consistent with this anecdotal evidence. These data continue to be collected and analyzed and will be reported in a future paper.

child welfare agency. The child welfare case was opened and soon after, the Smiths' 8-year-old daughter, Pam, became violent in the community and was hospitalized. Pam remained on the psychiatric unit for 6 weeks and was classified by hospital staff as "severely emotionally disturbed." At discharge, the hospital referred her for case management and outpatient mental health services. Child welfare also referred the family to a preventive service agency. In addition, child welfare arranged for the Smiths to receive family services and early intervention for their toddlers. Thus, all of the adults and children in the family were involved with different agencies and receiving treatment at different programs. Despite the influx of services, the Smiths faced another challenge in that the family was at risk for losing their Section 8 Housing and Public Assistance.

The FEP was a good fit for this family as it addresses the diverse needs of children and families by enhancing and coordinating the multiple services in which families are involved, and relying on a family centered and strength-based approach. For the Smiths, who were engaged with multiple providers and systems, the FEP could help structure all the various "helpers," and work to ensure that the Smiths were guiding the single agenda.

At the time of intake into the clinic, the Smiths were working with service providers spread across three different boroughs of New York City. In one day, the family could be expected to attend a public assistance meeting at 10:00 A.M. in one borough, a home visit scheduled at 1:00 P.M. in a second, and a medical appointment in a third. These expectations inadvertently set this family up for failure, as it was impossible to satisfy all of them. A second complication was that three different therapists, with diverse goals, were working with members of this family. Although the three children were seen by the same therapist for family therapy, Mrs. Smith was referred for individual therapy at a second agency, and the whole family was mandated to attend family therapy sessions at a third agency. All of this, combined with daily involvement with a parent advocate, resulted in extreme role confusion, fragmentation, and inefficiency for family members and providers alike.

Due to their multisystems involvement, the therapist informed Mr. and Mrs. Smith about the FEP team. The family decided to participate. At the first meeting that the family attended, and in response to the family's chief concern that services were too fragmented and that they felt they were being set up for failure, a collaborative decision was first made to transfer the children's and mother's cases to a single family centered clinician at one agency. Second, Mr. and Mrs. Smith were linked to a parent advocate who was of the same racial and socioeconomic background. This was done at the request of the family and in order to help mitigate the healthy suspicion that the Smith family expressed during the intake at the clinic. Third, a linkage was established between the family and the FEP's entitlements specialist, who supported them in negotiating the Section 8 and Public Assistance processes. Last, the family decided whom they wanted to participate in future meetings. The monthly FEP meeting acted as a consistent venue for the family to effectively communicate with and pull together self-identified resources.

These initial meetings became a platform for Mr. and Mrs. Smith to increasingly take ownership of the helping process. For example, though Mr. and Mrs. Smith were actively encouraged from the beginning to participate, it was not until the second and third meetings that Mr. and Mrs. Smith increasingly contributed agenda items and verbalized concerns. When Mr. Smith was not able to attend a meeting, he initiated calling in from work. The collaborative work of the family and providers mobilized the strengths, wisdom, and resiliency inherent in the family. The family gained the strength and support they needed to positively impact change in their lives.

Multisystemic Collaboration

First and foremost the Smiths are a family—one in which each member was in distress. An immediate concern was to alleviate this distress through the provision of concrete services. The tension experienced by the family over competing, albeit necessary, appointments was addressed through monthly team meetings at which Mrs. Smith, the internal FEP team, and relevant outside providers and supports were able to meet together. At these meetings, the team and Mrs. Smith engaged in a mutual exchange of ideas, identified target goals and objectives, and coordinated service delivery. Through this process, and through daily contact with the Smiths' parent advocate, Mrs. Smith became increasingly confident and hopeful about her family's future and achieved a sense of ownership of the process. This was evidenced when Mrs. Smith increasingly came to the meeting with an agenda, identifying areas for discussion, posing questions to service providers, and establishing priorities for the team. Mrs. Smith also began to present as less depressed, both through her ability to focus the FEP agenda, and through her increased range of expression and care in her appearance. Mr. Smith maintained sobriety and employment, and parent advocacy also guided family involvement in workshops on parent training and support groups. Entitlements assistance was provided to help stabilize the family in terms of their housing and finances.

FEP team meetings facilitate communication and greater understanding and synchronization among providers who often are siloed in different systems—for example, family advocates, clinicians, and child welfare staff—together with the family. While coordination of care is an essential feature of the FEP team, it is the synergistic interplay among the family members, parent advocates, clinicians, and entitlements specialists that is the most powerful element of this multisystemic intervention. Within this interplay, a family centered framework, open and respectful dialogue, empathic resonance, and appropriate boundary setting create the conditions conducive to learning, skill acquisition, collaboration, and follow-through. In the case of the Smiths, the initial emphasis was on establishing mutual priorities in the face of multisystemic demands, such as facilitating the family's involvement in a monthly family night, engaging their older daughter in an after-school mentoring group at the Family Resource Center, and advocating for the family at school meetings. These supports bolstered social connectedness and the Smith family's capacity to navigate multiple service systems. The level of direct involvement and support provided by the FEP team enables families to sustain their involvement in the sometimes emotionally demanding family therapy process, while building empowerment and family self-confidence.

Benchmarks of Positive Outcome

At the third monthly team meeting, which included service providers internal and external to the agency, Mr. Smith was unable to participate due to his job, but provided Mrs. Smith with a list of questions. At this meeting, the family's progress was immediately apparent. Mrs. Smith confidently relayed her husband's questions, and asked for clarification about specific aspects related to the family's case status. Mrs. Smith maintained consistent eye contact throughout the meeting. The family successfully secured housing and medical benefits, and was regularly attending all therapy appointments; in addition, the two therapists working with the family were engaged in ongoing collaboration. The team members reflected their observations of family progress, and Mrs. Smith echoed this sentiment. Pam was engaged in treatment, her aggression levels had decreased, and school attendance, homework completion, and behavior had improved for all of the children in the family. In addition, the family had been present consistently for weekly home visits with providers. The children were attending school regularly and were exhibiting improved behavioral functioning in the classroom.

For the Smith family, the multisystemic intervention described in this chapter resulted in the following outcomes as assessed by both professional observation and family feedback:

- Increased coordination of services.
- Greater access to concrete services (e.g., food stamps, disability, housing, legal aid).
- Increased daily living skills such as hygiene and time management.
- Improved parenting and household management.
- Decreased experience of mental health symptoms.
- Family preservation.
- Family ownership of the change process.
- Access to needed family resources via emergency funding provided by city and/or state contracts.
- Increased attendance at family therapy sessions.
- Increased involvement of important persons in the family's lives (e.g., ministers, coaches, other family members).

The outcomes experienced by the Smith family are consistent with the outcomes of other families that have chosen to utilize the FEP. Future steps for enhancing the FEP include synthesizing data from more diagnosis-specific outcomes measures, formally integrating family feedback, and incorporating legal and housing support.

Conclusion

This chapter has described the multisystems model and coordination of interdisciplinary care. It is our experience that this perspective, coupled with a collaborative, strength-based approach with our clients, can empower clinicians and clients alike in addressing complex treatment issues, especially those faced by poor clients and families.

The FEP is an evolving intervention that adapts the latest research (Carpinello et al., 2002; P. Minuchin, Colapinto, & Minuchin, 2006; Szapocznik et al., 2003) to the clinical needs of the families served and to the training needs of the participating staff. Its unique blend of multidisciplinary input provides a context that seeks to foster change in both the external and internal domains of multistressed urban families. While pulling together the component parts of a system that has an inherent complexity, there is simplicity in utilizing existing resources within a system in order to partner with families and match their expressed needs. By reducing barriers that interfere with engagement and treatment retention, and developing partnerships among system members, staff feel empowered to provide clinically sound and culturally sensitive services that are responsive to the family's needs. Families in turn are able to own and direct their involvement in treatment and to benefit from the supportive capacity of multiple systems.

CHAPTER 12

Group Therapy

Introduction

Given the productivity pressures that many clinicians and agencies experience today, this chapter addresses the process of group treatment for adults and adolescents and emphasizes the value of groups in real-world practice. Clinicians in some settings may find that they are one of few treatment providers in their clinics with an enormous caseload of clients. Groups can provide the opportunity to offer excellent treatment within the reality of these high-need and productivity situations. In addition, groups are helpful for clients with mental health problems, who may be isolated from social interaction and relationships. Groups can also be an excellent support for clients who are reducing or ending individual therapy sessions after their goals have been reached (see Chapter 9).

Although many clinicians run groups in their practices, clinics, hospitals, and agencies, it has been our experience that few have had ongoing training in this area, and often little training even within graduate programs. With this in mind, this chapter first explores the different types of groups. We then discuss the importance of the prescreening process and establishing group cohesiveness in the initial phase of a group. The key techniques for group facilitation are reviewed, including the ROPES model, incorporating motivational interviewing techniques, inspiring mutual ownership, following the affect, reflecting, and bridging. Real-world challenges as they relate to forming and maintaining effective groups are then addressed. Last, we examine the intricacies of effectively running groups with adolescents.

Types of Groups

There are a wide range of group practices within the mental health field. They can take the form of traditional therapy groups, structured and targeted psychoeducational groups, and more open "community meeting" formats. It is well beyond the scope of this chapter to cover all group types. Therefore, this chapter extracts areas of commonality across groups and offers real-world examples that will be most useful to practicing clinicians.

The early writing on group psychotherapy focused on long-term supportive outpatient group treatment. Yalom's (1995) work has had a major impact on the process of group treatment. His work is still relevant and widely used today. Yalom (1995) and Yalom and Leszcz (2005) have emphasized the following factors as critical components to effective group process:

- Instillation of hope.
- Universality (seeing that I'm not alone or have unique problems).
- Imparting information (educational).
- Altruism (unselfish giving).
- Corrective recapitulation (reenactment of family dynamics in a safe environment).
- Development of socializing techniques.
- Healthy imitative behavior.
- Interpersonal learning.
- Group cohesiveness.
- Catharsis (expression of pent-up feelings).
- Existential factors (accepting personal responsibility for one's life).

In addition to Yalom's work (Yalom & Leszcz, 2005), groups of various kinds have also been an important part of outpatient, inpatient, residential, and day treatment programs. Many have focused on educating clients and their families about their illnesses and ways in which they can improve their functioning. CBT groups have had a major impact on the field by providing clinicians with evidence-based treatment manuals for a wide range of group treatments (Freeman, Schrodt, Gilson, & Ludgate 1993). Examples of evidence-based groups include Seeking Safety, a manualized group treatment available in multiple languages for people with PTSD and co-occurring substance use (Najavits, 2002; *SeekingSafety.org*); Wellness Self-Management, a group curriculum for people who have had experience with mental health problems and are looking to take more control of their lives (Salerno et al., 2008a, 2011); and groups for depression (Gallagher & Thompson, 1982) and substance abuse (Godley, Godley, Dennis, Funk, & Passetti, 2007). Some research centers also publish group therapy materials and manuals that are evidence based. The UCLA/RAND National Institute of Mental Health Center for Research on Quality in Managed Care is an example of one such site where manuals for group therapy for depression are provided free of charge in both English and Spanish *(www.hsrcenter.ucla.edu/ research/wecare/CBTmanuals.html)*. Additional group manuals with empirical support can be accessed from the SAMHSA Knowledge Application Program website *(http://kap.samhsa.gov/products/manuals)*.

Pregroup Preparation and Screening

Whenever possible, it is important that an assessment and screening of individual clients take place before they are placed in a group. This serves two purposes: (1) it allows the clinician(s) to assess the client's readiness for group, and (2) it gives the group leader(s) an opportunity to establish a connection with the client prior to the beginning of the group. This can contribute to group cohesion and can significantly impact the client's ability to stay engaged in the ongoing group process. It can also have an impact on a member's satisfaction with the group (Riva, Wachtel, & Lasky, 2004).

In the real world with extensive demands on clinicians' time, a full screening session may not be possible, but even a 10-minute meeting with clients before the first group session can be advantageous. This is true even in inpatient, residential, and day treatment programs, where all clients may be assigned to groups and the screening function may not be as relevant. Even in these situations, however, the opportunity for the therapist(s) to meet briefly with each client before the first group session can have a major impact on the ability to establish trust, safety, and group cohesion. In the assessment phase of pregroup preparation and development, the therapist(s) works to (1) identify the clients' needs, expectations, and commitment; (2) address myths and misconceptions; (3) convey information about the group; and (4) screen the person for group fit (DeLucia-Waack, Gerrity, Kalodner, & Riva, 2004; Riva et al., 2004). Throughout this process, it is important that the therapist(s) assumes a supportive role, conveys empathy, and uses this process to establish therapeutic rapport with each client. By doing this, the therapist(s) becomes a bridge, helping each client to feel connected to someone in the group before group cohesion is established. This can greatly reduce the dropout rate (DeLucia-Waack et al., 2004).

Initial Group Session
and the Development of Group Rules

The initial group sessions are an opportunity for therapists to introduce or reintroduce themselves to the group members, to review the
purpose of the group, to have each person introduce him- or herself
and say something about him- or herself, and to begin the development
of group rules and norms. Group rules must be established to ensure
the development of trust, confidentiality, safety, respect, and honesty.
To accomplish this, common group rules should include punctuality,
attendance at all sessions, respect for each other, confidentiality, and
early notification if members are unable to attend. Equally important
are group norms that encourage participation, speaking, and involvement; turn taking and having only one person speak at a time; not
interrupting; and the use of "I statements" (DeLucia-Waack et al.,
2004; Riva et al., 2004).

   Yalom and Leszcz (2005) have emphasized the importance of
group rules and what can happen when they are violated. They assert,
for example, that continued tardiness and absence by group members
can threaten and compromise the cohesiveness of the group. They note
that subgrouping and scapegoating can also undermine the group process.

   In Yalom and Leszcz's (2005) model, they also raise a concern
about "disruptive extragroup socialization" (p. 118). It was this concern that led many early group leaders to prohibit socialization by
members outside of the group. The groups presented in this chapter,
however, are conceptualized with the real world in mind. Unlike traditional therapy groups, the groups presented in this chapter are viewed
as therapeutic support groups that assume outside contact between
members and encourage them to bring their issues and experiences into
the group discussions. This is particularly helpful for isolated clients,
who may not have family or friends to support them in their process
of change.

   The benefits of eliciting rules from group members are numerous.
Writing down rules suggested by group participants can increase a sense
of ownership and group cohesion, and can initiate an atmosphere of
self-enforcement where participants can remind other members of the
rules when they are violated. With populations that may find the group
setting challenging, the participants may decide to agree on a tardiness
policy that is more flexible. For example, members may agree to allow a
10-minute window after which if a member is late, it becomes up to the
group participants (rather than the group leader) to uphold and enforce
this rule.

The Leader's Role in Developing Group Cohesion

The group facilitator enters the experiential field alongside clients and is in a unique position to lead the way in creating and fostering an atmosphere conducive to the transformative experience. Through modeling, consistency, and predictable follow-through, the group leader sets the tone for subsequent group experiences. In addition to being a vehicle for the dissemination of information, the practitioner also acts as a model for containing difficult affect. One of the most important roles of the leader(s) is to build and maintain a positive and therapeutic group climate. This involves developing group cohesion by helping to foster a climate that is safe, positive, supportive, and strong enough to handle charged emotions (DeLucia-Waack et al., 2004; Riva et al., 2004; Yalom, 1995; Yalom & Leszcz, 2005). Skills that are expanded upon below, such as use of reflection, bridging, and validation, are critical to invoking increased group cohesion.

The leader's role is to encourage the development of positive relationships among all group members and between the leader(s) and the clients. To accomplish this goal, the posture of the leader toward the clients must include concern, acceptance, genuineness, and empathy. In emphasizing the importance of this way of relating between group leaders and members, Yalom and Leszcz (2005) have stated that "nothing . . . takes precedence over this attitude" (p. 117). It is central to the therapist's use of self in this treatment modality. Another role of the group leader(s) is to establish the group norms regarding communication and feedback. In initial group sessions, it is often helpful to place more of an emphasis on positive feedback and building strengths.

It may be hard for some group members to hear feedback and/or respond to group material in the early phases of a group, particularly when it is negative. "Members are more likely to hear negative feedback if it follows positive feedback or is sandwiched between two positive statements" (Riva et al., 2004, p. 42). An example of a group leader modeling such a process:

> "Maria, clearly what you are saying has a lot of meaning and importance. The way that you are communicating it right now seems to be keeping the other group members from truly hearing what you are trying to express. Do you think you could try to rephrase what you are saying in a way that the other members of the group can truly hear the hurt and need rather than just the anger?"

The leader is responsible for shaping the norms of the group and creating a positive group culture. Yalom and Leszcz (2005) have shown that this process of culture building is facilitated if honesty and open expression are encouraged.

The leader sets the tone for the group by displaying nonjudgmental acceptance and an appreciation of others' strengths as well as challenges. It is essential that the leader models interpersonal honesty and spontaneity for group members. This can create a safe space in which members are free to interact with each other. In this regard, it is also important that the members are encouraged not to "direct all of their comments to or through the leader" (Yalom & Leszcz, 2005, p. 124). Increasingly, during ongoing group sessions, the leader should encourage group members to take ownership of the group process.

The Clients' Roles

Once group rules have been established with the help of all participants, group members can play an important role in encouraging each other to keep these rules. Facilitators should foster and encourage other members to enforce norms, as this is the basis of a new experience and a powerful example of self-modeling. Members of the group often reenact past experiences by testing limits and structure. While on the surface, structure might be appealing, for some of our clients it is something unfamiliar and even frightening. The process of believing that the group is going to be a supportive vehicle for change requires trust. The challenge for the group facilitator is to be empathic and accepting of all members, while also enforcing the established structure.

A group is a microcosm that mirrors clients' real-world experiences. Many of our clients have histories that may be interpersonally fragmented and/or inconsistent. For example, an adult client who grew up with an alcoholic single parent may display behaviors that are consistent with the way he or she learned to manage and survive in such an environment. For instance, he or she may present as tentative, reluctant to assert him- or herself, and overresponsible to other group members at the expense of his or her own needs. The group leader can make this dynamic explicit within the group process by gently encouraging and challenging the participant to expand his or her interpersonal repertoire. This modeling can inspire and encourage other group members to do the same.

Techniques

Group Structure: The ROPES Model

Establishing and maintaining a firm yet flexible group structure is essential to creating the conditions for clients to have a safe and grounded experience wherein unresolved interpersonal conflicts can be safely expressed and worked through. There are many different models of group psychotherapy (Yalom & Leszcz, 2005), and theories of structure differ among them. One that is particularly helpful in real-world settings is the ROPES model (Nemec, McNamara, & Walsh, 1992; Salerno et al., 2008b). This model was originally developed to support recovery-oriented groups that focused on skills acquisition (Nemec et al., 1992). The model has since been expanded to address group facilitation and process as well (Salerno et al., 2011).

ROPES stands for Review, Overview, Presentation, Exercise, and Summary (Nemec et al., 1992; Salerno et al., 2011). It provides a structured approach to facilitating educationally focused groups that work well in real-world settings. It is our experience that the ROPES model provides clinicians of all experience levels with a user-friendly framework to organize the often complex group process and to effectively facilitate groups. The five components of the ROPES model are described below using an example of a group addressing substance use.

Review

At the start of the group, a review of the last group is elicited from participants. This gives the group an opportunity to reestablish the rapport and more easily pick up where they left off at the last meeting. In addition, follow-up is requested on any items that were to be completed or addressed between the two groups. If it is the initial session of the group, the review portion covers the goals and purpose of the group. The following example illustrates this process.

> "Last week we spoke about the pros and cons of continuing to use substances. We talked about the positive effects of using substances such as reducing symptom intensity and providing constancy in an unstable world, as well as an opportunity to relax and socialize. We also spoke about the negative aspects of use, such as risks associated with drug interactions, withdrawal, unstable finances, potential decompensation, and the need to take increasingly more. You engaged in an exercise where you were able to examine your own personal pros and cons and were encouraged to think about these pros and cons in relation to your goals and values. At the end of the last group you were asked to think about how substance use serves as a barrier to getting closer to the things that are important. Who would like to share their reflections and experiences?"

Overview

In this portion of the group, the facilitator conducts a brief overview of the activities that will take place in that day's group. The group leader may ask the group members about their existing knowledge of the day's topic and engage the group in a brief discussion about the importance of the topic. For example:

> "Today we will be examining the degree to which substance use impacts your ability to move forward in the direction of your values, for example, family, work, school, and religion. We will cover some factual information about values and substance use and then participate in an exercise that will allow you to reflect on your individual needs and how these needs are filled or not filled with continued substance use."

Presentation

The next step is getting into the details—presenting the specific content and material for the current session. Group members must have the opportunity to react and give their own impressions of, or experiences with the topic under discussion, otherwise, the risk is that buy-in will not be gained from the participants, and/or the topic will not be incorporated into the participants' experience. For example, a group leader directing the group to think about the pushes and pulls of ongoing substance use might invite members to read from a handout on this topic, and engage the group in a discussion about need, substance use, and personal values as they relate to these push/pulls. The group leader might then engage members in a discussion of the difference between immediate need and long-term need. As a way to get the conversation going, he or she might begin by highlighting that an immediate need may involve using substances to quell ongoing shame and anxiety connected to reestablishing family relationships, whereas a long-term need may involve developing a broader repertoire of ways to address and manage this anxiety so that substance abuse does not act as a barrier to reestablishing important relationships in one's life.

Exercise

Once group members have responded to the materials presented, it is helpful if group members can do an exercise together that helps to illustrate the topic under discussion. The main goal of the exercise portion of the group is to provide an opportunity for group members to personalize the day's content. Sometimes this can take the form of asking group members to take turns describing their own experiences in this area or their feelings about it. Or the group leader may involve the group participants in an experiential exercise, such as pairing off to share answers to specific questions, or completing a worksheet that is then shared with the rest of the group. This is the part of the group where group leaders can get creative and skills such as storytelling and role playing can greatly enhance the process. For example, the group could be broken up into small groups and members encouraged to identify one value that they hold dear. They would then be asked to share with the group the degree to which substance abuse moves them closer or further away in relation to this value. The group would reconvene and share salient points.

Summary

A brief summary brings together all of the discussion points and captures the essence of what was addressed during the session. This supports ongoing learning in that it provides group members with a "take away," or something they can leave the group thinking about and continuing to process. Positive feedback can also be incorporated into the summary by focusing on specific aspects of the day's lesson. This portion of the group should encourage group members to think about how to apply the skills and lessons learned from the present group discussion to their everyday lives outside of the group. This promotes continuity of and applicability between group sessions, particularly as the Review portion of the following group reminds participants of the content, discussion, and skills of the prior group, and asks group members to reflect on how they applied the knowledge gained in the last group to their lives. For example:

> "In today's group, you all had the opportunity to examine the role of substance use in relation to your values. I'd like to commend you all for engaging in a discussion that can at times be difficult. You were provided with factual information regarding the difference between immediate and long-term needs and were asked to reflect on your own needs, and how your methods of filling your needs relate to substance use and values. Robert, you were very open about the shame and frustration that you feel about being stuck in a pattern of filling your needs with substances. Your courage is appreciated and can hopefully serve as a model for how to move forward in life in the face of difficult feelings. Barbara, you found it difficult to think about other ways to have long-term needs filled independent of substance use. You gave voice to a struggle that is consistent with many other group members' experiences, and I want to thank you for remaining in the group even though it may have been more comfortable for you to leave. Between now and the next group, I'd like for you to think about one alternative way to satisfy a need other

than substance use when you feel compelled to use. We will reflect on your experiences at the beginning of our next group."

In summary, the ROPES format is another vehicle through which the following key elements to effective groups can flourish:

- Safety.
- Continuity.
- Predictability.
- Modeling.
- Expectations.
- Collaboration
- Follow-through. (Salerno et al., 2011)

Using Motivational Interviewing in Groups

The MI stance (W. R. Miller & Rollnick, 2002, 2013; see Chapter 6 in this book) helps members feel heard and supported, and fosters a positive environment in which therapists and clients collaborate to produce change. Researchers have established a growing evidence base for incorporating MI principles in groups (Wagner & Ingersoll, 2013). In their book on *Motivational Interviewing in Groups,* Wagner and Ingersoll (2013) have presented a four-phase model of motivational tasks for sequential group sessions.

The first phase involves *engaging the group* by helping members connect to each other, establishing group cohesion, and creating a group structure that fosters therapeutic interactions (Wagner & Ingersoll, 2013). The second phase, *exploring perspectives,* helps members better understand their own and others' difficulties and life circumstances, and identify areas of their lives in which they feel stuck. Clients are also encouraged to formulate and explore the values, goals and identities that are important to them. Emphasis throughout is on the client's present life. Exploration of past experiences is included only in the service of helping the client to move forward (Wagner & Ingersoll, 2013).

In the third phase, *broadening perspectives,* MI is used to help members incorporate new perspectives into the preexisting views of their lives and difficulties. Members start to consider how they can begin to live a more fulfilling life and build the confidence they need to make the changes they desire. In the fourth and final phase, *moving into action,* group members work with each other to plan for and implement the steps necessary to initiate change in their lives. Members then help each

other to maintain these changes once they have been made (Wagner &
Ingersoll, 2013).

MI recognizes that group members may be at different stages of
change and present with varying degrees of ambivalence (Wagner &
Ingersoll, 2013). W. R. Miller and Rollnick (2013) have noted that it
is important to mobilize change talk, particularly when clients focus
on sustain talk, which is the opposite of change and helps to maintain
the status quo (see Chapter 6). However, through the inclusion of MI
techniques such as OARS, providing feedback, rolling with resistance,
developing discrepancy, avoiding the expert stance, and emphasizing
personal responsibility, group facilitators can more readily honor and
work with each participant based on his or her stage of change and
ambivalence (W. R. Miller & Rollnick, 2002; see Chapter 6 in this
book).

Although W. R. Miller and Rollnick (2013) in recent years have
distanced MI from its original emphasis on the stages-of-change model,
we have found it particularly useful to educate group members on these
stages (DiClemente & Velasquez, 2002; Prochaska & DiClemente,
1982) as a way of normalizing and universalizing the change process (see
Chapter 6). Group discussions about ambivalence are often productive,
as they give participants the opportunity to openly discuss the dynamic
tension between wanting to change and wanting to stick with familiar
behavior patterns. With the facilitator modeling empathic exploration,
the discrepancy between the desire to change and presenting behaviors,
and consistent affirmation, participants can begin to challenge each
other and provide feedback around barriers to pursuing their own needs
and values, while still supporting each other's self-efficacy. The following example illustrates this process.

Myron, a 33-year-old male who struggled with depression, frequently complained of life being too painful to get out of bed. This impeded his desire to
engage in satisfying activities with his family and to progress in his employment. Though medication had been repeatedly recommended by his treatment team, Myron continued to resist going on medication out of a desire
to "do it himself." After multiple group sessions wherein the facilitator validated Myron's experience and explored his desire to connect with his family
and his reluctance to take his medication, Sally, a 37-year-old female in the
group, challenged his repeated complaining and urged him to reconsider
taking medication so that he could actively take a role in addressing his
depression. Sally was able to relate to Myron's ambivalence and draw from
her own experience with medication to support Myron and communicate a
belief in his ability to change.

Mutual Ownership

Facilitators can promote mutual ownership of the group by speaking to and honoring members' "best-perceived self"—the part of them that wants change (Hayes, Strosahl, & Wilson, 1999, 2002). The facilitators in a substance abuse recovery group used the following statement to address past patterns of group disruption and encourage support for mutual ownership of the group norms:

 "This program is about your recovery, and it is important that we all hold true to this idea. This group is an opportunity for change and we don't want anyone to miss out. Therefore, we want to pull for everyone's commitment to attendance, punctuality, remaining focused, and not interrupting one another."

By emphasizing each group member's responsibility in his or her own recovery, group members are made aware of their contribution to their peer's recovery as well. The following case illustrates this principle.

Constance, a 28-year-old female who struggled with bipolar disorder, was talking in group about her past experiences with an abusive father. When she noticed that group members were having a side conversation, she brought attention to it and demanded their respect and attentiveness and stated, "Excuse me, what happened? I'm talking here and you need to listen!" The facilitator framed Constance's assertion as honoring and taking ownership of her group experience and then elicited feedback from other group members about the interaction that had just taken place.

Follow the Affect

When group members present personal experiences, it is our role as facilitators to validate members' contributions and then generalize them in order to best harness the potential power of the group. Following the affect (W. R. Miller & Rollnick, 2002) leads the group closer to shared experiences and mutual healing. Additionally, it can assist facilitators with focusing on context, which lends itself to the universal human experience, rather than content, which can lead to individual problem solving or possibly "therapy with an audience" (Salerno et al., 2008a, slide 42). Below are examples of responses that group facilitators can use to lead groups in this direction:

"How does that affect you personally?"
"I hear the frustration in your voice, can anyone else relate to what he is expressing?"

"One of the things that I pick up on is an extreme lack of trust. Can other group members relate to this experience?"
"How did you feel when that happened?"
"It must make you sad and frustrated to realize how difficult this has turned out to be."
"Tell us more about it."

Reflections, Bridge Statements, and Redirection

A key technique in MI (Miller & Rollnick, 2002, 2013; see Chapter 6 in this book) is reflective listening and reflections. These involve an empathic re-telling of the client's statement by the therapist. They help the client feel understood and often include affect. Reflections can be combined with bridge statements that are then directed to the rest of the group. Reflections can foster universality and further exploration and mutual support from group members. The following is an example of combining reflection and bridge statements in a group process:

> "Diane, you feel isolated in the house, and you feel that this isolation affects your ability to focus on recovery. [reflection] Who else in the group can relate to feeling lonely at times? [bridge statement]"

At the same time, despite the use of reflections and bridge statements, some clients may have difficulty staying on topic. Other clients may attempt to stay on topic, but given their symptomatology, it may sometimes be difficult for the group leader(s) to realize this. It is the facilitator's role to extract meaning from a client's statement and bridge to the larger group as the example above illustrates. If this proves difficult, the therapist can redirect while validating the client as shown in the following example:

> "Mr. Johnson, I think that we can all tell that your story means a lot to you. Thank you for sharing it with us. [validation] I wonder if there is a way that we can relate your story to our discussion of [redirection]. . . . "

Collaborative Brainstorming

The promotion of brainstorming instills a sense of mutual aid, empowerment, and hope. A solution-based, problem-solving approach encourages all group members to share their ideas (Wofsy & Mundy, 2011a). This can increase motivation and decrease feelings of hopelessness and helplessness. The following statements can be used to help members brainstorm alternatives to their present difficulties:

"Have you spoken with your psychiatrist about your concerns?"

"During these difficult times, what have you been doing to take care of yourself as best you can?"

"Sometimes we feel like we're trapped in a bad situation. We've been considering the problem from our usual way of looking at things. But these are unusual times, and maybe a different way of looking at things is needed. Let's ask others in the group if they've had a similar problem and what they did."

" 'One day at a time' sounds like good advice, Pat. But so we can better understand exactly what you are recommending, can you give a specific example from your own personal experience of a specific time that you've taken this advice and used it?"

"Does anyone else find themself focusing on the negative thoughts and feelings all the time? How would your life be if you were to focus on what you can do and can be?"

The combination of (1) following the affect → (2) reflecting → (3) bridging → (4) eliciting collaborative brainstorming is a powerful intervention that can foster altruism, hope, and optimism among group members, and ultimately provide the foundation for a transformative experience. The following case illustrates this process.

Louise, a 27-year-old female participating in a 10-week trauma-focused CBT group, was sharing her experience of not being able to walk down her street after seeing a person who resembled an abusive partner from her past. She lamented over the fact that it had been 5 years since this relationship and that she was still easily triggered. The facilitator reflected back Louise's feelings of disappointment, futility, and hopelessness and elicited from other group members whether they shared similar feelings and experiences. Another member, Alicia, spoke about never feeling quite at ease while commuting to her job. The facilitator touched on the commonality of the shared experience and invited the group members to engage in a collective discussion about specific ways to identify and manage triggers. Another group member, Samantha, related to the group a conversation she recently had with a friend who was an alcoholic in recovery and felt triggered when passing a bar or in the presence of alcohol. Samantha's friend talked about coming to terms with the fact that she would likely have to manage these types of triggers—to varying degrees—her whole life. Samantha wondered if this level of acceptance could be applied to PTSD symptoms.

Observing the Process

Sometimes no matter how hard we try as leaders to keep a group focused, there will be instances when members have difficulty connecting with or staying on topic. If all attempts at promoting a focused group fall short, do not be afraid to stop the group and address the process that you are observing by saying, "What is troubling us today?" or "I think it may be time for us to have a discussion about how this group can serve us better."

Remember too, that in running groups, silence is also a communication (Yalom & Leszcz, 2005). In cases where a group has fallen silent, it may be helpful for the facilitator to reflect:

"The group seems silent today. Does anyone have any thoughts on what might be on our minds?"

The Challenges of Group Therapy in the Real World

Conducting effective groups in the real world is challenging, particularly for clinicians who have been trained primarily in a long-term, outpatient psychodynamic model. Therapists facing the demands for productivity have found that they are often forced to incorporate a more short-term, focused approach. While this represents a shift in actual implementation, many have found that their earlier training is still useful in understanding group process, particularly when disruptions occur. This section presents a number of common issues faced by therapists running groups, including the panic or challenge a group leader might feel when one group member repeatedly monopolizes the focus, several group members pull the group in every direction but the topic at hand as a way of having their individualized needs met, or when one individual becomes particularly symptomatic and displays psychotic thinking or behavior. While the techniques described earlier in this chapter can assist group facilitators with such real-world challenges as maintaining the focus of the group, promoting participation, handling large groups, maintaining attendance and punctuality, "getting stuck," and managing psychiatric heterogeneity, the following techniques serve as more situation-specific interventions.

Group Size

When running groups in the real world, facilitators can often find themselves overwhelmed by an unusually large number of group participants.

This often occurs on inpatient units, in residential programs, day programs, and in schools. Many settings do not have sufficient groups to meet the needs of their client population. Facilitators, who find themselves alone and overwhelmed, can utilize a number of possible strategies. One possible approach is to enlist colleagues, including case managers, other therapists, and interns or students who may be eager to learn and to have an experience facilitating groups. Often in groups, a particular member may emerge as a cofacilitator. For example, the Wellness Self-Management group model (Salerno et al., 2008a, 2011), an evidence-based approach described above, systematically encourages members to rotate filling the cofacilitator role if they feel comfortable doing so. The added benefit of this approach is that it reinforces mutual ownership and actualizes the recovery-oriented perspective that everyone has skills and traits that are valuable and helpful. In some programs, particularly day treatment, partial hospitalization, and rehab programs, a graduate of the program may serve as a cofacilitator. Additionally, breaking the group into small groups to cover a particular topic and then reunite as a group so that each subgroup can share their experiences with the rest of the group is another way to effectively manage large group size. Simple tools such as writing on newsprint or a whiteboard can also assist members with maintaining focus in a large group.

Recruitment

Recruitment is another important process in developing a group that is often overlooked in the literature. Many facilitators have found that the development of groups requires active outreach. This can be particularly challenging in outpatient programs where the outreach extends into the community. Offering food at the beginning or end of sessions usually increases recruitment and attendance. In settings where some group members are continuing from a previous year (e.g., in schools) or where other clients are members of a particular program, the use of testimonials by others, who have been in prior groups or who have "graduated" from the group process, can be helpful.

Maintaining Focus

As we indicated earlier, it is often helpful to write group rules on a large sheet of paper and post them on the wall at the beginning of each group. This can serve as a reminder to all group members. It can also be a helpful tool if a member becomes disruptive or breaks one of the rules. Sometimes multiple group members may be agitated and disruptive on a particular day. If attempts to focus on the process are unsuccessful, it is sometimes helpful to break into smaller groups to brainstorm or to conduct an activity. Sometimes pointing out the lack of focus of the group and engaging members in either a centering exercise or physical activity, such as getting up and stretching, can assist members with either calming down or improving energy and concentration.

Psychiatric Heterogeneity

In real-world settings it is not always possible to screen and select candidates so that the group composition lends itself to structure and focus. Due to productivity requirements and large caseloads, groups are increasingly heterogeneous in their makeup. For example, while the ideal group size is about 8 to 10 members, an integrated dual-disorder treatment group in a day program setting may have as many as 20 to 25 participants, all of them spanning the different stages of change and degrees of psychiatric symptomatology. It is important to remember that each client has his or her unique set of clinical circumstances that need to be understood in the biopsychosocial context of that individual. It is up to the treatment team, including the group facilitator, to systematically evaluate and support the psychiatric stability and mental health needs of each client. For example, Jack might be sleeping in group for any of these reasons:

- Medication.
- Loud roommate.
- Sleep apnea.
- Substance use.
- Boredom.

The treatment team must be proactive in creating conditions conducive to treatment responsiveness, including the use of case conferences, psychiatric consultation, and multisystem integration, as well as mobilizing the client's natural support system. There is no one-size-fits-all approach; it is up to the provider to reach out and support the group member with maximizing the potential benefits of the group. The interventions for working with the difficult client described below can also assist in working with psychiatric heterogeneity in groups.

Working with Difficult Clients

Many clients have difficult and painful histories. People often reenact their stereotypical response patterns in the group setting (Yalom & Leszcz, 2005), which can result in repetition of past interpersonal difficulty. The challenge for the group facilitator is to provide a new restorative experience by empathically responding to the client, setting appropriate clinical limits, and involving the rest of the group in a helpful way. As stated above, there can be different degrees of psychiatric symptomatology at any given time that can make the group process difficult to manage. We have found the following strategies useful in addressing the needs of the difficult client and maintaining the focus and continuity of the group.

Use of the Client–Therapist (or Client–Caseworker) Relationship

As stated above, it is paramount to establish and maintain an individual relationship with each group member. This allows for the opportunity to conduct pre- and postgroup check-ins with group members who can present as difficult and disruptive to the other group members.

Alfred, a group member who struggled with attentiveness and frequently stood up, walked around, left the room, and then rejoined the group, was asked to meet with the facilitator at the conclusion of the last group. The group leader shared his observations and expressed concern about the impact his frequent disruptions have on both him and the other group participants. He validated Alfred's contributions to the group and underscored the contributions he was further capable of making. He also reflected Alfred's difficulty with focusing. The group leader expressed that he would not be fulfilling his role as an effective facilitator if he didn't challenge Alfred and support him in addressing these disruptions. Alfred acknowledged that sometimes the group became overwhelming for him. The group leader and Alfred established a plan to meet right before and after each group in order to assist Alfred with remaining focused and utilizing the benefits of the group.

Creative Seating

The value of maintaining a strong individual relationship with each group member can extend to the group process itself via the use of creative seating. Whether it is sitting across from the group leader to maintain eye contact, sitting next to the group leader to create a sense of safety and containment, or requesting members who often side talk to sit apart, creative seating can be a powerful strategy for softening disruption and helping members to integrate more cohesively into the group. This can be done by asking permission or requesting willingness to consider changing the seating arrangement.

During one particular group, the group leader noticed that Alfred was having a difficult time staying focused and present for the group. When discussing Alfred's experience in the postgroup follow-up, Alfred noted that he often felt unsafe, overwhelmed with anxiety, and worried that he was going to have a panic attack. The group leader validated Alfred's experience and shared with him that, in encountering similar situations in the past, group members had found it helpful to sit close to the group leader. The leader explored with Alfred if he thought that this would be helpful, and Alfred responded that it would.

For the group members who struggle with maintaining concentration and focus, in addition to creative seating, predetermined and gentle cues such as a soft tap on the shoulder or a key word can recapture the group member's attention and remind him or her of the importance of the group and his or her participation in it.

VERB Strategies

Most clinicians with experience running groups have encountered a group member who presents as perseverative and difficult to contain despite multiple promptings. We have found that the following VERB strategies (Wofsy & Mundy, 2011a), when woven together, have often proven effective with these types of encounters.

Validate/Contain

There is always something of value in even the most difficult and complex perseverations. They may be hidden and eclipsed by complicated presentation (e.g., paranoia and psychosis), but it is up to the group leader to extract the value and meaning beneath the surface.

Empathic Reflection

Though situations like those described in the brief case examples above can often be frustrating for the group leader, it is important for the group leader to maintain his or her equanimity and empathically reflect back the affect and need expressed by the client. Tone of voice is a critical component of this intervention.

Request Willingness

We have found that people do not like being told what to do, nor do they appreciate being silenced in the midst of expressing themselves. In an effort to meet the client's need while meeting the needs of the group, the group leader can request permission from the client to allow feedback from other group members.

Bridge

Bridging provides the opportunity to expand the client's experience to that of the other group members. For example:

> "Mr. Johnson, I can tell this is really important to you, and you are making a really good point. I'm picking up on your anger and frustration. Would you be willing to sit back and let your peers take a crack at offering a response to your words so far? Can anyone else relate to what Mr. Johnson is saying?"

This set of strategies, when combined with the use of creative seating, pre- and postgroup check-ins, and pulling the treatment team together, can go a long way in maintaining group cohesiveness and efficiency.

Working with Mandated Clients

Many clinicians new to the field express difficulty in working with mandated clients. This population can be particularly challenging, in that they are often in the precontemplation stage of change and are there only because someone is telling them to be there. We have found that a values-based stance that emphasizes choice and personal responsibility and seeks to translate external motivation (e.g., a court order) to internal motivation (e.g., valuing one's freedom) can help the practitioner create a stance that allows him or her to disengage from the power struggle and puts the onus for change and continued participation in the hands of the client. Mandated group members may be upset about their presence in the group. However, they did choose to be present and, by emphasizing the client's choice, then validating his or her choice to be present, the facilitator:

- Highlights the part of the group member that can be accessed to reflect on goals and values.
- Highlights the power of the participant to make changes in his or her life.
- Paves the way for honoring and exploring the group member's ambivalence.
- Creates a dynamic tension within the participant by shifting the focus from interpersonal dynamics to internal dynamics.

This stance promotes the exploration of values. The literature in this area is now pointing to the need to support people getting connected with their values, their goals, and what they want their lives to represent (Corrigan, Mueser, Bond, & Drake, 2009; Hayes et al., 2011; W. R. Miller & Rollnick, 2002).

Introducing the concept of values and eliciting a group discussion around this topic can soften group resistance and put clients directly in charge of their lives. An important concept in working with mandated clients is to empathically work with them to identify some meaningful experience they can derive from this group

> GROUP MEMBER: This is bull shXX! I don't need to be here. I'm only here because that stupid judge says so.

> GROUP FACILITATOR: Right, I hear that you don't want to be here, and I hear that you are resenting this judge's order. Did I get that right? *(Client nods.)* But, you are here, and I'm wondering if part of you has decided to get out from underneath this judge. So given that you're going to be here for the next 10 weeks, what would help maximize this time for you? How can you walk away from this having gotten something meaningful?

Working with Adolescents in Group Treatment

Many of the guidelines presented above in our discussion of adult groups are also relevant to our work with adolescents in groups, especially the ROPES model. Given the special developmental issues presented by adolescents in groups, however, further discussion of this age group (13 to 18) is warranted. A number of researchers and therapists have addressed the needs of this population (Batista, 2009; K. G. Dies, 2000; K. R. Dies, 1992; Glodich, Allen, & Arnold, 2002; MacLennan, 2000; D. B. Miller, 1995; Nichols-Goldstein, 2001).

In many ways, group treatment is an ideal intervention for adolescents, particularly given the importance that they often place on peer relationships and support. In fact, adolescents may be able to hear constructive feedback or alternative points of view more easily from their peers (Abraham, Lepisto, & Schultz, 1995; Batista, 2009). Group therapy can provide an opportunity for adolescents to address these common developmental challenges and also to address the issue of interpersonal relationships, which are a central part of this developmental stage (Batista, 2009; Calhoun, Bartolomucci, & McLean, 2005). Garrick and Ewashen (2001) have indicated that group treatment "enables healthier perspectives that empower adolescents to be active agents of change in their lives" (p. 169). Many of the group treatment models for adolescents were originally adapted from adult models. With this in mind, a number of therapists have called for careful development of group therapy models tailored to the special needs of adolescents (Batista, 2009; Garrick & Ewashen, 2001).

K. G. Dies (2000) has documented the stages in adolescent group development. She has developed five stages in addition to an initial pregroup preparation stage. As we indicated above, this pregroup screening is an extremely important part of the group therapy process. Batista (2009) and MacLennan and Dies (1992) have emphasized that this pregroup preparation stage is particularly helpful to adolescents who may be self-conscious about speaking in a group. In addition to the value of screening to assess the appropriateness of an adolescent for group treatment (Batista, 2009), K. G. Dies (2000) describes two other purposes of this pregroup preparation phase: "(1) to establish basic criteria for admission to the group, and (2) to educate the prospective group member about the workings of the group" (p. 101). After this stage, the five phases include (1) initial relatedness, (2) testing the limits, (3) resolving authority issues, (4) work on self, and (5) moving on (K. G. Dies, 2000).

After this initial pregroup process, the first phase is *initial relatedness* (K. G. Dies, 2000). In this stage the group leader works to establish a connection among the adolescents in order to create an atmosphere that is safe for them and that will promote therapeutic change. In this stage, group leaders serve as role models for the adolescents, demonstrating interpersonal skills (K. G. Dies, 2000). An extremely important role of group leaders in this phase is the creation of a safe and positive climate for the group (K. G. Dies, 2000). K. G. Dies describes the following characteristics of an effective group leader in this initial phase. "Leaders who are able to demonstrate the ability to actively listen, make eye contact, provide support, avoid 'shoulds,' and take risks will provide effective models for members to emulate" (p. 103). She gives the following example of selective self-disclosure on the part of a group leader during this initial phase:

> No matter how many groups I have done, I always have a little sense of tension that I can actually feel in my shoulders at the beginning. But I have learned that there is so much positive from groups like this that I just take a deep breath and trust what we will be able to do together. (p. 103)

She then opens the question up to other group members by asking: "Do any of you have a sense of tension about what is going to happen in the group?" (p. 103). This opens up the topic for group members' comments and models an openness to discuss feelings.

In the second phase, adolescents often begin *testing the limits* (K. G. Dies, 2000). Many new therapists are often surprised to discover that adolescents "are able to view setting the limits as evidence of caring" (p. 104). Teenagers will often test to see whether the group leaders will still be there for them if they act out or test the limits. This is particularly important when one realizes that for many adolescents today, their families and schools may not provide this dependable limit setting (K. G. Dies, 2000). The challenge for leaders of adolescent groups is that they "require a degree of flexibility and a capacity to negotiate with members in order to convey a commitment to structure without the rigidity that turns teenagers off" (K. G. Dies, 2000, p. 104).

Resolving authority issues is the third phase (K. G. Dies, 2000). Group leaders must walk a fine line between showing tolerance while maintaining firm boundaries particularly around authority issues. In the fourth phase (K. G. Dies, 2000), *work on self,* group leaders help members to work on themselves. They use group exercises and experiences to help the adolescents examine how they relate to others. In the fifth phase, *moving on* (K. G. Dies, 2000), the group leaders review the process and the things learned over the time of the group in preparation for termination.

Therapists often struggle with the testing-the-limits phase. The following example illustrates the challenging situations that group leaders may encounter in this phase and questions about duty to report ethical issues.

In a session of a violence prevention group of adolescent boys in a middle school, one of the boys, Martin, reported that he was expecting to be "jumped" by gang members after school. When the group leaders expressed their concern and asked how he planned to protect himself, he pulled out a stiletto knife. After the group leaders recovered from their shock, they asked for the knife, which the boy reluctantly gave to one of the group leaders. The group leaders then asked the other boys for their input. They also expressed their concern and encouraged their group member to "not go looking for trouble." This led to an enlightening discussion of the pressures of gangs in their community and how difficult it was to avoid trouble.

During the session, the group leaders struggled with questions of "duty to report." They had discussed confidentiality with the boys, but they had also discussed the types of things that they would not be able to keep confidential. The group had discussed the rule that no weapons were allowed in school or in the group and the leaders had discussed with the boys the fact that they would have a duty to report if they felt that they were a danger to themselves or to others. They told Martin that they appreciated his honesty and the fact that he had turned in the weapon, but that they would have to report this to the school authorities. Initially, Martin was angry. The group leaders offered to go with him to the principal's office so that they could let her know the special circumstances and their concerns about not leaving him defenseless if he was attacked by gang members.

In the week following this incident, the group leaders met individually with Martin and with the other members of the group to discuss their feelings about the incident. This represented a painful group "rupture" but their bonding with the group leaders and with each other had been strong enough to survive a difficult limit-setting experience.

This example captures the realities of therapy in the real world. Adolescents are often prone to take risks; judgment and decision making can be impaired when they are faced with an anxiety-producing situation, such as a threat of gang violence. Many inner-city adolescents live with these realities on a daily basis. This example illustrates the ironic fact that adolescents are often grateful for the limits, if they are given in a caring, supportive way (K. G. Dies, 2000). Although Martin and the other boys were initially angry that his disclosure would need to be reported, they were aware of the limit and ultimately recognized that the group leaders had their best interests in mind.

Conflict Resolution Strategies

One of the common fears often expressed by new clinicians is the fear that a conflict might erupt in the group. Many of these therapists are afraid that they will not know how to handle such a conflict and that it will escalate out of control. It is important for clinicians in this situation to remember that they do not have to resolve everything in that session. Sometimes, clinicians have found it helpful to end a session and to tell group members that they would like to talk with them to help resolve the conflict in the period before the next group session. The following example illustrates this process in an adolescent group.

In the sixth session of an adolescent trauma group in a day treatment program, one participant "told a lie on" another group member and mocked his past traumas. This caused a heated verbal argument that almost led to a physical fight. The group leader, a social work intern, ended the group early that day. This group leader spent the following week validating the group members' feelings about the incident and discussing it as an opportunity to learn how to move forward without letting disturbing incidents interfere with one's goals and values. The group leader cited and commended specific contributions that each member had made to the group. The person who had been the target of the lie agreed to meet one-on-one with the member who had insulted him, and the group leader. The result was a heartfelt discussion about fear, feeling threatened, and abuse.

Everyone attended the next scheduled group. The two members spoke openly and honestly and an apology, which had been made in the one-on-one meeting, was repeated. Through this proactive, open, validating, and respectful commitment to each member and to the group itself, a disturbing event came to be the greatest contributor to positive group cohesion that the group experienced.

Implementing and Supporting the Development of Groups within Clinics, Hospitals, and Agencies

Clearly, groups are extremely helpful in addressing the issues presented in the real world; however, many clinicians, administrators, and programs feel apprehensive about developing groups in their settings. In addition, many clinicians find that they need help and support in working with clients who challenge the group process. The strategies discussed above capture some approaches. In addition, just as engaging peers as cofacilitators can support group process, it can also be useful to engage staff in peer learning. Peers have a shared experience and respect each other's opinions and knowledge. Therefore, a senior staff member who obtains further training, or a peer team of clinicians who implement groups and provide follow-up training to staff, can often produce a greater impact than a presentation by administration or a one-shot training without follow-up. Ultimately, clinicians will need further supervision and support in learning new methods, and the supervisor and program director must take on the challenge of follow-up around new strategies in order for them to be incorporated into the culture and repertoire of a program.

Conclusion

Groups can be enormously effective in the real world as they bring together individuals in a collaborative context that promotes universality, hope, optimism, and mutual aid. In today's climate, however, group facilitation with a diverse client population can be an incredibly complex and challenging task.

This chapter has provided an overview of group treatment interventions for adults and adolescents across various treatment settings. We discussed the process of developing groups with a particular emphasis on the realities clinicians face and presented the ROPES model as a comprehensive approach that can be helpful in working with clients with a wide range of diagnoses and presenting issues. The particular challenges of conducting groups with adolescents, including conflict resolution strategies, were also addressed. Finally, we explored the challenges in implementing and supporting the development of groups within clinics, hospitals, agencies, and schools. It is our hope that this chapter will be helpful to new and experienced clinicians, as well as supervisors or administrators charged with creating groups within their clinics and treatment facilities, as we have found this modality extremely helpful for a wide range of clients and presenting problems.

PART IV

Risk Assessment and Crisis Intervention

CHAPTER 13

Risk Assessment
and Suicide Prevention

Introduction

One of the realities of the mental health field is that anyone working with clients will experience people in acute distress. Graduate training often does not address risk assessment in great detail, and clinicians are often left with a limited tool kit to aid them in responding to these situations. With this in mind, this chapter provides a comprehensive overview of the key elements of a clinical risk assessment, including common types and indicators of risk and a framework for responding to these indicators. We then provide an in-depth exploration of the elements of suicide assessment and clinical response, and discuss how to preserve the therapeutic relationship following a psychiatric hospitalization. Last, this chapter reviews the Clinical Risk Consultation Team, an agency risk management model that can aid clinicians with the often challenging decisions regarding these clients.

Risk Assessment

Heckart, as cited in Wofsy, Mundy, and Tse (2009), indicates that risk can occur any time there is a *heightened potential* for harm to the well-being, functioning, or stability of an individual. It also refers to the potential for harm to others. The following list illustrates many of the different kinds of risk that can present in clinical situations:

- Suicidal ideation, intent, or behavior.
- Homicidal intent or behavior.
- Aggressive/assaultive behavior.
- Self-injurious behavior.
- Sexually abusive ideation, intent, or behavior.
- Fire setting.
- History of/or current victimization status.
- Uncontrolled active psychotic symptoms.
- Involvement in a clinical emergency situation. (Wofsy et al., 2009)

Red Flags for Potential Risk Situations

One helpful strategy for clinicians in preparing for risk situations has been to begin to understand the "red flags" that may indicate the potential for heightened risk. The following are some examples:

- Disengagement from treatment or program services.
- Sudden change in behavior or uncharacteristic behavior.
- Recent life changes.
  - □ Significant loss.
  - □ Relationship, marital, family, job, or environmental stressors.
- Changes in or poor hygiene and grooming.
- Isolation from friends, family, and/or support system.
- Withdrawal (e.g., not getting out of bed).
- Change in usual activities or routines.
- Change in attitude (e.g., irritability, frustration).
- Substance use or abuse.
- Stopping the use of medication.
- Emergence of new symptoms (e.g., voices, depression, insomnia, disorganized behavior). (Wofsy et al., 2009)

Responses to Indications of Risk: When in Doubt, Check It Out

Experienced clinicians often develop an ability to recognize the indicators of increasing risk potential in clients before they reach the crisis level. For beginning clinicians, it is important to begin to develop a strategy for identifying these indicators and responding with a more thorough assessment. In teaching students and young clinicians, we have adopted a "when in doubt, check it out" strategy. If you are a supervisor working with a new clinician, it is extremely important to validate his or her "gut feeling" that something might be wrong with a client.

Clinicians can learn to ask more appropriate questions in order to assess the level of risk. These might include:

- How long has the client been feeling this way?
- How many times in the last week?
- How strong is the behavior or impulse?
- How is the client coping with these feelings?
- What supports or protective factors are in place or could be put in place? (Wofsy et al., 2009)

Never Do This Alone

Throughout this chapter, we discuss many aspects of clinical risk assessment. We incorporate strategies for clinicians who are addressing these urgent issues. Before we begin, we would like to emphasize an extremely important aspect of these risk assessments. It is essential that clinicians (even those with a great deal of experience) not attempt to make these assessments alone. For relatively new clinicians, it is important to contact one's supervisor for guidance throughout the process. Since many of these episodes occur late in the evening when supervisors are not available, clinicians are encouraged to speak to a more senior therapist or the psychiatrist on staff. If these supports are not available, clinicians should contact their local emergency room or local mobile crisis team for advice during the process. (We recommend having these numbers in advance so that they are readily available in times of crisis.)

Challenges of Working with Suicidal Clients

Many clinicians, both new and experienced, report that working with suicidal clients is one of the most stressful and anxiety-producing tasks in their practice (Rudd 2006; Toth, Schwartz, & Kurka, 2007). Even clinicians with many years of experience report that the assessment and treatment of suicidal clients are the most challenging aspects of their clinical work (Toth et al., 2007). In the real world, it is therefore important that therapists regularly update their knowledge of suicide risk factors, assessment, and treatment.

Demographics of Suicide Risk Factors

Toth et al. (2007) provide an excellent overview of populations at risk for suicide including such issues as gender and age. According to the Centers for Disease Control and Prevention (CDC), more than 30,000

Americans commit suicide each year. It is, in fact, the eighth leading cause of death for males and the 19th leading cause of death for females (CDC, 2006; Toth et al., 2007). Additionally, suicide is the third leading cause of death for youth between the ages of 15 and 24, with a 3:1 male-to-female ratio among suicide completers (National Institute of Mental Health, 2001). Toth et al. (2007) have indicated that adolescent suicides have been increasing, however, with teenage girls showing more vulnerability (Lewinsohn, Rohde, Seeley, & Baldwin, 2001). Adolescents who present with depression and substance abuse are at an even greater risk for suicide (Gould & Kramer, 2001).

Toth et al. (2007) have also demonstrated that elderly white males over the age of 65 are the most at-risk group (CDC, 2006). Many of these suicides have involved gun use (75%), a particularly lethal method (Frierson & Melikian, 2002). Toth et al. have speculated that

> at this age, the elderly are struggling with physical and mental depreciation, as well as the loss of friends and family members, leading to a mild or moderate depression that they may never have experienced before. Therefore their coping strategies may be inadequate (CDC, 2006; Maris et al., 2000). (p. 2)

Gender is also an important risk factor in completed suicides (Toth et al., 2007). As Toth et al. have indicated, "There are four male-completed suicides for every one female-completed suicide, but there are three female-attempted suicides for every one male attempt (CDC, 2006). Simply stated, more men complete suicide, while more women attempt it" (Toth et al., 2007, p. 2).

Shea (2002) has shown that serious mental illness accounts for 95% of all completed suicides. According to the American Association of Suicidality (AAS; 2005), persons with major depressive disorder are 20 times more likely to commit suicide than the general population. Although serious depression is a major factor, other serious mental illnesses, such as schizophrenia, bipolar disorder, and borderline personality disorder can also be risk factors for suicide (Maris, Berman, & Silverman, 2000; R. C. Schwartz & Rogers, 2004; Shea, 2002; Toth et al., 2007). Alcoholism and drug abuse can increase the likelihood of a completed suicide (Maris et al., 2000; Toth et al., 2007; Westefield et al., 2000). All of these clients should be regularly and carefully assessed by a psychiatrist and monitored in ongoing psychotherapy (Jobes, 2006; Shea, 2002; Toth et al., 2007).

Another at-risk group is composed of persons living with serious medical illness or chronic pain (Toth et al., 2007). These individuals may feel hopeless and see suicide as a way out of their ongoing distress (Jobes, 2006; Schwartz & Rogers, 2004; Shneidman, 1993; Toth et al., 2007).

A previous history of suicide attempts in combination with current suicidal symptoms are also among the most important predictive factors (Indart, 2008; Jobes, 2006; Shea, 2002). According to Toth et al. (2007):

> The three most critical at-risk factors for suicide assessment are the number and severity of previous attempts, a family history of suicide, and current suicidal ideation (Jobes, 2006; Maris et al., 2000; Peruzzi & Bongar, 1994; Rogers & Soyka, 2004). . . . Research by Packman, Marlitt, Bongar, and O'Connor-Pennuto (2004) found that multiple attempters possessed a greater overall baseline risk, indicating that [prior] suicide attempts increase the overall vulnerability for future suicide completion. (p. 3)

Suicide Risk Assessment

In order to give clinicians an overview of the most helpful models of suicide risk assessment, this chapter explores Shawn Shea's (2002, 2004) Chronological Assessment of Suicidal Events (CASE) approach. Readers are also encouraged to explore David Jobes's (2006) Collaborative Assessment and Management of Suicidality (CAMS), and the Aeschi Conference Group's guidelines for clinicians working with suicidal clients *(www. aeschiconference.unibe.ch)*. These are among the most helpful models for eliciting suicidal ideation and conducting suicide risk assessment.

Shea (2004) emphasizes the significance of eliciting suicidal ideation as an important part of any suicide risk assessment. In the real world of clinical work, this is extremely important because a client may be seen over time by different outpatient therapists, a crisis intervention specialist, an emergency room resident or therapist, and a psychiatrist and other clinical staff on an inpatient unit (Shea, 2004). It is extremely useful, therefore, to have careful assessments of the client's suicidal ideation at different points in time and of previous suicidal gestures and attempts. Shea indicates the value of this information in future situations where a clinician may be meeting a client for the first time in an emergency room, for example.

The CASE Approach (Chronological Assessment of Suicidal Events)

The CASE approach (Chronological Assessment of Suicidal Events) (Shea, 2002, 2004) gives therapists a clinically sensitive, empathic approach for eliciting suicidal ideation. Shea (2004)[1] has indicated that this approach can often create a "positive interpersonal experience" for clients during the assessment (p. 387). Ironically, this sensitivity in and of itself can have a positive impact for clients. It often creates a sense of safety and comfort that can lead them to seek help in the future when contemplating suicide (Shea, 2004).

As indicated above, Shea (2004) has stated that in the real world,

> complicated suicide assessments have a knack for occurring at busy times, such as in the middle of an extremely hectic clinical day or in the chaotic environment of a packed emergency department. . . . In many suicide-assessment scenarios, we find a harried clinician performing a difficult task, under extreme pressure, in an unforgiving environment. It is understandable why mistakes are made. (p. 388)

With these realities in mind, Shea (2002, 2004) has developed a model that attempts to reduce the large number of issues that a clinician must remember in these often difficult assessment situations. There are four techniques that comprise the CASE approach: (1) the behavioral incident, (2) gentle assumption, (3) denial of the specific, and (4) symptom amplification (Shea, 2004). These techniques are helpful not only in suicide assessments but also in other "traditionally sensitive areas, such as sexual history, physical and psychological abuse history, alcohol and drug abuse histories, and violence and antisocial behavior histories" (Shea, 2004, p. 389).

The Behavioral Incident

Clients dealing with suicidal ideation are often uncomfortable discussing these issues with a clinician. Shea (2004) lists the following reasons why clients might distort information: "anxiety, embarrassment, protection of family secrets, unconscious use of defense mechanisms, or conscious attempts at deception" (p. 389). Since many aspects of client reports are subjective, Shea argues that it is more helpful for the clinician to focus on specific behavioral details and facts. For example, the therapist might ask the client "How many pills did you take?" or simply ask the patient to describe "What did you do next?" (Shea, 2004, p. 389). This technique can be extremely helpful to an interviewer because it gradually opens up the story of a suicide attempt through a series of behavioral incidents (Shea, 2004).

---

[1] Excerpts from Shea (2004) are reprinted with permission from Slack, Inc.

Shea (2004, p. 389) gives the following examples of behavioral incidents:

"Did you put the razor blade up to your wrist?"
"When you say that 'you taught your son a lesson,' what did you actually do?"
"Have you ever missed a day of work because of a hangover?"
"What did your father say then?"
"Tell me what happened next."

Gentle Assumption

The gentle assumption technique is particularly helpful when a clinician is addressing a taboo topic with a client. As Shea (2004) indicates, "With gentle assumption, clinicians assume potentially embarrassing or incriminating behaviors are occurring and frame their questions accordingly, using gentle tones of voice" (p. 389). It is important for the clinician to first take the time to establish therapeutic rapport with the client and to assume a gentle, nonaccusatory tone of voice in this process. For example, rather than asking a suicidal patient if he or she has considered other forms of suicide, which might lead to an immediate denial, the therapist might ask, "What other ways have you thought of killing yourself?" (p. 390). Shea warns clinicians to be cautious when using this tool:

> Gentle assumptions are powerful examples of leading questions. The clinician must use them with care. They should not be used with patients who may feel intimidated by clinicians or with patients who are trying to provide what they think clinicians want to hear. (p. 389)

Denial of the Specific

Shea (2002, 2004) has developed a technique that is helpful in cases where a client may initially deny an entire category of behavior following a gentle assumption. In these cases a list of specific questions may be used. Shea (2004) describes the process as follows:

> For example, if a patient responds to the gentle assumption "what other ways have you thought of killing yourself?" with a blanket "no other ways," the clinician may use the following series of questions concerning common ways in the patient's culture that may have been contemplated by the patient but not yet mentioned:
> - Have you thought of shooting yourself?
> - Have you thought of overdosing?
> - Have you thought of hanging yourself?

It is important to frame each denial of the specific as a separate question, pausing between each inquiry and waiting for the patient's denial or admission before asking the next question. The clinician should avoid combining the inquiries into a single question such as "Have you thought of overdosing, shooting, or hanging yourself?" A series of questions combined in this way is called a cannon question, which frequently leads to invalid information because patients only hear parts of them or choose to respond to only one question in the string. (p. 390)

Symptom Amplification

Patients often minimize problematic behavior. For example, they may describe less frequent drinking behavior or less of a feeling of suicidality than they actually experience. Shea (2004) indicates that a clinician can bypass this tendency by setting the upper limits of the feeling or behavior at a high amount. When the client subsequently minimizes the feeling or behavior, it is often then closer to the actual amount. Shea gives the following example:

For example, a clinician may ask, "How much liquor can you hold in a single night—a pint or a fifth?" The patient may respond, "Oh no, not a fifth, I don't know maybe a pint." The clinician is still alerted that there is a problem despite the patient's minimizations. (p. 391)

A similar approach can be used in the case of suicidal thoughts:

"On the days when your thoughts of suicide were most intense, how much of the day did you spend thinking about killing yourself—50%, 80%, 90% of the day?"
Clinicians must be careful not to set the upper limit at such a high number that it seems absurd or even creates the appearance that the interviewer doesn't know what he or she is talking about. (p. 391)

Critical Elements of Suicide Risk Assessment: Ideation, Plan and Intent

There are three critical elements of any suicide risk assessment: (1) ideation, (2) plan, and (3) intent (Jobes, 2006; Shea, 2002; Wofsy et al., 2009).

Assessment of Ideation

The discussion of suicidal ideation begins when the client first expresses thoughts involving ending his or her life. There are three main aspects of the assessment of these thoughts. The first relates to the *duration* of the thoughts. The clinician should ask the client, "How long have you been having these thoughts?" The *frequency* of the thoughts refers to the question "How often do these thoughts occur?" The third aspect of the suicidal ideation refers to the *intensity* of the thoughts. To ascertain this, the therapist should ask, "How strong and intrusive do you experience these thoughts?" It is also important for the therapist to validate the client for sharing his or her thoughts and experience. This honest reporting is a potential protective factor. Sharing feelings of suicidality may indicate that there is some ambivalence on the client's part and that he or she wants help. Further, once the client makes the clinician aware of the client's suicidal ideation, the clinician has the opportunity to intervene and further support the client in how he or she responds to these feelings.

Assessment for a Suicide Plan

The plan refers to the method of self-harm. The first question in this part of the assessment should explore whether the client has a plan for self-harm. The therapist should then explore that plan in detail. Once this has been done, the clinician should assess the following three characteristics of the plan (Jobes, 2006; Shea, 2002): (1) accessibility (Does the client have access to the stated method?), (2) lethality (How severe is the method?), and (3) feasibility (How likely is this to occur?).

Assessment for Intent

Intent refers to the question of whether the client has the motivation and desire to actually carry out this plan. The two examples below illustrate low intent versus strong intent:

- *Example of low intent:* "I hate my life, and I often feel like not waking up, but I would never really do anything because of my children."
- *Example of strong intent*: "I cannot go on. I can't guarantee that I could be safe overnight."

Other Aspects of Suicide Risk Assessment

There are five additional areas that should be addressed as a part of a suicide risk assessment. These include (1) precipitating factors, (2) medical condition, (3) past history of depression and suicide attempts, (4) medication considerations, and (5) substance abuse (Wofsy et al.,

2009). Precipitating factors refer to any life events that may have led up to or contributed to the suicidal ideation. The possibilities are idiosyncratic to each client but they may include the loss of a relationship, trauma or the reexperiencing of a traumatic event(s), or the death of a loved one. Chronic or life-threatening medical conditions (e.g., cancer) or ongoing experiences of chronic pain can also lead to suicidal ideation.

It is also important to assess the past history of depression and suicide attempts. Has the person had suicidal thoughts or ideation in the past? If so, when and what were the precipitating factors? Has the person attempted suicide in the past? What was the nature and the degree of this attempt(s)? Was the person hospitalized? Is there a neurobiological vulnerability to depression or to bipolar disorder? Has the client been feeling profoundly depressed? For how long? It is also important to explore whether there is a family history of suicide attempts.

Clients who have been taking medication may be vulnerable if there has been a change in their medication recently. It is necessary to assess whether the client has been on medication in the past and whether or not they have been taking their medication. If not, it is important to inquire as to how long they have not been taking their medication. Substance use and abuse is also a serious risk factor as it can lead to increased impulsivity that may underlie an attempt. The clinician should therefore inquire about current and past substance abuse including the substance(s) of choice.

Assessing the Degree of Suicidal Risk

If all three critical elements—ideation, intent, and plan—are strongly positive, the degree of risk is high (Jobes, 2006; Shea, 2002; Wofsy et al., 2009). In this case, interventions designed to stabilize the crisis and keep the client safe (i.e., calling 911, seeking an assessment in an emergency room, and hospitalization), should be the first line of response. As we have stated throughout this chapter, clinicians in this situation should never do this on their own. They should utilize and rely on the support of supervisors, senior administrators, and clinicians who are experienced in suicide risk assessment.

The challenge, however, is that the degree of risk becomes less clearly defined when the client does not endorse all three critical elements. In these circumstances, clinical judgment and targeted safety planning become paramount. It is also important to assess the degree of family and/or friend support that might be available to the client. If possible, it is helpful to obtain phone numbers and addresses for those individuals.

Case Example

Susan, a 14-year-old White female struggling with depression, was new to treatment. She was in her therapist's office for her second session following an incident at school where she submitted a poem to her English teacher with themes of death and dying. In the session, she reported that she felt emotionally and socially isolated from family and peers. She noted that she regularly woke up in the morning feeling that "life would be better if I were not here."

Assessment of Suicidal Ideation

There was a history of depression and suicide on Susan's paternal side of the family. When asked if she had ever had thoughts of hurting herself, she stated that sometimes she had thoughts of taking a handful of Tylenol. Susan denied any previous suicide attempts and stated, "I could never do that to my family." The therapist validated her honesty and asked her to tell him more about those thoughts. When asked how long she has been having these thoughts, she stated that she has had them "on and off for over a year." The therapist then explored what might have happened around the time that she had begun having these thoughts. Susan stated that her parents had started really fighting and were talking about divorce. She indicated that their relationship had been "a roller coaster" for the last year but that they had actually separated last month. Susan admitted that she was feeling the loss of her father who had recently moved out.

The therapist then explored the frequency with which Susan had these thoughts. She reported that usually they did not occur often but that in the last month since her father moved out, she had experienced them about once per week. When the clinician explored how strong and intrusive these thoughts were, Susan explained that they would occur at different times. She had found herself thinking about them during her English class as she was writing the essay on death and dying. She repeated again that she would never do this to her family.

Assessment of the Client's Plan

The nature of Susan's plan was assessed next. She was vague but she mentioned again that she had thought about taking Tylenol. When asked how many she would take, she reported that she had no idea. The therapist then asked about the accessibility of Tylenol in her home. Susan reported that she had not checked but that she was pretty sure she could find some.

Although this plan was vague, the therapist was concerned about the feasibility because of the ready availability of Tylenol.

Assessment of the Client's Intent

In assessing for intent, the therapist explored Susan's motivation to carry out this plan. Susan responded that she did not really want to die but she felt so down and depressed since her parents' separation that she didn't feel like continuing to live.

Validation of the Client's Strengths

The therapist validated Susan's strengths and told her, "It was really important that you felt empowered and safe enough to come and speak with me about this." He also validated that this seemed to be a very upsetting time for her. He observed that there seemed to be many different feelings that she was having and many different parts of those feelings. He then aligned with Susan's strengths and the part of her that wanted help by saying, "The part of you that came here today is that part that is reaching out for help. I know that you are feeling really bad right now, but I would like to partner up with the part that got you here today to support you in being safe."

The therapist then told Susan that he really cared about her and was concerned that she might hurt herself because she was feeling so sad.

Therapist Calls His Supervisor and Clinic Psychiatrist

The therapist told Susan that he would like to get some more help for her and that he would phone his supervisor and ask the supervisor to come down and talk with them about this. He called his supervisor and stepped outside of the room briefly in order to update her on his discussion with Susan.

The supervisor then joined the session and repeated the assessment of her ideation, plan, and intent. At the end of the session, the supervisor told Susan that she shared her therapist's concern and that they would need to meet with Susan's parents in order to figure out how to keep her safe. The supervisor asked for both of Susan's parents' phone numbers and the therapist called and asked them to meet her at the clinic as soon as possible. In the meantime, the therapist asked the psychiatrist to also conduct an assessment of Susan.

Assessment of Risk, Triggers, and Protective Factors

The therapist and psychiatrist then explored the risk and protective factors in Susan's life. They first explored the risk factors and asked about the triggers that had led her to feel suicidal. A fight between her parents was a large trigger and one had occurred the day before. When asked to describe it she stated that her father had come to the house to talk with her mother about visitation with Susan and her younger sister. An angry verbal argument ensued. Susan denied domestic violence between them. Susan denied substance abuse but acknowledged again that Tylenol might be readily available in her home.

They then explored the protective factors. She reported that she loved her family including her sister, father, and mother, and that the thought of the divorce was "tearing her apart." She denied suicidal intent.

Family Involvement

Susan's mother and father arrived at the clinic in separate cars about an hour later. The therapist and his supervisor met with Susan and her parents. The therapist helped Susan to tell her parents what she was experiencing. They were shocked at the degree of her depression and her suicidal thoughts.

They began arguing about whose fault this was. The therapist interrupted and acknowledged that they seemed angry at each other. He shared, however, that he sensed that they both loved Susan a great deal. He told them that their daughter desperately needed them to set their differences aside for the moment and work with them to address her depression and suicidal thoughts and to come up with a plan for her safety. They both agreed.

The therapist asked both parents to agree to come for family therapy so that these issues could be addressed with Susan. He also made an agreement for daily individual sessions with Susan in order to monitor her feelings over the next week.

Contract for Safety with the Client and Her Family

The therapist and his supervisor then spoke with Susan about whether she felt that she could make a contract for safety with them. They explained the process to her and she agreed. They also asked her parents whether they would agree to help to implement the safety plan for her. Susan, her parents, and the treatment team all agreed to the following plan:

1. Susan agreed not to attempt to take her life.
2. Her parents agreed to a 24-hour suicide watch in which one of them was always with Susan during that time.
3. Susan agreed to see her therapist each day for the next week and to continue ongoing individual therapy sessions.
4. The parents agreed to meet together with Susan and her sister as a family the next day in order to discuss these issues further.
5. The parents also agreed to ongoing family therapy sessions.
6. Both parents agreed to search their apartments and to remove all pills and place them in a locked area.

7. Susan agreed to contact her therapist and her parents if she began to have the suicidal thoughts again.
8. Susan and her parents agreed to go to the local emergency room should the feelings intensify in off-hours or when they were unable to reach the therapist.
9. Susan and her parents agreed to discuss and identify precipitating events and known triggers before the next session and to share them with the therapist in the next session.

Follow–Up

Although Susan was not hospitalized, the therapist continued to assess and monitor her suicidal potential on an ongoing basis throughout the course of therapy. He encouraged her to continue to be open and honest regarding her suicidal impulses and reassured her regularly of his own and her family's caring and concern. Ongoing treatment led to a lifting of her depressed mood and she no longer reported suicidal thoughts.

Family treatment continued and Susan was able to address her emotional upset to her parents about their separation and her fears about their divorce. In a later session, she was able to indicate to her parents with her therapist's help that she was afraid that she had done something to cause their separation and pending divorce. The therapist normalized these feelings and helped the parents to clearly state to her that she was not responsible in any way for their separation and divorce and that they both loved her and would always be there for her.

Preserving the Therapeutic Relationship Postpsychiatric Hospitalization

Although the case example above did not result in a psychiatric hospitalization, risk assessments of suicidal ideation can often lead to this outcome. The emergency room is a useful intervention for situations where there is immediate risk and danger to self or others. This may lead to a psychiatric hospitalization. In these cases, clients are often angry with the therapist for this hospitalization. It is important that the therapist work to express care and concern directly to the client and to ally with the part of the client that wants to survive. The following case illustrates this process.

Ronald, a 56-year-old African American man, came into a session with his therapist and reported strong suicidal ideation. He was a former police officer, had a gun, and had thought about "blowing his brains out."

Assessment of Suicidal Ideation

The therapist explored this suicidal ideation and asked how long he had been having these thoughts. Ronald reported that it was the anniversary of the death of his partner on the police force. They had been ambushed one night and Ronald's partner was killed. Ronald was wounded and was unable to save his partner's life. This incident had occurred 1 year ago and this was the first anniversary of the event.

When the therapist explored how long he had been having these thoughts he said that he had experienced them since the beginning of the month and that they were becoming stronger as he approached the anniversary of his partner's death. The therapist explored the frequency of these thoughts and Ronald reported that he had been "haunted by these thoughts constantly for the last month." When the therapist explored the strength and intensity of these thoughts, Ronald reported that they were strong.

Assessment of the Client's Plan and Intent

Ronald was very clear that his plan was to go home, take out his gun, load it, and "eat the bullet" (shoot himself through the mouth). He indicated that he had his service revolver in a box in his closet at home. Given that this method was lethal, and that the plan was clear and seemed feasible, the therapist was concerned that Ronald's potential for committing suicide was great. The therapist felt that Ronald's intent was strong and he was so depressed that he would commit suicide.

Validation of the Client's Strengths

The therapist validated Ronald's strength in coming in for the session. He indicated that he understood the intensity of the feelings that he was having and his reasons for wanting to kill himself. He also indicated that he cared about Ronald and did not want to see him die.

Exploration of Risk and Protective Factors

The therapist explored the risk factors and was clear that having the gun in the house increased the likelihood that he would commit suicide. He explored Ronald's network to see if he had any supports. Ronald reported that he was isolated and the only person in his life was his son, who "had his own life" and "checked in" on him every few months. He also indicated that this son had a key to his apartment and would come in even if he refused to answer the door. The therapist asked for his son's phone number and told Ronald that he was really concerned about him. Ronald was angry and said that he did not want his son involved.

The Therapist Contacts His Supervisor and the Client Is Hospitalized

The therapist told Ronald that he was so concerned that he wanted to ask his supervisor to step in and meet with them. Ronald refused. He became agitated, stormed out of the office, and left the building. At his supervisor's suggestion, the therapist called the mobile crisis unit and asked them to go immediately to Ronald's home. They intervened and transported Ronald to the emergency room at the nearby psychiatric hospital and he was hospitalized. The therapist then contacted Ronald's son and asked him to remove the gun from the closet in his father's apartment.

The Therapist Contacts the Psychiatrist on the Inpatient Unit

Because of the seriousness of his suicidal ideation, Ronald was hospitalized. His therapist contacted the inpatient psychiatrist and arranged to have a meeting with Ronald before his discharge. Ronald was still angry about the hospitalization but he agreed to the meeting. During the meeting, the therapist explored Ronald's feelings about the hospitalization. He reported that he was actually glad now that he had not committed suicide but that he was angry about the therapist's intervention of sending the mobile unit to hospitalize him. The therapist acknowledged Ronald's mixed feelings about his suicidality and his anger at the therapist about his hospitalization. The therapist aligned himself with the part of this client that wanted to survive. The therapist acknowledged that there was a part of Ronald that wanted to commit suicide but there was also a part of him that was reaching out for help—that part had brought him to the clinic to meet with the therapist. The therapist added, "I care about you and I know that you are angry with me but I don't want to see you die; I want to see you live." By the end of the session, although still angry about the hospitalization, Ronald agreed to return and continue to work with the therapist in outpatient therapy.

Contract for Safety

Ronald agreed to contract for safety before his discharge from the hospital. The therapist, the inpatient psychiatrist, and Ronald discussed the following agreement:

1. Ronald would commit to attending a day treatment program within the clinic where the therapist worked.
2. He would see his outpatient therapist three times during the first week after discharge and twice per week in subsequent weeks.
3. Ronald agreed to continue taking the antidepressant medication that he had received on the inpatient unit after his discharge.
4. He agreed to tell his therapist if his suicidal feelings returned.

5. He agreed to go to the emergency room at the hospital if those feelings returned.
6. The therapist explored Ronald's network with him. He agreed to participate in some family sessions with his adult son and the therapist.

Follow-Up

Ronald attended the day treatment program for the next 3 months. His therapist continued providing individual therapy twice per week during this time and after his discharge from the day treatment program. Ronald continued on antidepressant medication and was able to work in therapy to resolve the guilt that he felt about his partner's death.

Clinical Risk Consultation Team (CRCT) and Clinical Case Conferences or Roundtable Discussions

As mentioned throughout this book, clinicians at varying levels of experience and training often find themselves in difficult clinical situations where they must evaluate the acute or ongoing risk presented by clients. This is often an extremely stressful aspect of clinical work and one for which many new clinicians are not adequately prepared. In order to support clinicians in the ongoing process of risk assessment, we have found that the development of an agencywide *Clinical Risk Consultation Team* (CRCT; Blady & Cleek, 2010; Blady, Cleek & Kamnitzer, 2009; Campanelli, 2010; Pappas & Howard, 2009; Wofsy et al,, 2009) is one of the most helpful interventions. It is important to note that this section describes one model for the management of clinical risk; it is our hope that different agencies will choose to incorporate some of these ideas and adapt this model to their own needs and staffing requirements.

The CRCT is a time-sensitive, multilevel crisis response team designed to support clinical and other program staff with focused, agencywide expertise around high-risk cases (Blady & Cleek, 2010; Blady et al., 2009; Wofsy et al., 2009). This team is composed of two standing members, who are senior supervisors or clinical staff with a high degree of expertise, who have had many years of experience in providing risk assessment and management. It is important to note that in some instances, the CRCT serves a debriefing function after the emergency aspects of the crisis have been addressed and the client is safe from harm. In these situations, it provides an opportunity for staff to learn from the experience and develop treatment plans for future interventions.

The first function of the CRCT is to respond to crises in a time-sensitive manner. The goal is to provide case disposition, recommendations, and preliminary support within 48 hours of receiving the referral. (In emergency cases, the therapist and supervisor may have already taken action.) When a referral is received from a clinician or supervisor, one of the standing team members reaches out to the person making the referral. A full team is then convened with members whose expertise is most applicable to the needs of the client being presented. Program-specific clinical consultation and crisis intervention can then be conducted. (Blady & Cleek, 2010; Blady et al., 2009; Wofsy et al., 2009). This clinical consultation might include the referring therapist and supervisor, other clinicians and senior staff in the agency, and in some cases, the client, family, and outside agency participation, if necessary.

Another focus of the CRCT is the opportunity for ongoing learning and support for clinical staff. Clinicians and trainees throughout the agency can be invited to present at case conferences or clinical roundtables. At these meetings, cases requiring a risk assessment, or cases where a risk assessment has occurred and debriefing is necessary, are presented. This process provides a valuable opportunity to learn from and reflect on risk and crisis cases (Blady & Cleek, 2010; Blady et al., 2009; Campanelli, 2010; Pappas & Howard, 2009). Clinical roundtables can also provide an opportunity for clinicians and staff to brainstorm with other colleagues, clinical experts, the client, and the client's significant others including spiritual leaders, family members, and/or other loved ones in a different context or environment. Depending on the need and the time available, these meetings can be scheduled on an "as needed" or ongoing basis for clinical support and learning. Some clinics have established an ongoing case conference time in which all clinical and case management staff meet to discuss challenging cases (Wofsy & Mundy, 2009).

This process can be an excellent opportunity for staff training and can create a collaborative and supportive approach to continuing education for everyone. It can also be a part of an agencywide initiative to provide preventive and treatment guidelines for managing acute and ongoing risk. Over time, this can lead to more clearly defined policies that map out risk reporting procedures.

Administrative Support for Staff

In our experience, the development of a Clinical Risk Consultation Team (CRCT) and a Clinical Case Conference Roundtable are two of the most important investments that an agency can make in quality assurance in terms of client care. They are also an antidote to staff burnout and provide clear support for "front-line" clinicians and supervisors by conveying a strong message that they are not alone with these difficult risk assessments and clinical decisions. This overall administrative philosophy is particularly important in the current environment in which productivity requirements clearly impact agency and program survival in this time of economic pressures (Pappas & Howard, 2009). It provides clinical staff with additional tools and strategies to support the integrated and coordinated assessment and intervention of clinical risk for all clients. This can improve the lives of persons served by our clinics and hospitals whose diagnoses and life circumstances predispose them to a higher risk of harm to self and others. It can also reduce the risk that agencies and staff assume in working with the most vulnerable clinical populations.

The CRCT and Clinical Case Conference Roundtables can also improve communication within an agency and within and between programs, as well as among clinicians, case managers, supervisors, and administrators. These clinical forums also provide excellent opportunities for training and consultation and the creation of a culture of responsibility that empowers all staff to develop strategies to intervene early and effectively (Campanelli, 2010).

The following section provides case examples of the use of a CRCT in supporting clinical and program staff working with high-risk cases. Because so many of the cases in this chapter have focused on risk assessment for suicide, we have chosen three cases below to illustrate the use of the CRCT that involve other forms of risk. The first case illustrates the use of the CRCT for a dual-diagnosed client engaging in a number of risky behaviors related to her alcohol abuse. The second case provides an example of the use of the CRCT with a client who has recently begun cutting again and for whom a risk assessment is done to rule out suicidal ideation. The third case examines the efforts of the CRCT team following an incident of homicidal ideation and intent. (See Chapter 14 for a more in-depth examination of crisis management around violence and homicidal risk and behaviors.) It is important to note that in each of these cases, the CRCT was utilized by the primary therapist and clinic staff to support treatment efforts and provide clarity during and following a high-risk situation.

Clinical Risk Consultation Team: Case Example 1

Dual Diagnosis: Risky Behaviors Related to Alcohol Abuse

Isaura, a 45-year-old Latina diagnosed with schizoaffective disorder, was referred to an outpatient clinic by her congregate residence for persons struggling with dual diagnosis, (i.e., mental illness and substance abuse). She had a significant history of homelessness, trauma, and alcohol abuse.

She was sexually abused by her stepfather and older brother throughout her childhood. At age 17 she ran away from home, and began engaging in a cycle of homelessness, transitioning in and out of shelters, rehabilitation programs, and residential treatment centers. Her only family contact since that time had been inconsistent phone calls with a sister who lived in another state. Initially, Isaura was engaged in therapy and attended consistently. The therapist became concerned when Isaura's attendance started to decrease. At this time, the case manager at the residence informed the therapist that Isaura's alcohol use had increased to the point of daily intoxication. She was panhandling on the subway, and recently had to receive emergency medical care due to a late-night fall while walking home inebriated. The case manager alluded that there was also some indication that Isaura was engaging in potentially risky sexual behavior while intoxicated. When confronted empathically by the therapist about these behaviors, Isaura verbalized that these were the behaviors of someone with a death wish.

The Therapist and Supervisor Call for a CRCT Meeting

Upon hearing this statement, the therapist consulted her supervisor and they decided to refer the case to the CRCT. The client was invited to the CRCT meeting but she refused to come. The therapist arranged for the client's case manager and the residence director to participate in the CRCT meeting via telephone. The CRCT also secured the presence of the clinic's substance abuse specialist.

At the meeting, a comprehensive case description was presented and areas of risk, strengths, and protective factors were identified and explored. The first area of concern for the program staff was how to respond from a harm reduction perspective to someone who was choosing to put herself in danger while in a treatment program. Though Isaura's behavior was increasingly reckless, she always presented as competent and willing to engage in a discussion. The participants in the meeting struggled with the question of how to respond when the element of risk is high, yet the client is exercising a level of choice and autonomy. After a careful group discussion in which it was decided that Isaura was competent, lucid, and not presenting any imminent danger to herself or to others, the team agreed that hospitalization was not an option.

This meeting allowed for divergent perspectives on the case to enter the conversation and created an increased appreciation for the client's self-determination and stage of change. This perspective had a softening effect for both the therapist and the case manager, who were concerned about the client and about their role in trying to help her. Both the therapist and the case manager were given the green light to pull back and not "overfunction" in reaction to the client's continued "underfunctioning." It was also decided that motivational interviewing strategies were needed to reconnect the client with her values and meaning in life. At the CRCT meeting, individuals not involved in the case asked the therapist and case manager what was important to the client. Both the therapist and case manager identified the client's relationship with her sister as a core value. The team then provided the therapist with ideas and strategies to engage the sister and procure her involvement. It was agreed that if the sister attended the next therapy session either in person or by phone that it would increase Isaura's motivation to utilize services and engage in safety measures.

Involvement of the Client's Family Member

Following the CRCT meeting, and with Isaura's written permission, the therapist reached out to Isaura's sister. The sister agreed to participate via phone in a session with the case manager present. Isaura was curious about the sister's involvement. In the session, the therapist and case manager echoed the sister's concern and emphasized the importance of avoiding life-threatening situations. The therapist utilized MI to develop the discrepancy between Isaura's expressed desires to move on with her life and one day go back to school versus her current high-risk behaviors. Because it was felt that the first priority was to stabilize her alcohol use, the therapist and case manager suggested rehab. The client, in tears, agreed to enter a rehab program and was admitted later that day.

Discussion of CRCT Interventions

Through the CRCT, the therapist and case manager were able to access support from individuals with varying levels of expertise who collectively provided insight and strategies that would otherwise not be available. The therapist and the case manager left the CRCT meeting with concrete next steps and specific clinical interventions to facilitate these next steps. The case discussion deepened the work and provided members of Isaura's treatment team with requisite anxiety management and the strategies to utilize recommended interventions effectively.

Clinical Risk Consultation Team: Case Example 2

Cutting and Self-Harm

Martha, a 21-year-old African American female client, who had been in treatment at an outpatient clinic for 6 months, reported to her therapist that following a fight with her boyfriend the night before, she had locked herself in the bathroom and cut herself with a razor blade. She had made six cuts on the inside of her left arm. She had no history of suicide attempts but had a long history of cutting.

Exploration of the Cutting

All six cuts were surface cuts that resulted in bleeding. She pulled up her sleeve and showed her therapist. She denied any suicidal intent and explained that she actually enjoyed cutting and did not want to stop. When the therapist pursued the function of Martha's cutting, she explained that it helped her to deal with the anger and pain around the fight with her boyfriend and allowed her to feel more in control. She also stated that she felt calmer and relieved after the cutting.

The therapist then explored the role of the self-harm in more detail. She asked if this was something that Martha did often. Martha replied that she did it only when she was extremely upset. The therapist then asked how often Martha had cut, and she reported that she had not done it in the last year. She stated that, as a teenager, she cut herself more often because it was a stressful time for her. The therapist explored in detail what Martha used to cut herself, and Martha stated that it was consistently a razor blade.

When the therapist explored what she was thinking about while cutting herself, Martha mentioned the pain of the fight with her boyfriend, which had resulted after a friend had revealed that she had seen Martha's boyfriend "hanging out" with another woman. When Martha confronted her boyfriend, an angry fight ensued that resulted in Martha cutting when she returned home.

Exploration of Suicidal Ideation, Plan, and Intent

The therapist then carefully returned to the question of suicidal ideation. The client denied all suicidal ideation and reported that she did not want to die, she just wanted to get control of her feelings and cutting helped her do that. Martha denied a plan to kill herself. She reported she knew how deep to cut so as not to "go too far."

Exploration of Risk and Protective Factors

The therapist and Martha explored current risk factors for cutting, including the availability of razor blades, which Martha described as only "a drug store away." Martha also lived alone and had been isolating herself from her support systems. In terms of protective factors, it was clear that even though she was upset, Martha had a good relationship with her therapist and had been able to get herself to her appointments. She was talking openly with her therapist about her feelings around the argument and cutting incident. Although Martha had been isolating over the last few weeks, she did have a sister, whom she was close to, and a number of friends who were a support to her.

The Therapist Consults Her Supervisor and the Psychiatrist

The therapist explained to Martha that she was concerned for her and wanted to ask her supervisor to meet with them in order to discuss ways to keep Martha safe. The therapist then called her supervisor, who joined the session. The supervisor questioned Martha carefully about the cutting and did another suicide risk assessment. The supervisor told Martha that she would also like to have the clinic psychiatrist join them. Following their discussion with Martha and the therapist, the supervisor and psychiatrist did not feel that Martha needed hospitalization but were concerned for her safety.

Contract for Safety

The therapist, supervisor, and psychiatrist asked Martha for written permission to contact her sister. They discussed her plans for the weekend and asked if she could stay with someone so that she would not be alone. Martha agreed to stay with her sister and to turn over all razor blades and contract for safety. She also agreed not to cut herself or harm herself over the weekend. The therapist arranged for Martha to wait at the clinic until her sister arrived and the therapist then reviewed the safety plan with Martha and her sister. Her sister was given the number of the psychiatric emergency room at the closest hospital and was encouraged to call 911 if she became concerned about Martha over the weekend. Martha and her sister also agreed to meet with the therapist in the coming week for a family session.

Martha agreed to see her therapist and the psychiatrist on Monday morning. For the next month she was seen in twice-weekly therapy and met with her psychiatrist on a weekly basis.

Clinical Risk Consultation Team Meeting

Because of the seriousness of Martha's case, the therapist and her supervisor agreed to present the case to the CRCT and encouraged all of the staff and supervisors in the clinic to attend in order to debrief on this difficult case. The psychiatrist, a member of the CRCT, began the discussion with a presentation on cutting and self-harm as well as the need for a suicide risk assessment. The therapist then presented Martha's case. The clinical staff benefited from the opportunity to explore the relevant risk and protective factors in Martha's case, and the ability to discuss how to make differential assessments of self-harm versus suicidal risk.

Clinical Risk Consultation Team: Case Example 3

Assessment of Homicidal Risk

Jordan, a 16-year-old White male, was being seen by a therapist in outpatient therapy due to his increased oppositional behavior at home and at school. In the past 3 months, he had been breaking into houses and getting high with his friends. He had also missed multiple therapy appointments.

During one of his therapy sessions, he reported that the night before, after getting into an argument with his stepmother, his father had threatened to send him away to military school. Jordan reported that he had no intention of going to military school and that he would rather kill his family than "allow that witch to kick me out of the home." During the previous night, he had thoughts of stabbing his parents while they were sleeping.

Exploration of Homicidal Ideation, Plan, and Intent

When the therapist explored Jordan's thoughts about his parents, it was clear that he was still in a rage at them. In response to the therapist's questions, he described how he had thought of using a kitchen knife and had actually brought one into his room the night before. It was clear that he would have easy access to kitchen knives at his home. Throughout the session, Jordan's rage at his parents continued and he continued to state clear homicidal ideation.

Therapist Calls in an Experienced Clinician

As this session occurred at 6:00 P.M., after the therapist's supervisor and clinic psychiatrist had left the building, the therapist called a senior colleague whose office was a few doors away. The senior therapist met with the client and the therapist and helped to make the decision to call 911 to transport the client to the emergency room. The therapist called the client's parents and asked them to meet him at the emergency room. He then called the psychiatric emergency room, gave them the necessary information on the client, and told them that the client would be arriving shortly.

Emergency Room and Hospitalization

At the emergency room, the therapist briefed the staff and stayed with the client until he could be evaluated by the psychiatrist on call. The psychiatrist made the decision to hospitalize Jordan. The psychiatrist and Jordan's therapist then met with the parents and discussed the events of the evening and the decision for hospitalization.

During his first month in the hospital, it was clear to the staff that Jordan's anger at his parents had not lessened even after intensive individual and family therapy sessions. The clinical staff made the decision that he should remain in the hospital until an application could be made for a residential treatment center that had a good family therapy program. The family agreed to be involved in his treatment.

Clinical Risk Consultation Team Meeting

The clinical decisions in this case had to be made quickly within a crisis intervention framework. Once again, the purpose of the follow-up CRCT meeting was to debrief with clinical staff and to establish clear guidelines for emergency-room referral with a client with clear homicidal ideation, plan, and intent. Involving the clinical staff and trainees in this debriefing process helped to underscore the high risk in this case. They were also able to discuss processes and procedures related to decision making in similar situations. For example, they reviewed the process of accessing help from clinic supervisors and senior clinicians when the person's usual supervisor was not available, and decision making regarding the need for hospitalization when homicidal intent was involved.

Conclusion

This chapter has reviewed the real-world risks that surface in clinical work and has offered specific ways to view these risks and intervene when a client exhibits a heightened potential for harm. Clinicians should never feel alone in these kinds of situations, and best practice is to always consult with others, whether that involves a supervisor, psychiatrist, or senior staff member. We also recommend that agencies address risk in a coordinated, multisystemic way so that clinicians and other staff can feel supported in working with high-risk clients. Addressing risk in a more formal process through case conferences and clinical risk consultation teams can provide a forum for agency dialogue around high-risk situations and can serve to empower clinicians who face similar client situations (Campanelli, 2010). This proactive stance can lay a strong foundation for risk assessment and management among therapists and clinic staff, and can serve to minimize risk in the future.

CHAPTER 14

Crisis Intervention in Clinics, Schools, and Communities

Responses to Violence, Suicide, and Homicide

Introduction

Crisis intervention and management as well as posttrauma interventions have become an important and increasing component of therapy in the real world. When traumatic events occur, clinic or hospital staff, parents, school administrators, and community members typically turn to mental health professionals, guidance counselors, psychologists, social workers, licensed professional counselors, family therapists, clergy, and pastoral counselors for help in managing the aftermath of the tragedy. Few clinicians, however, have received explicit training in such posttraumatic interventions.

Unlike the individual risk and suicide assessments discussed in the last chapter, this chapter addresses the process of managing the aftermath for the survivors of sudden traumatic experiences or loss related to violence, suicide, and homicide in clinics, schools, and communities (Underwood & Dunne-Maxim, 1997; Underwood et al., 2010). Many of the principles discussed in this chapter—such as elements of the emotional response to violence, administrative responses following traumatic events, and prevention—can provide a framework for addressing other forms of violence or sudden traumatic loss, including those following natural disasters, terrorism, and school shootings, such as Columbine and Sandy Hook Elementary School.

Underwood and Dunne-Maxim (1997) recommend a "proactive

planning process" through which "wise administrators put in place policies that address the procedures to follow during a crisis" (p. 15). If your clinic, school, or community has not yet had to address the issue of a sudden trauma or traumatic loss, this chapter will give you the information you need to advocate for the creation of a crisis response team. In a clinic or mental health center, this team might include senior supervisors and/or administrators. Within a school district, this might include the superintendent, principals of different schools, and representatives from guidance departments, child study teams, and crisis response teams found in the broader community (e.g., hospitals, community mental health centers, local psychologists, psychiatrists, social workers, family therapists, and members of the clergy). The group can pool resources in terms of training utilizing Underwood and Dunne-Maxim and Underwood et al.'s (2010) work as policy guides.

With this in mind, this chapter presents three different examples of postcrisis intervention responses in different traumatic circumstances. The first addresses a violent incident in a clinic and the subsequent responses to help staff and clients process this experience. The second involves the suicide of a young adolescent in a middle school and the subsequent interventions to help the students, teachers, counselors, administrators, parents, and families at the school. The third example involves a homicide in the community in which mental health professionals, school staff, a local minister, and community members work together to address the crisis.

Responses to Violence

One aspect of our work in the mental health field that is rarely discussed is the risk that our clients can sometimes present in terms of the potential for violence. With this in mind, some inpatient units are now providing training for staff on the identification of and appropriate responses to violence (North Shore Long Island Jewish Healthcare System-Syosset Hospital, 2012). It is still unusual for many outpatient clinics or mental health centers, however, to even discuss this possibility with staff or to provide explicit training in this area. The following case example illustrates the traumatic experience of violence within a clinic setting and the helpful and appropriate administrative and clinical response.

Following a traumatic event at an outpatient mental health facility, the Director enlisted the support of two senior supervisors, a psychologist and a social worker, to assist staff with processing their stress. Supervisory staff were encouraged to make time available for all staff to convene and process the previous night's events both as a group and, if need be, individually.

Upon the arrival of the two supervisors at the clinic, it was revealed that a clinician was violently assaulted in the waiting room of the facility, resulting in the calling of Emergency Medical Services (EMS). This individual was admitted to the hospital for 24-hour observation after being punched in the head from behind. As expected, clinic staff at all levels were feeling shaken and vulnerable. Though authorities were called as soon as the clinician was assaulted, the assailant immediately fled after the event and was still at large. In processing the event with the clinic supervisor, the two senior supervisors learned that the assailant was known to the clinic as he was the stepfather of a daughter and husband of a mother with open charts at the clinic.

As the senior supervisors talked with the staff, they reconstructed the following series of events. In a session the previous week with the assigned therapist, the mother had encouraged the daughter to speak openly about being inappropriately touched in a sexually suggestive manner by her stepfather. The clinician consulted the supervisor and was immediately advised to contact child protective services (CPS). When CPS arrived at the house, the stepfather absconded. Upon investigation of the allegation, CPS assessed that there was risk and the authorities were contacted. The mother and child were relocated to stay at a cousin's house, and the stepfather was nowhere to be found. The stepfather had been an unstable presence in the family treatment. He attended therapy inconsistently, presented as volatile at times, and was noted to have a history of violence.

Four days following the call to CPS, the stepfather entered the clinic and informed front desk staff that he was there to see the family therapist. He presented as calm, and was told that the therapist was in session and that he was free to wait. He sat in the waiting room. When the therapist finished her session, she escorted the client to the reception desk to schedule a follow-up appointment, at which point the stepfather approached her from behind and hit her in the head with a closed fist. She fell to the ground and the stepfather kicked her before yelling a threat to all staff and running out of the clinic. The therapist was taken away in an ambulance and staff spent the rest of the evening working with the clients who had witnessed the event. Over the next week, staff members who were treating clients who had witnessed the event met with their clients again to help them to process this traumatic event. These clinicians received direct supervision and advice from the two senior supervisors. In addition, while the clinician was in the hospital, another supervisor in the clinic worked with the mother and child whose stepfather had been responsible for the attack. They were especially traumatized by this experience as they were still processing the revelation of the sexual abuse that had occurred.

It was determined after hearing this account that the initial need was for staff to convene and process the event from the night before. Staff members were feeling vulnerable, at risk, and not taken care of. The group convened and the supervisor, with the support of the two clinical supervisors, detailed the precise, known facts of the events that had transpired, and the subsequent safety measures that had been put in place. The police had been notified and made commitments to drive by the clinic every hour in their pursuit of the individual. All staff in the building were informed to be on the lookout for this individual and instructed to call the authorities and notify the supervisor should this individual appear.

The senior clinical supervisors then facilitated a group discussion with all staff, where they were given the opportunity to engage in mutual aid and support and to collectively process the previous evening's attack. Common themes included the discomfort of sitting with uncertainty and unpredictability, feeling isolated, angry, and looking to blame upper administration. In an effort to keep the dialogue constructive, the specialists normalized staff reaction and reframed the event as something that had happened to every employee and client at the clinic. The senior supervisors assured staff that measures would be put in place to avoid future assaults like this, but also recognized that there is a level of risk involved in this line of work. After reminding staff of the Employee Assistance Program (EAP) resources at their disposal, they made themselves available for the rest of the day for any staff that would want to utilize one-on-one support. A few staff members took advantage of this resource. The front desk staff member most involved with the event was concerned with his role in the attack, and a fellow clinician who had remained in her office out of fear during the event was struggling with her guilty feelings about this. Yet another staff member was struggling with feelings tied to a previous trauma triggered by this episode. The senior supervisors normalized these reactions, provided empathy and support, encouraged ventilation, and recommended utilization of EAP.

The two senior supervisors continued to meet with the staff weekly, both individually and in a group, and to consult on high-risk cases regularly over the next 2 months. They provided a supportive and comforting presence for the staff. Upon a subsequent, clinical review of the case, additional opportunities for risk assessment and intervention were identified. Specifically, they addressed the mechanism for the assessment and review of collateral risk. As a result, clinic policies were updated and staff members were subsequently trained.

This case illustrates a number of important aspects of intervention after a traumatic violent incident. It is the responsibility of the clinic director or senior management or supervisory staff members to ensure that everyone receives help in processing this event. The following list of steps may serve as a helpful guide to directors, leaders, supervisors, and clinicians in these situations:

1. Appoint senior supervisory staff (or a trusted outside consultant) to intervene as quickly as possible with all staff.

2. Give the message that this violent or other traumatic event happened to everyone. Emphasize that everyone experienced this event in different ways and may all have been shaken by this threat to their safety and security.

3. Emphasize the need for everyone to work together to help fellow staff and clients through this process.

4. Give all staff the opportunity to tell their own story of the event in a group.

5. Frame the staff meeting addressing the incident as an opportunity to learn more about the traumatic event and not to "point fingers" or to assign blame.

6. Take time to talk with staff members (both clinical and administrative) individually.

7. Refer staff members who are particularly traumatized by the event to the Employee Assistance Program (EAP) or an outside clinician for treatment.

8. Talk with the staff openly about the process of addressing these issues directly with the police or other investigative bodies.

9. Identify gaps in the agency's or clinic's ability to respond and attempt to fill them so that all of the staff members feel more secure.

10. Conduct a risk management assessment and explore further security needs.

11. Decide as a group how to address these issues with clients.

12. Intervene with clients in helpful and appropriate ways to help them feel safe in the clinic once again.

13. Continue to have senior supervisory staff come to the clinic on a weekly basis over several months. This can be an important intervention because staff members often feel abandoned if this intervention is a one-time event.

14. Assure staff members repeatedly of the different safety measures that have been taken to protect everyone.

15. Take into account the fact that clinics and other mental health agencies constantly evolve, and as a result, the needs and opportunities for improvement will also evolve. Although policies and procedures may already exist, take advantage of the types of experiences described in this chapter as opportunities for learning, growth, and evaluation.

Interventions to Prevent Future Violence and Ensure Staff and Client Safety

Training staff to recognize the signs of pending violence and to intervene to protect the safety of staff and other clients is an important strategy for preventing future violent incidents in a clinical setting. In addition, a common theme throughout the last chapter and this current one is the concept that no one should be left to cope with the challenges of risk assessment, or crisis intervention or management alone. As described in the last chapter, it is extremely helpful for clinics, schools, and communities to develop Crisis Response or Clinical Risk Consultation Teams (CRCTs) (Blady & Cleek, 2010; Campanelli, 2010; Pappas & Howard, 2009; Wofsy et al., 2009) that can discuss cases that present with some degree of risk on an ongoing basis. (See Chapter 13 for a more in-depth explanation of the CRCT.) These teams can be effective in helping staff to debrief following crisis situations and to develop policies that can guide responses in future situations. The next two sections of this chapter address situations in which a violent incident ended in death, and illustrate how the ensuing grief and loss responses were managed from a clinical, school, and community perspective.

Postsuicide and Posthomicide Interventions

Reactions to Loss and Death: Complicated Forms of Grief

Loss of a special person can be extremely painful and lead to intense grief and mourning. When death results after a long illness such as cancer, surviving family members and friends often have time to prepare for the impending loss. The process of grieving sudden death is even more complicated when the horror of violence, whether through suicide, accident, or homicide, is added. As clinicians we often "feel shocked that such a terrible thing could have happened. . . . Pervasive feelings of helplessness can overwhelm us as we realize that there was nothing we could have done to prevent the tragedy" (Underwood & Dunne-Maxim, 1997, p. 11). Everyone involved (e.g., family, friends, classmates, coworkers, teachers, administrators, community members) experiences feeling out of control (Underwood & Dunne-Maxim, 1997).

Multiple losses, either at the same time or in rapid succession, can flood our emotions and cause our capacity to grieve to shut down (Underwood & Dunne-Maxim, 1997). Catastrophic losses, such as those created by the terrorist attacks on 9/11, or the dislocation and deaths of

Hurricane Katrina, can be especially overwhelming and require additional therapeutic support. Similarly, when the cause of death may be subject to social stigma (e.g., suicide or AIDS), the event can become "unspeakable" and individuals can feel silenced or overwhelmed by rumors (p. 12).

Death of anyone who is young or that occurs before it is expected in the "normal" life cycle can be devastating (Underwood & Dunne-Maxim, 1997, p. 12), particularly for parents or grandparents who outlive their children and grandchildren. Also, children and adolescents who lose peers due to sudden death experience these losses as emotionally disorganizing and often fear for their own safety (p. 12).

Grief Reactions of Children and Adolescents

Children and adolescents respond to grief and loss with a wide range of reactions. Their responses may be partly related to their developmental age (as opposed to their actual, chronological age), their relationship to the deceased, and the reactions of the adults around them. It is important for adults (including parents, teachers, school counselors, and other mental health professionals) to provide a safe environment in which their reactions can be discussed.

Postsuicide Interventions in Schools

There has been an alarming increase in the number of suicides in the preadolescent and adolescent population (Underwood et al., 2010). Between 1980 and 1992, for example, the suicide rate rose 28% among youth ages 15 to 19 and 120% among youth ages 10 to 14 (CDC, 1995, as cited in Underwood & Dunne-Maxim, 1997). During the 1980s and 1990s, young Black males had the most rapid growth in suicide, with the rate increasing 283% and 165% among Black males ages 10 to 14 and 15 to 19, respectively. Experts assert that these reported rates could be in reality even higher as a number of youth deaths attributed to events such as accidents, being hit by a car, and so on, might actually be the result of suicide (Underwood & Dunne-Maxim, 1997).

In terms of the suicide of a student, Underwood and Dunne-Maxim (1997) point out that there are "few events in the life of a school that are more painful or potentially disruptive" (p. 2). They note that "Shock waves from the death reach out to touch those close to the victim, those merely acquainted with the victim, and sometimes even those who just heard about an event" (p. 2). Of particular concern in a school setting is the fear of suicide contagion or copycat suicides. While most incidents of suicide do not lead to contagion (Underwood & Dunne-Maxim, 1997), it is the concern for the peers of the victim that makes postsuicide interventions so important in schools and communities.

The Nature of the Response

It is important, when structuring a response to a suicide or any sudden, violent death of a student or other member of the school community, to consider the following components of any response: *support, control and structure* (Underwood & Dunne-Maxim, 1997, p. 7). In the case of a suicide, the following guidelines also apply:

1. Nothing should be done to glamorize or dramatize the event.
2. Doing nothing can be as dangerous as doing too much.
3. The students cannot be helped until the faculty is helped.
4. Maintain the structure and order of the school routine.
5. Facilitate the expression of grief in a controlled and organized way. (p. 7)

In the face of this type of crisis, structure and order are important to everyone involved. Underwood and Dunne-Maxim (1997) have indicated that the "regular routine of the school day provides a measure of support around which other activities can be organized" (p. 7).

One element that is essential to the healing process involves allowing students and faculty the opportunity to express their grief over the loss. These authors recommend that small classroom discussions be held rather than large general assemblies, as smaller, familiar groups can provide a more comfortable atmosphere for the expression of grief (Underwood & Dunne-Maxim, 1997, p. 7). They suggest that mental health professionals and other members of a crisis team be available to help classmates and teachers with the often difficult and intense discussions and make a special effort to monitor students who are in the same classes as the deceased. Underwood and Dunne-Maxim utilize the framework developed by Worden (1991) in identifying the tasks to be accomplished during the mourning period: (1) accept the reality of the loss, (2) work through the pain of grief, (3) adjust to an environment in which the deceased is missing, and (4) emotionally relocate the deceased and move on with life and adapt to a school environment without them.

TASK 1: ACCEPT THE REALITY OF THE LOSS

School administrators are often concerned about how to address the issue of a suicide or other sudden loss within the school. Underwood and Dunne-Maxim (1997) recommend the following:

Acknowledge the loss. Don't ignore what happened, but make sure it is talked about in a structured, controlled manner. Your taking active control is one way to minimize the situation's getting out of control.

Stick to the facts! Use written communication whenever possible to minimize speculation, rumors, or gossip about the death. Steer clear of making value judgments, offering explanations or attributing blame. Having data that is as factual as possible assists in helping people acknowledge that the loss has really occurred. (p. 10)

TASK 2: WORK THROUGH THE PAIN OF THE LOSS

Helping students and faculty work through the pain associated with the loss is also critical. Experts recommend providing students and staff with a time and place, in school, to express their grief. This can be done in an individual or small-group format. It is also important during this time to identify high-risk students, particularly those who were close to the deceased or shared classes with them, and to provide these students with assistance and connections to community resources. Underwood and Dunne-Maxim (1997) recommend thinking through the long-term grieving process as well and helping students and faculty to remember "to anticipate the critical times when the intensity of the loss might resurface (anniversaries, holidays, special school events)" (p. 10) and to reach out to the close friends of the deceased who may experience grief up to 6–9 months following the death.

TASK 3: ADJUST TO AN ENVIRONMENT IN WHICH THE DECEASED IS MISSING

In adjusting to an environment in which the deceased student is no longer there, staff and administrators are encouraged to recognize that "the empty desk, locker, or parking space left by the deceased student is a concrete reminder to the entire school of the loss" (Underwood & Dunne-Maxim, 1996, p. 10). Administrators and faculty should work together with students to decide how to honor and address these reminders without sensationalizing them (Underwood & Dunne-Maxim, 1997).

TASK 4: EMOTIONALLY RELOCATE THE DECEASED AND MOVE ON WITH LIFE

Schools, faculty, and students must be given the time to grieve so that they can eventually come to terms with and move on from the loss of the deceased. The "resolution of grief is a focus on the meaning of the life of the deceased, not on his/her death" (Underwood & Dunne-Maxim,

1997, p. 10). Schools and administrators are cautioned to be careful in choosing activities to memorialize the deceased, and to make sure to select ones that will not keep students stuck in the death or will serve as constant reminders of the trauma (Underwood & Dunne-Maxim, 1997). In this way it is hoped that schools and faculty can help students honor the deceased while gradually facilitating the return to everyday life.

Administrative Interventions in the Days Following a Suicide

If you are an administrator or have been called upon to advise school administrators or concerned members of the community after a suicide or other sudden traumatic loss, Underwood and Dunne-Maxim (1997) recommend that you conceptualize interventions in terms of the tasks required each day. They emphasize the importance of providing *"support, control, and structure"* (p. 7) during the crisis period.

DAY 1

The first step is to notify and mobilize the members of the crisis response team. If possible, a meeting should be called the day of the tragedy, the day after, or early in the morning of the first day in which the students have returned to school after the loss. If the school system does not have its own crisis response team, county resources can be requested or school administrators can seek the help of local mental health agencies or service providers.

An important action to be undertaken on the first school day following the death is the preparation of an announcement that can be presented to the teaching and counseling staff (Underwood & Dunne-Maxim, 1997). This communication should be a "statement of the facts" as they have been "*officially* communicated to the school" (p. 16). They caution school administrators to

> be extremely careful not to overstate or assume facts not in evidence. For example, if the official cause of death has not yet been ruled suicide, avoid making that assumption. There are also many instances when family members insist that a death that may appear to be suicide was, in fact, accidental. (p. 16)

DAY OF THE FUNERAL

Underwood and Dunne-Maxim (1997) emphasize that written permission must be obtained from a parent if a child will be attending a funeral with classmates under the auspices of the school, or that a parent accompany the child if the school has not organized student attendance. They also offer the following guidelines for the day of the funeral:

1. FUNERAL ATTENDANCE. If the funeral is scheduled early in the school day, many students may choose to attend directly from home. If it occurs midday, students may begin the school day and ask to be dismissed for the services. In some instances, entire classes or grade levels may want to attend. In these latter situations, some schools have used buses to transport students to and from the funeral, assigning crisis staff to ride on the buses to provide support and control for the students. Community resources including clergy and mental health professionals are often helpful as ancillary support at the service itself, especially if funeral attendance is large.

2. CLASSROOM COVERAGE. Letting faculty attend funeral services can sometimes create problems in class management. Some of the solutions employed by schools to allow as many faculty to attend as possible have included staffing classrooms with crisis team members from other district schools, consolidating classes, or using parent–teacher organization volunteers for coverage.

3. AFTER THE FUNERAL. If students return to school after the funeral, you can anticipate that many of them will have been affected by the services and resuming a regular school day will be difficult. Crisis stations where these students can talk individually or in small groups are an effective way to address their needs and not disrupt the routine of those students who want to remain engaged in classroom activities. (p. 19)

OTHER SUGGESTIONS

Underwood and Dunne-Maxim (1997) have also collected the following suggestions from administrators in schools that have experienced sudden deaths:

1. The school superintendent should be on-site throughout the first day as a show of support and to personally thank staff for helping the students make it through this difficult time.
2. Administrative staff members who answer the phones should be given direction on how to respond to inquiries. . . .
3. Recognize that the day of the funeral service may be the most difficult and have additional support available in case it is needed.
4. Schedule a substitute nurse to come in for the duration of the crisis to free up the regular nurse, who generally knows the students well and can be available to help grieving students.
5. "Scripting" announcements for the teachers to read to the

students or to be read by secretarial staff to parents who phone for information is helpful in creating a consistent and "singular voice" to disseminate information.

6. Establish a central clearing house for rumors, perhaps in the superintendent's office. This gives you some means of assessing which rumors might have some validity. . . . For example, in one school several students approached different faculty members with the rumor of a "suicide pact" between two other students. When these different sources of information were correlated by the superintendent, he was able to give added emphasis to his directive that these two students *must* be taken by their parents for a professional mental health evaluation.

7. Strongly insist in middle schools that only students who are accompanied by a parent or relative be allowed to attend the funeral. Because this may be the first experience with death for many of these children, the support and presence of a parent or relative is critical. . . .

8. The aftermath of suicide is not an appropriate time to implement suicide prevention curriculum in the classroom. Intense feelings are close to the surface and the unsettled atmosphere of the crisis will hang in the air for an unspecified length of time. Informal classroom discussions that focus on prevention strategies, help-seeking and the mental illness that are underlying components in all suicides are appropriate. Classroom teachers can be assisted by members of the crisis response team in managing these discussions. Local mental health professionals may also be available to participate in classroom activities that identify options for help and support that exist in the community. (pp. 19–20)

Case Example

John was a 13-year-old seventh grader who had moved in the middle of the school year from a nearby city. The transition to his new middle school had been difficult for him and the extensive level of conflict in his family made it impossible for him to derive any support from them. He had been the victim of bullying in school, particularly about his appearance, and cyberbullying on MySpace and Facebook. Although a few of his friends knew, he had not told any of his teachers or other school staff about these experiences. During the week of spring break, John committed suicide by hanging himself with a rope in the basement of his home. Later, it was revealed that the cyberbullying had continued even after his suicide. Initially, he had been rushed to the hospital after his mother discovered him hanging in the basement and she called 911 in shock. John remained alive in a coma for 2 more days. One of the adolescents from his school visited him in the hospital, took a picture of him in his hospital bed, still connected to tubes. To the horror of his friends and family, this picture was posted on MySpace and Facebook and quickly spread by text messages throughout the school. His friends were so incensed that they threatened to retaliate against the boy who had posted the picture and the other students in the school who had bullied their friend.

The principal and vice principals were notified by a family member and they contacted counselors, staff, and teachers through e-mail and an emergency phone tree that had been established for snow emergencies. The supervising psychologist and counselors of a school-based intervention program for at-risk students were notified by the principal of the middle school over the weekend that the suicide had occurred. At the suggestion of the director, the principal was advised to also contact a representative of a suicide crisis response team at a local community mental health clinic. All parties agreed to meet with the principal, vice principals, guidance counselors, substance abuse counselors, school psychologist, and child study team members the next morning at 6:30 A.M. at the school.

Although the staff at the school had never experienced this type of traumatic loss, they had received training on responses to suicide and had some ideas about how to proceed. The principal had written a very careful statement to be read at an assembly of teachers and counselors prior to the arrival of the students, copies of which were given to each teacher. Members of the crisis response team were introduced to the teachers and their availability to offer support to teachers and students throughout the day was stressed.

The decision was made by the crisis team and the principal to have a regular school day and to provide support in school, due to the fact that many of the adolescents had parents who worked outside of the home. A note was prepared for the students to take home to their parents explaining what had occurred and giving them a number to call if they had questions or concerns. In addition, the parents of the adolescents who were closest to the deceased received a personal telephone call so they could be prepared for their children's responses.

Two counselors were assigned to follow the deceased student's schedule for that day and to be available to help teachers and students in those classes with the greatest amount of contact with the deceased. The counselors met first with the teachers as a group to answer their questions and to help discuss the ways in which the teachers wanted the counselor to participate in their class. Some preferred that counselors be actively involved in classroom discussions, while others preferred to conduct the discussion themselves with the counselor available if needed. The teachers also identified the adolescents who they felt were closest to the deceased and those who may have had losses in their own lives that might be reactivated by these events. The counselors agreed to speak individually with such students.

A team of counselors from the school reached out to the family of the deceased and offered counseling support. Two of the counselors went to the home to offer grief counseling to the family and continued their visits for several months.

A crisis counseling station was created in the library. Throughout the day, individual and group sessions were held by the team with those who knew the deceased and a number of students especially upset by this loss came for counseling. For some, particularly those who were close friends of the deceased, the expressions of shock and grief were evident. In addition, some of the girls and boys blamed themselves for not having realized that he was so depressed and that he was feeling suicidal. Counselors also helped John's friends to discuss the anger that they felt at the students who had bullied and cyberbullied him. This intervention helped to avoid further violence directed at those who had bullied John.

Concerned about the possibility of "copycat" suicides, the counselors helped these adolescents to talk about the "signs" that they felt that they had seen (in retrospect). They shifted the focus to learning from this tragic experience and working together as a group to support each other. The importance of "telling someone" if they were even a "little concerned" was stressed. The adolescents identified school guidance counselors, teachers, and family members, as well as members of the crisis response team who they would call.

At the end of the day, the crisis counselors held a debriefing session with the principal, school administrators, counselors, and teachers. This was an open meeting that allowed everyone to express concerns, feelings, or questions. The crisis team members also made themselves available at the end of the day for individual teachers or other school personnel.

Many of the boy's friends expressed a desire to attend his wake and funeral. The school sent a letter to parents informing them that only students accompanied by a parent would be excused from school to attend the funeral. Counselors were also available in the school after the funeral in order to offer support to adolescents and their parents.

One lesson learned from this experience was the importance of preparing children or adolescents for the emotional impact of a wake or funeral. The family of the deceased, in keeping with their cultural and religious tradition, had decided to have an open casket at the wake and the funeral. Many of the adolescents who attended had never seen a dead body before and were traumatized by the experience. Sessions were held with the students and their families. In addition, follow-up groups were held with the students over the next few weeks where they talked about the experience and did a number of exercises including writing a letter of good-bye to their friend and participated in art therapy sessions.

The crisis counseling team was available in the school for the remainder of the week and one member continued to follow up on "at-risk" youth during the next 2 months. In addition, many of John's friends were a part of ongoing group and individual therapy interventions provided by a school- and community-based mental health program for the remainder of the school year.

ADDRESSING THE ISSUE OF GUILT

The issue of guilt raised by some of John's classmates and friends was an important concern that merited further consideration. There were many forms of guilt expressed by students. Some adolescents were haunted by negative encounters that they had with the deceased prior to his death. Another theme, common among his friends, was guilt caused by a failure to recognize the "warning signs" of his depression and intent to commit suicide. Underwood and Dunne-Maxim (1997) offer the following guidelines in addressing both forms of guilt:

> Help children see that the causative factors were not related to their behavior; that no matter what we think or feel, we don't have the power over another person's death. Reiterate that every relationship includes negative as well as positive feelings, but again, our feelings cannot cause another's death. Also, clearly give permission to children to go on enjoying life and living. (p. 14)

Many of John's friends were helped by their counselors to use art to express their feelings of grief and loss. Three of these students also volunteered to take part in a school assembly (discussed below) in which students were taught that bullying can have serious consequences.

ADDRESSING THE ADOLESCENTS RESPONSIBLE FOR THE BULLYING AND CYBERBULLYING

In the 2 days following John's death, the school officials did a thorough investigation and identified the students (ages 13 to 14) who were responsible for the bullying and cyberbullying. Two boys (including the one who had posted the picture from the hospital) and two girls were questioned by the principal and their parents were called in for meetings with the school administrators. Because of the seriousness of the cyberbullying and its tragic result, the students involved were suspended from school for 10 days. All four of these adolescents expressed a great deal of remorse for their actions. It was clear that they were stunned by John's suicide. When they returned to school, they were required to attend a schoolwide assembly that addressed the issue of bullying. They were also given counseling to continue to address the seriousness of their behaviors and were mandated to attend an antibullying program.

THE ROLE OF CYBERBULLYING, THE INTERNET, AND SOCIAL NETWORKING WEBSITES

One extremely important lesson learned from this experience for the school and all of the crisis counselors was a growing awareness of the role of communication technology in the lives of these adolescents, specifically text messaging and Internet sites such as Facebook, MySpace, and Twitter. John had begun to develop a growing group of friends despite his difficulty adjusting to the new school, yet these friends were an insufficient protection against the pervasive teasing in school and cyberbullying on Facebook and MySpace.

In addition, the crisis intervention revealed that most of the students knew about the suicide, which had occurred over spring break, before their return to school. Many had communicated through the Internet, specifically MySpace, Facebook, and text messaging, along with telephone calls. Even students who did not have access to a computer or a telephone had learned from their friends. Ironically, the medium that had contributed so greatly to John's despair offered a venue in which he was mourned and memorialized—there were a number of "R.I.P." (Rest in Peace) messages on his MySpace and Facebook pages.

In the months after this tragic incident, the school held a number of training sessions for counseling staff and teachers about cyberbullying and an assembly was later held for all the students. It is important for teachers, school counselors, mental health professionals, parents, and families to learn more about the role of the Internet, text messages, and websites such as MySpace and Facebook in the lives of their children and to be alert to the potential for cyberbullying. Counselors are encouraged to discuss these issues openly with students.

Involving Parents and Families and Addressing Their Concerns

There are primarily two groups of parents or family members to be considered: (1) parents of the victim and (2) those of the other children (Underwood & Dunne-Maxim, 1997). In the case above, school counselors and members of the crisis team reached out to the parents and family of the deceased. Family therapy sessions were helpful to them because they provided support for all family members, not just the parents. It was also important to include the siblings of the deceased, cousins, or other relatives in the school. As mentioned above, the adolescents who were close to John were seen in individual and group counseling sessions at their school.

Special counseling and support for siblings in these situations should be made available whether or not they attend the same school as the deceased. In some cases, it may be possible to request that counselors on the crisis response team or local mental health professionals provide grief counseling and family therapy for the family. In addition, depending on the family's religious or spiritual beliefs, it may also be appropriate to request that local clergy become involved. Family members may also be provided with contact information for other supports and survivors' groups in the community.

It is also important to anticipate the concerns of other parents in the school and community who may be concerned about their own children's responses (Underwood & Dunne-Maxim, 1997). Parents should be notified as soon as possible. In schools where parents have provided e-mail addresses, a prepared statement can be sent out. Another means of transmission would be utilization of a preexisting phone tree, often facilitated by class parents or parent–teacher-organization members, set up to be used for emergencies, such as snowstorms. If this method is used, it is important to give volunteers a prepared statement and discourage them from speculating on additional details. In many cases, however, where it would be difficult or impossible to reach most parents during the day, a carefully worded letter can be sent home with each child. Some schools have opted for a compromise in which someone is assigned to contact all of the parents in the deceased child's class or grade directly by phone, and letters are sent home with the rest of the children in the school. When teachers or counselors are aware of other children in the school who may be impacted by the death, such as friends of that child's siblings or the family, these parents should also be called directly when possible.

Parents can be offered the opportunity to talk directly with a school administrator or a member of the crisis response team. Sometimes a schoolwide informational meeting for parents is helpful, particularly if it can be scheduled in the evening after work hours, and babysitting can be provided. Underwood and Dunne-Maxim (1997) offer the following caution in scheduling these meetings:

> You must be careful in scheduling parental meetings after a particularly sensational death when community sentiment may be running high. While a large meeting may require fewer resources and seem easier to plan, it can also get out of control. Smaller parent groups which may require more staff support, also provide parents with more support. Several schools have handled the challenge of scheduling a parent meeting by assigning crisis team staff to facilitate parent groups. As parents enter the school, they are divided into smaller groups which meet in individual classrooms. (p. 36)

Posthomicide Interventions in Communities and Schools

There are many communities in the United States where youth homicide, largely through gang and drug activity, has become a common and tragic reality (Boyd-Franklin, Franklin, & Toussaint, 2000; Underwood & Dunne-Maxim, 1997; Underwood et al., 2010). In recent years, these issues have expanded beyond what had previously been primarily an inner-city phenomenon to impact a much broader range of communities, representing all socioeconomic levels. Thus, the experience of sudden traumatic death due to homicide is a potential reality for many schools and communities. Jenkins and Bell (1994) have addressed the post traumatic stress disorder (PTSD) that can be experienced by children and adolescents who have multiple experiences of tragic death due to homicide in their communities. Many of the guidelines addressed above for schools dealing with suicide will be applicable to dealing with homicide.

When considering youth homicide, schools and communities must remember that both the victim and the perpetrator may be students in their schools and may be known and/or related to other students. It is essential in these situations to reach out to the parents and families of the perpetrator, as well as the victim, to offer support and counseling. Also, families of the friends of these individuals should also be contacted to offer support in handling their children's feelings and discussing possible future developments, including the intrusion of the media. Guidelines for schools and communities coping with homicide are listed in Box 14.1.

Case Example

On a Sunday night in May, Michael, a 17-year-old African American high school junior, was standing on a street corner near his home. Suddenly, shots rang out and he fell over, gravely wounded. He was the victim of random violence between two gangs and was hit by a shot that was intended for someone else. A nearby store owner called the police and emergency services. He was rushed to a local hospital by ambulance. Neighbors called his mother and rushed with her to the hospital. In a panic, she called the minister of her church and asked him to meet her at the hospital. They prayed together and held Michael's hand as his life slipped away. His mother was devastated. He was her only child and a "good kid," who played basketball and did well in school. He had had hopes of gaining a scholarship to college in the next year. Now, all of those hopes had died with him.

A crowd of Michael's friends had gathered in the hospital waiting room. They became increasingly angry and many were threatening retaliation against those who had shot their friend. Michael's mother and her minister

BOX 14.1. Coping with Homicide in Schools and Communities

1. Anticipate that the death will generate a great deal of media interest and design a proactive response strategy. Media usually request permission to interview close friends of the victim (and/or perpetrator), no matter how young; be prepared to respond to this request. Realize that the interview may take place regardless of whether you identify and or give media access to students so providing a structured context for such interviews may give these students maximal structure, control and support.

2. Be sensitive about how the circumstances of the homicide may impact survivors. Recognize the complications inherent in the identity of the perpetrator, i.e., someone who is known to students may provoke side-taking or retaliation by survivors. An unknown perpetrator may expose children to an overload of fear and apprehension that can paralyze the entire community. If the homicide has included additional violent circumstances like abduction or sexual assault, its impact will be exacerbated.

3. In the event that the climate in the school feels like it is getting out of control, consider using uniformed police presence to provide an immediate atmosphere of support and control. Many schools have successfully applied this technique, especially if news of the homicide is received during the course of the school day.

4. Be sure to reach out to the family of the alleged perpetrator [as well as those of the victim] if either that child or his/her siblings attend district schools. Devise plans for continuing support for [both of] these families after the initial crisis; use community resources to supplement what the school cannot provide.

5. Recognize the long range effect on the families of both victim and perpetrator. Expect that the trial will reactivate the crisis for the families and close friends of either party.

6. Plan specific outreach activities for any children who witnessed the event. Collaborate with local community mental health resources to respond to the posttraumatic stress needs of this high-risk group of survivors.

7. If your school is in a community that is plagued by violence, consider using this event as an opportunity to actively pursue discussion with students about alternatives to violence. Some inner-city schools, for example, have used a student homicide to engage students in classroom problem-solving around the question "What's worth dying for?" or in devising strategies to avoid similar situations in the future.

(continued)

BOX 14.1. (*continued*)

8. Appreciate that parental response will effect the way younger children handle this trauma. Structure ways to educate parents about how to help their children. Ways to do this include handouts sent home, small group meetings, or crisis counselor availability.

9. Lastly, recognize that school staff may also need additional support and education to deal with the trauma. Unless your school has frequent exposure to homicide, staff may remain extremely unsettled by the experience. And even when violence and trauma seem like a way of life, staff can benefit from the opportunity to share their feelings and concerns. Rely on the resources of your community crisis team to assist with this and remember that the children cannot be helped if the staff members are not helped first.

From Underwood and Dunne-Maxim (1997, p. 67).

came out and talked with the group. They shared their sadness and anger but his mother begged them: "Don't tarnish his name by continuing the violence. You know that he would not want that. Please stop the violence."

A community member contacted the school principal. He arranged for a crisis intervention meeting at the school early the next morning. A number of local mental health professionals and Michael's minister were asked to attend. In addition, a crisis team at a local mental health center was asked to participate. All of the teachers and counselors in the school were contacted via a phone tree used for emergencies and were told about his death. A meeting was held before the school day started, with the principal, all of the administrators, teachers, and counselors in the school in attendance.

The principal had prepared a statement regarding the facts of Michael's death and the school staff processed their shock and sadness about his loss. The principal shared the news with all of the students gathered in a school-wide assembly. Students were then divided into smaller groups by grade and meetings were held in different classrooms throughout the day to help the students process what had occurred. The mental health workers, the minister, and the members of the crisis team stayed throughout the day and worked with the teachers and the counselors to help the students cope with this tragedy. In addition, crisis counseling stations were established in the guidance office for any student or teacher who needed additional help and support.

Two crisis counselors worked directly with Michael's friends who had witnessed the homicide and helped them to process what had occurred. They were upset and angry and were still threatening retaliation against those who were responsible for their friend's death until one boy spoke up and reminded the group of Michael's mother's words the night before. Her plea had had a profound effect on each of them.

By now, the newspapers had carried the story and reporters were attempting to enter the school. The principal, with the superintendent's support, decided that none of the students or school personnel would speak to the press at that time. The principal held a news conference where he read a statement expressing the sadness of the entire school at the news of Michael's death and expressed his sympathy and concern to Michael's mother and his family. He explained that the school would be offering grief counseling all day and he requested that the press respect the privacy of the students and school staff as they tried to deal with their shock and sorrow. He then answered a few brief questions.

Because an autopsy was necessary, the funeral was delayed for a number of days. The arrest of an 18-year-old from the community had sparked increased anger. The local mental health professionals and members of her church reached out to support Michael's mother and her family. Grief counseling sessions were held. In addition, the crisis team reached out to the members of the accused perpetrator's family.

During that week, a teacher at the school gathered Michael's friends and classmates and they organized a memorial in his honor. They read poems expressing their anger and sadness. They wrote about their positive memories of their friend and read them aloud at the memorial service.

On the day of the funeral, so many of the students, parents, teachers, and school personnel wanted to attend the service that the school was closed for the day. Many of the members of the church and the community came to support Michael's mother and to pay their respects to him. The minister gave a moving eulogy to the full church. At the end, he returned to the words of Michael's mother and called for an end to the violence. At the altar call, he asked for everyone in the community who had a weapon to come forward and lay it at the foot of the coffin and stand together to stop the violence. Young men from all over the church came forward and laid down their weapons. He called for a gang summit to address the violence in the community.

Over the ensuing weeks, the crisis team continued to work with the school and the community to provide counseling and support for students, their families, and members of the community. In the next few months, there were a number of difficult periods, particularly when the trial of the accused perpetrator began. This was a trying time for a number of the students in the school, who were called to testify, and their families. Counseling and support continued throughout this period.

This case illustrates the power of utilizing support systems in a community including a minister, local mental health professionals, school personnel, parents, and the members of a crisis team from a mental health center, to address the tragedy of a homicide in the community.

Conclusion

Throughout this chapter, we have emphasized the importance of having a crisis plan and a team in place before tragedies occur. Having pre-established policies and organizational structures that include a crisis response team can help agencies, schools, and communities to more effectively intervene in crisis situations. As we have stressed throughout this chapter, postinterventions should never be done in isolation and are best conducted when mental health centers and clinicians partner with schools and communities to build crisis teams to support individuals and communities facing traumatic loss. Helping clients and communities to cope with sudden death resulting from suicide, homicide, violence, terrorism, or natural disaster can be one of the most overwhelming and challenging clinical experiences. It is our hope that this chapter will empower mental health providers and agencies with the knowledge to structure interventions following such tragedies so that they can help clients and communities move through the grief process.

PART V

Challenges of Clinical Work, Clinician Self-Care, Supervision, and Training

The Benefits and Challenges of Clinical Work and the Importance of Clinician Self-Care

Introduction

The mental health field attracts many individuals with a unique capacity for compassion toward those who are experiencing psychological distress. The process of establishing a therapeutic bond and empathic connection with clients that leads to empowerment and the alleviation of suffering is tremendously gratifying for many therapists. Witnessing clients' growth can be a source of inspiration for many clinicians and can sustain them through difficult times.

One challenge can occur, however, when therapists, particularly those beginning their careers, discover that so many clients present with traumatic life experiences. These clinicians often have had no preparation for working with clients who have been exposed to devastating and abusive circumstances, and had no plans or training to become trauma counselors. Some clinicians, unaware of the positive aspects of doing psychotherapy with this population, may find themselves caught up in their client's distress and feel overwhelmed. The demands of doing this work are not just limited to beginning therapists, and can present difficulties for even the most seasoned clinicians.

This chapter provides helpful information on the potential benefits and risks for therapists working with those who have suffered trauma.

It draws on the extensive trauma literature to help therapists understand the possible consequences of bearing witness to the pain and trauma of a client, including strong negative countertransference, empathic strain, vicarious and secondary traumatization, compassion fatigue, and burnout (Dass-Brailsford, 2007). The signs of vicarious traumatization, compassion fatigue, and burnout are explored in order to help therapists become more aware of their symptoms and impact.

This chapter also explores "vicarious posttraumatic growth" (Arnold, Calhoun, Tedeschi, & Cann, 2005) and "vicarious resilience" (Hernandez, Gangsei, & Engstrom, 2007), and the positive benefits that therapists can experience in witnessing the growth and resilience of their clients in response to trauma. Finally, issues of clinician self-care are addressed. Examples of preventive strategies are presented that therapists may employ when working with trauma survivors or in coping with the demands of large caseloads and the pain of clients.

It is our hope that new and experienced clinicians reading this chapter will become proactive in their own personal and professional self-care. We would also encourage agencies, clinics, and other mental health organizations to offer more support for front-line clinicians. Chapter 16 presents strategies that these organizations can utilize in order to provide training and supervision as antidotes to burnout for their staff. In addition, Chapter 16 also builds on the self-care concepts discussed below and offers strategies for clinicians across a variety of treatment settings, who may feel isolated in their work and want to build their own networks of support.

Clients' Traumatic Experiences

There has been extensive research and clinical literature on different kinds of trauma, including terrorist attacks (Boscarino, Figley, & Adams, 2004); mass violence (Straussner & Philips, 2003; Tosone & Bialkin, 2003); natural disasters (Boyd-Franklin, 2010; Dass-Brailsford, 2007); combat (Maxwell & Sturn, 1994); torture, political repression, and violence (Comas-Diaz & Padilla, 1990; Hernandez et al., 2007); child sexual abuse (McCann & Pearlman, 1990; Neumann & Gamble, 1995; Pearlman & MacIan, 1995); physical abuse or physical assault (C. R. Hartman, 1995; Parson, 1994); rape and domestic violence (C. R. Hartman & Jackson, 1994; Josephs, 1996); serious illness and disability (Sinason, 1991); and the Holocaust (Auerhahn & Laub, 1998; Danieli, 1998). In addition to these forms of trauma, therapists may also be called upon to work with survivors, families, mental health agencies, and communities following a traumatic event, including a suicide (Ting,

Sanders, Jacobson, & Power, 2006), homicide, or experience of random violence. (See Chapter 14 for examples of all three of these postintervention experiences.)

Many clients and families have experienced multiple traumas. The collective impact of hearing continual stories of trauma can profoundly affect mental health providers over time. One danger many providers face is becoming so inured to hearing about such horrific occurrences, that they do not recognize the profound impact that working with these clients can have on their physical, emotional, psychological, and even spiritual well-being. There is extensive literature exploring the consequences experienced by providers working with such clients and families, including countertransference, secondary or vicarious trauma, compassion fatigue, and burnout (Dass-Brailsford, 2007). Becoming familiar with these concepts can be helpful to all clinicians working with traumatized clients throughout the mental health field, whether or not they have identified themselves as "trauma counselors."

Poverty, Homelessness, Community Violence, Gangs, Racism, and Systemic Trauma

It is common in nonprofit agencies and clinics for mental health providers working with those living in poverty to encounter clients for whom survival is a daily challenge. These clients' lives may involve repeated traumatic experiences, such as multiple periods of homelessness, drug and alcohol abuse, racism, sexism, homophobia, and ageism. In addition, many clients in urban areas have experienced systemic trauma through negative interactions with the outside agencies and organizations ever present in their lives including schools, police, courts, prisons, the probation system, child welfare and child protective services, welfare and housing authorities, and health and mental health systems.

Clients in urban areas often experience the trauma of physical violence in various forms, whether they themselves are victims or have lost family members or close friends. As the case example in the last chapter indicates, frequent gang violence may be a fact of life in their communities. The fears this gives rise to in many children, adolescents, and parents can be severe. Jenkins and Bell (1994) have documented that the trauma of community violence may result in PTSD for a large number of children in urban areas. An additional source of PTSD in clients is the accumulation of experiences with racism (Butts, 2002; Franklin, Boyd-Franklin, & Kelly, 2006; Sanchez-Hucles, 1998).

Mental health providers are often drawn to the field because of their commitment to social justice issues and their desire to make a difference in the lives of clients who are poor and suffer discrimination. These therapists, particularly those who come from middle-class families and may not have had to deal with the multisystemic levels of trauma that large numbers of their clients confront every day, can frequently find themselves feeling overwhelmed and discouraged. They may begin to believe that they cannot make a difference in the lives of the clients, families, and the communities in which they work. Some handle this discouragement by becoming proactive and advocating on a systems level for policy changes. Others can experience vicarious traumatization, a sense of helplessness, and even demoralization (Dass-Brailsford, 2007). Unfortunately, these consequences may not be recognized by therapists, supervisors, and agencies as symptoms of compassion fatigue and/or vicarious or secondary traumatization and burnout.

Common Reactions of Clinicians to Client Trauma

Countertransference

Therapists are, first and foremost, human beings with their own experiences, including painful and traumatic ones. Although the concept of *countertransference*, a term first used by Freud (1957) to describe a therapist's unconscious reaction to a client, has fallen out of favor in view of the current preference for evidence-based treatment, it is useful in understanding the uniqueness of each therapist's relationship with each client. More recent therapists (Dass-Brailsford, 2007; Figley, 1995) have understood countertransference as "a normal reaction to a client and a reflection of the counselor's personal life experiences" (Dass-Brailsford, 2007, p. 293). Dass-Brailsford[1] presents a comprehensive analysis of the concept of countertransference and the pitfalls of the failure to recognize it:

> Countertransference refers to the feelings and reactions that therapists have toward their clients as a result of a therapeutic relationship (McCann & Pearlman, 1990). These feelings and reactions are produced by the therapist's personal and professional experiences and are capable of influencing the therapist's attitude and behavior toward a client (Dass-Brailsford, 2003). The counselor's negative feelings are due to resolved and unresolved conflicts within the clinician (McCann & Pearlman, 1990). Awareness of these feelings is an important first step; discussing them in supervision is a necessary second step to prevent countertransference from having a deleterious effect on the client. If countertransference is left unattended, it

---

[1]Excerpts from Dass-Brailsford (2007). Copyright 2007 by Sage Publications. Reprinted by permission.

can contribute to a counselor's vulnerability to secondary or vicarious trauma. Counselors who are unaware of the effects of secondary trauma may lose their sense of optimism and overidentify with clients. (p. 293)

Clients' Traumatic Experiences as Triggers for Clinicians

For some clinicians, listening to clients' stories of trauma can sometimes serve as triggers, bringing up feelings they had around traumas they experienced, or even reliving the trauma (Dass-Brailsford, 2007). For example, therapists who have experienced physical or sexual abuse or who have witnessed domestic violence against a loved one may be retraumatized by hearing a client's account of a similar experience. It is important for therapists who find themselves in this situation to seek help, either through their own therapy or through consultation with a trusted supervisor. Sometimes both of these interventions will be necessary to help a therapist through this challenging process, as illustrated by the following example.

Monica, a 23-year-old student, had just entered a psychology doctoral program. During her first year, as a component of her assignment to an outpatient program, she worked with children, adolescents, and families that had experienced physical, sexual, and emotional abuse. As a new clinician, she was quickly overwhelmed by the traumatic stories that she heard from her clients and their families.

She was particularly drawn to Mary (age 13), who had been sexually abused by her father when she was a young child. This experience triggered a strong reaction in Monica, who had also been sexually abused as a child. As the weeks went by, Monica began to feel depressed and felt disillusioned about her work. She became hesitant to go to school and work. Her supervisor noticed the change in her and began to explore her feelings. She let Monica know that working with clients who have had such traumatic experiences, particularly as children and adolescents, can be overwhelming for therapists, particularly those who are new to this work.

Gradually, as Monica began to trust her supervisor, she revealed that listening to Mary's story triggered her own feelings about the sexual abuse she had experienced as a child by her now-deceased father. Her supervisor was supportive and helped to normalize Monica's reaction to her client's story. She also encouraged Monica to seek her own treatment as a way of getting ongoing support for herself as she did this difficult work.

As this example illustrates, therapists who find themselves in the situation of having a client's traumatic experiences trigger their own should recognize that this is a normal reaction under the circumstances.

As discussed above, clinicians should not feel embarrassed about seeking help either from a trusted supervisor or colleague. Another strong recommendation is that they pursue their own therapy. In fact, the process of seeking one's own therapy during a time when one is seeing clients can be among the most important learning experiences for a therapist. It is important to remember that traumatic experiences can be retriggered at any point in life, so that even if a therapist has already been through therapy for a particular issue, he or she should not hesitate to seek help at other points in his or her career if painful memories reemerge.

Compassion Fatigue

Most therapists and other mental health providers enter the field with a strong desire to help their clients. Many have a natural gift in providing empathy, caring, and compassion and communicating these traits to their clients. Working with clients who have traumatic experiences and life stories, particularly children, adolescents, and adults who have been physically, emotionally, or sexually abused or tortured, can be painful and difficult for therapists. This difficulty may be magnified when large numbers of clients have undergone such experiences. The natural caring and empathy can sometimes become so overwhelming that a therapist begins to feel *compassion fatigue*, a term first introduced by Figley (1995). Dass-Brailsford (2007) has described this phenomenon:

> Compassion fatigue is a consequence of listening to a client's traumatic history and the negative reactions that derive from such empathetic contact. When counselors are unable to maintain a psychological distance from clients' traumatic material, they may feel as if the trauma were happening directly to them. In effect, the counselor takes on the clients' trauma as his or her own. (p. 295)

It is important for clinicians who begin to experience compassion fatigue or vicarious trauma (described below) to realize that these reactions are not pathological (Cunningham, 2004; Pearlman & Saakvitne, 1995) but that they are a "consequence of a sensitive therapeutic interaction . . . when counselors engage empathically with a client's traumatic material" (Dass-Brailsford, 2007, p. 294).

Vicarious Trauma or Secondary Traumatic Stress Reactions

It is extremely common in the average clinical caseload for clients to have experienced physical, sexual, or emotional abuse. Although the field of trauma treatment has expanded greatly within the last 30 years, and there is a growing literature on the ways in which ongoing work with a traumatized population can affect a caring clinician (Dass-Brailsford, 2007), many clinicians have not been specifically trained in trauma work. Therefore, it can be helpful for all clinicians to understand the impact of vicarious trauma or secondary traumatic stress reactions, which are defined as "the change that occurs within the therapist as a result of empathic engagement with a client's trauma experiences" (Pearlman & Maclan, 1995, as cited in Dass-Brailsford, 2007, p. 293) and the therapist's reactions to these experiences (Tripanny, White Kress, & Wicoxon, 2004).

Munroe (1995), Pearlman and Maclan (1995), and Dass-Brailsford (2007) have indicated that vicarious trauma may be a risk related to a therapist's work with traumatized clients. Dass-Brailsford has cited the following factors as leading to possible vicarious trauma: "a therapist's personal trauma history, the meaning attached to traumatic life events, psychological and interpersonal style, current stressors and support systems (Pearlman & Maclan, 1995)" (p. 293).

Burnout

Burnout is one of the most debilitating, long-term issues faced by mental health providers. Vicarious traumatization is conventionally attributed to a reaction to the treatment of clients with traumatic experiences. Ironically, burnout is more likely to stem from external systemic factors in the mental health field (Dass-Brailsford, 2007). These might include "large client caseloads, lack of adequate supervision, isolation in doing trauma work, and other institutional and bureaucratic factors" (Dass-Brailsford, 2007, p. 296). The following excerpt from Dass-Brailsford describes the components of burnout:

> Burnout is defined as a general malaise, psychological stress, and a "chronic tedium in the workplace" (Jenkins & Baird, 2002, p. 425). Burnout due to psychological depletion is accompanied by feelings of physical exhaustion, helplessness, hopelessness, disillusionment, negative self-concept, and negative attitudes toward work, people, and life itself (James & Gilliland, 2005).
>
> Some of the other danger signs of burnout are difficulty leaving home in the morning, frequent clock watching, an inability to concentrate or focus on tasks, high absenteeism, increased pessimism, and cynicism about the workplace.
>
> A sense of being overloaded and overextended dominates the counselor's reactions. Feelings of burnout tend to develop gradually over an extended period and do not derive from a specific or identifiable incident; rather, the stress of working under unrelenting pressure

and with little support appears to have a cumulative effect. The slow progression of burnout eludes early detection. (p. 296)

The next chapter explores supervision, training, and organizational or administrative support as antidotes to burnout and strategies individuals, agencies, and organizations can adopt to prevent or ameliorate the issue.

When Personal Life Stressors and the Demands of the Job Combine

Therapists, like all human beings, are particularly vulnerable to burnout when the demands of the job coincide with personal life stressors. These experiences can occur at any time in a clinician's life and circumstances and reactions may vary greatly among individuals. One particular difficulty arises when clients are reporting and attempting to cope with the same stressors as the therapist. For example, a marriage and family therapist with a large caseload of couples found that when angry arguments between husbands and wives occurred in the course of treatment, it was challenging for her to retain a professional demeanor given that she was in the middle of an angry and contentious divorce process and custody battle herself.

Boyd-Franklin (2010) and Dass-Brailsford (2010), in their work in New Orleans after Hurricane Katrina, noted the difficulty of some clinicians, teachers, health professionals, and ministers when they repeatedly heard or witnessed the trauma of their clients. Many of these counselors and other helpers had lost their family members as well as their homes; many were living in trailers like their clients. Trying to help others cope with the trauma of the hurricane and its aftermath, while they were trying to cope with so much grief and loss themselves, reactivated for some their own traumatic experiences.

Therapists who work with clients experiencing traumatic grief and loss may function well with no adverse affects for many years. This can change abruptly when stressful circumstances occur in a therapist's life, such as personal injury or illness or that of a family member; anticipatory loss, death, or periods of mourning; stress related to concerns for one's own family members, etc. It is helpful in these instances for therapists to seek their own therapy (see discussion below). There are also ways in which caring supervisors, coworkers, or administrators can make this situation less stressful, such as by making a temporary adjustment to the counselor's caseload. Sometimes this can take the form of fewer clients; in other circumstances, the supervisor may limit the number of similar or particularly traumatic cases until the personal situation has begun to resolve. Since there is no timetable to predict when large caseloads and clients who have had traumatic experiences will combine with painful and difficult personal realities, the need for therapist self-care as a regular part of our lives and work is strongly advised.

Warning Signs for Therapists

Dass-Brailsford (2007) has identified a number of "red flags" for therapists as warning signs of vicarious traumatization, compassion fatigue, or burnout. These reactions, which may parallel the responses of trauma victims, fall into five categories of responses: physical, psychological/ emotional, cognitive, behavioral, and spiritual. *It is important for clinicians to understand that these are normal responses to experiences of vicarious or secondary traumatization and should not be ignored.*

Physical Responses to Trauma

Just as clients often respond to traumatic experiences with physical symptoms, counselors and therapists may have physical reactions as well. Clinicians, however, may not respond to these manifestations properly, either by ignoring or minimizing them, or by being unable to connect them to their own experiences of compassion fatigue, vicarious or secondary traumatization, and burnout. Dass-Brailsford (2007) lists the following physical responses that are common reactions to trauma:

> change in sleep patterns, shallow rapid breathing, headaches, increased heart rate, fatigue, chest palpitations, changes in appetite, dizziness, pain or tension in the body, stomach upset, sweating/rapid pulse rate, nightmares/night terrors, inability to remove oneself from the event (emotionally or physically), and tearful and crying for no reason. (p. 302)

It is important to note, however, that these physical symptoms are not only responses to stress but can be indications of potentially serious medical conditions, so therapists should refrain from diagnosing themselves and schedule a thorough physical exam.

Psychological/Emotional Warning Signs of Trauma

The timing of psychological and emotional responses to trauma cannot be predicted. Sometimes these are cumulative and occur gradually over time; sometimes these responses are more immediate after working with a client or clients who have presented with severe trauma. Dass-Brailsford (2007) describes a range of psychological and emotional responses, including the following:

> shock or numbness; feelings of fear/terror/disbelief; guilt and frustration; feeling unsafe and vulnerable; feeling helpless and hopeless; anger and rage; anxiety; anger toward others involved; depression, sadness and loneliness; feeling powerless or worthless; being on an emotional rollercoaster; fear of ongoing victimization. (p. 302)

Some clinicians have also expressed a fear of the negative reaction that might result were others to become aware of their psychological or emotional distress (Dass-Brailsford, 2007).

Cognitive Responses to Trauma

Traumatic experiences may also impact a therapist's cognitive ability. Many counselors have excelled in school and have relied on their cognitive strengths throughout their careers, and thus may be frightened when this type of reaction occurs. Dass-Brailsford (2007) discusses the following possible cognitive responses that are often generated by participants in her secondary trauma and self-care workshops:

> confusion; lapses in memory; distorted thoughts; slowed thinking; thoughts about dying; intrusive images; difficulty concentrating; difficulty making decisions; too many thoughts at once; thinking the world is unsafe; flashbacks and replaying the event repeatedly. (p. 302)

Behavioral Responses to Trauma

Therapists may also notice a range of behavioral responses as they attempt to cope with the trauma of their clients. Dass-Brailsford (2007) has identified the following:

> easily startled; jumpiness; angry outbursts; crying; fear of being alone; conflict in relationships; critical of others; increased conflict with others; withdrawal from others; nervous energy or hyperactivity; the tendency to overwork; difficulty trusting; false generalizations about others; doubts about others; irritability; clinging to people; decreased energy; sense of aloneness; alienation; avoidance of places that evoke the event; strong reactions to a small change (i.e., in routine or in the environment); inability to perform easy tasks; changes in sexual activity; disruption of daily routine; increased use of alcohol or medications; lower productivity. (pp. 302–303)

Spiritual Responses to Trauma

In the process of ascertaining responses to trauma experienced by participants in secondary traumatization workshops, Dass-Brailsford (2007) found that a number of clinicians discussed their spiritual responses. These included "loss of faith; questioning old beliefs; [experiencing] life [as] meaningless; a sense of the world being changed; spiritual doubts; despair; and withdrawal from church or community" (p. 303). Hearing or bearing witness to traumatic material can cause a counselor to question his or her belief in God or to wonder why bad things happen to good people. One therapist, who struggled with this dilemma after learning that a child she had been treating was killed soon after being reunited with his birth parents, described her process as one of "spiritual warfare." She struggled with feelings of guilt for having helped with the reunification, and her strong spiritual beliefs battled with her sense of hopelessness, helplessness, and anger at God because this had occurred.

The Positive Experience of Working with Trauma

Vicarious Posttraumatic Growth

As indicated above, there is an extensive literature on the potential negative effects for clinicians working with traumatized clients (Dass-Brailsford, 2007). More recently, researchers have begun to focus on the benefits for clinicians doing this type of work. Arnold et al. (2005) have identified a positive aspect of trauma work as providing *vicarious posttraumatic growth* for the therapist. Arnold et al. assert that clinicians treating trauma survivors

> sometimes perceive important work-related benefits or rewards including gains in relationship skills, increased appreciation for the resilience of the human spirit, the satisfaction of observing clients' growth and being a part of the healing process, personal growth, and spiritual well-being (Brady, Guy, Poelstra, & Brokaw, 1999; Herman, 1992; Pearlman & Saakvitne, 1995; Schauben & Frazier, 1995). (p. 243)

It should be understood, however, that even such positive reactions may pale in comparison to the overwhelming negative ones (Arnold et al., 2005, p. 243). Allowing for this disparity, Arnold et al. nevertheless investigated the positive sequelae for therapists working with trauma survivors.

In a qualitative research study on this topic, Arnold et al. (2005) reported that although all of the therapists interviewed experienced some negative responses (e.g., intrusive thoughts, sense of personal vulnerability, exhaustion), most reported that these were transient and disappeared within a few days. When participants discussed positive responses to trauma work (Arnold et al., 2005), a number of themes emerged. For example, some therapists reported a heightened awareness of the positive aspects of their own lives, more optimism about the future following their observations of clients' growth after traumatic experiences, and an impact on their own spirituality (Arnold et al., 2005). This last area of positive impact is particularly interesting. Some therapists reported that their sense of spirituality had grown, while others found that their work with trauma survivors broadened their spiritual perspective by exposing them to different spiritual belief systems (Arnold et al., 2005).

Vicarious Resilience

Another concept that may be particularly helpful to clinicians is the concept of *vicarious resilience,* which is defined by Hernandez et al. (2007) as a "process . . . characterized by a unique and positive effect that transforms therapists in response to client trauma survivors' own resiliency" (p. 237).[2] Drawing on the work of Masten and Coatsworth (1998) and Walsh (2006), the authors defined resilience as "the way in which trauma survivors access adaptive processes and coping mechanisms to survive and even thrive in the face of adversity" (Hernandez et al., 2007, p. 229). Their research is particularly compelling because they interviewed therapists who worked with victims of political violence and kidnapping, many of whom were torture survivors. The intensity and graphic nature of many of these clients' narratives made listening to them in therapy particularly painful. The authors give the following summary of their results:

> All subjects described ways in which witnessing their clients overcome adversity affected or changed the therapists' own attitudes and emotions. Witnessing and reflecting on human beings' immense capacity to heal and reassessing the dimensions of one's own problems were common themes. . . . Understanding the role of spirituality and religion and seeing clients as sources of learning were also typical responses. (Hernandez et al., 2007, p. 234)

Therapists reported that they were touched by and benefited from their clients' ability to transcend tragedy and find meaning in uniquely difficult situations. One clinician in the study shared the following case experience which helped her to find hope in her work:

---

[2]Excerpts from Hernandez, Gangsei, and Engstrom (2007). Copyright 2007 by John Wiley and Sons. Reprinted by permission.

I had a case of a client whose husband was kidnapped. He spent four and one-half years in captivity. She was a person with many resources, able to analyze and see facts clearly. She believed that her children could learn from her strengths and survive this situation. . . . It was discovered that she had cancer. She never recovered from it and died three years later while her husband was still captive. I accompanied her until she died. She taught her children about finding and using their strengths and about coping with loss. I learned about how human beings have so many resources to face tragedy, the importance of spirituality, tolerance and the ability to survive. She left that message clearly to her sons and they survived well for eight more months until the father was released. She called me to the hospital the day she died and thanked me for teaching her how to die by talking with her about life. While everybody else spoke to her about death and dying, she said that I taught her and her children about life. (Hernandez et al., 2007, pp. 236–237)

This case confirmed for this therapist the belief in the power of the therapeutic process to instill hope in a client and demonstrated that this clinician was sustained in her work with other victims of trauma through the vicarious resilience gained from this experience.

Through their exploratory research in the area of vicarious resilience, Hernandez et al. (2007) have added to our knowledge of the ways in which therapists can cope with and be enriched by their work with trauma survivors. They argue that this concept is a "useful tool to counteract deeply fatiguing processes in which therapists may come to see themselves as 'victims' of those who have been victimized" (p. 239). Another important point that these authors emphasize is that "awareness of VR [vicarious resilience] processes may strengthen the experiences that already reinforce the motivation and persistence of therapists who work with survivors" (p. 239).

Container of the Hope

Many clients, especially those who have been traumatized, present first with their problems and traumatic experiences. Some may have lost the hope of moving beyond their pain, particularly when surrounded by family members and others in their lives who reinforce their feelings of hopelessness. In this circumstance, the therapist can often provide the "container for the hope" for the client. This theory envisions an interactive process that can provide mutual benefits. While the therapist works with such clients to generate positive changes in their lives and access their capacity for survival and resilience, this process can help to produce the experience of vicarious resilience in the therapist

(Hernandez et al., 2007). The case above is an excellent example of the container for the hope theory: the client held on to her hope despite the challenges of her husband's imprisonment and her own cancer and this client's resilience and strength had an enormous impact on the therapist.

Therapist Self-Care

Many authors have addressed the issues of self-care for therapists working with traumatized clients (Dass-Brailsford, 2007; Hunter & Schofield, 2006; Neumann & Gamble, 1995). In our experience, however, self-care is a necessity for every therapist and counselor. Neumann and Gamble view self-care as an ethical responsibility of all therapists. Clinical work is extremely rewarding but it is also demanding, particularly during times like those described above when the therapists are experiencing stressful issues in their own lives.

Once again, the trauma literature and research can provide guidance for all therapists with its emphasis on specific self-care measures and activities.

   • *Setting firm boundaries around one's work and home life.* This has been identified by a number of researchers and trauma therapists (Dass-Brailsford, 2007; Hunter & Schofield, 2006; Neumann & Gamble, 1995). In their study, Hunter and Schofield found that the idea of "having a balance between the personal and the professional aspects of life was seen as one of the most valuable coping strategies for restoring a sense of perspective and maintaining emotional stability" (p. 126).

   • *Relaxation, meditation, and self-nurturing.* In their research, Hunter and Schofield (2006) cited these three strategies as extremely important to participants in their study. These strategies can of course be unique to the counselor. For example, "some describe having a bath with scented oils, meditation, massage, reading novels and other escapist literature" (p. 126).

   The types of activities that can be relaxing can vary greatly. For example, Dass-Brailsford (2007) has noted that when she does secondary traumatization and self-care workshops, she is always struck by the wide variety of suggestions that she elicits for self-care activities. Some participants have described doing a load of laundry or cleaning the house as a symbolic activity representing cleansing the mind and letting go of upsetting feelings.

- *Close relationships, social activities with family and friends, and social support* have been cited by many researchers (Hunter & Schofield, 2006; Neumann & Gamble, 1995). A fulfilling personal life is often a protective factor for some therapists (Neumann & Gamble, 1995). These researchers have emphasized the importance for therapists of having their own social network. Dass-Brailsford (2007) has indicated that there may be cultural differences in terms of which family activities counselors found the most relaxing. For some therapists, cooking a family meal or visiting with family members may be helpful in reducing stress.

- *Physical activities* have also been mentioned as an extremely useful form of stress management and reduction. Counselors in Hunter and Schofield's (2006) study recommended going to the gym, walking, jogging, manual labor such as mowing the lawn, playing sports, dancing, and swimming.

- *Taking care of oneself physically.* Dass-Brailsford (2007) discusses eating healthy meals and the importance of sleep. She recommends doing something relaxing before retiring for the night such as listening to soothing music, taking a bath, or reading. It is often not helpful to look at news programs depicting a number of traumatic events just before bedtime.

- *Avoiding drug and alcohol use and abuse.* Although counselors may initially feel that use of substances helps them to cope with stress, use of drugs, alcohol, nicotine, and other stimulants and depressants can lead to addiction and other psychological problems (Dass-Brailsford, 2007).

- *Engaging in fun activities.* Dass-Brailsford (2007) discusses the ways in which laughter and humor can be tension releases. Some counselors find that sitcoms or film comedies will lift their spirits and help them to relax.

- *Take regular vacations, holidays, and weekends off.* This is a crucial proactive self-care strategy that can help therapists to renew their energy and keep their enthusiasm for their work.

Spirituality

Research has shown that some therapists find working with traumatized clients deepens their own personal sense of spirituality (Hernandez et al., 2007); others rely on their spirituality to help them to cope with hearing traumatizing material and as a way to renew themselves in the process of doing ongoing clinical work. In their research, Neumann and

Gamble (1995) found that some therapists who work with trauma survivors draw on their spirituality as a way to stay positive and avoid cynicism and negativity:

> This work inevitably raises questions of good and evil for the helper and many trauma therapists find themselves, perhaps for the first time in their lives, searching for ways to make spirituality a more serious part of everyday life. Becoming involved in activities that restore a sense of meaning, connection, and hope are all ways of caring for the soul and combating VT [vicarious traumatization]. For some, participating in organized religious practice is restorative, while for others sacred depth is found in meditation and reflection, creating art, spending time in nature, or working with others in the community for social change. In addition, each therapist will have to work out ways to remain open and aware of the totality of experience without becoming lost in negativity. (p. 346)

These findings are equally valid for counselors and clinicians who are not trauma therapists. Each therapist needs to craft a strategy for rekindling hope and for restoring energy in this work.

Personal Therapy for the Clinician

One strategy that is uniformly recommended in the trauma literature has been the process of encouraging therapists to seek their own therapy (Dass-Brailsford, 2007; Hunter & Schofield, 2006; Neumann & Gamble, 1995). Personal therapy can offer therapists the opportunity to process their reactions to their clients' material and discuss memories of losses or traumatic experiences in their lives that have been triggered by clients. It also provides a safe, protective, confidential environment where they can express doubts about their work and the systemic and organizational stressors that can lead to burnout. It can also serve as an invaluable preventive step for all therapists and counselors if they begin to experience any of the cognitive, emotional, psychological, physical, behavioral, or spiritual signs of stress described above.

We recommend that training programs in the mental health field urge students to engage in their own ongoing therapy, as they once did in the past. We believe that this is important both in terms of training clinicians in the process of therapy and for its ongoing benefits to therapists throughout their careers. This is, of course, essential for trauma therapists, but even clinicians who do not specialize in trauma treatment are still likely to work with some clients who have experienced severe trauma. Therefore, it is important for all clinicians to view their own treatment as a preventive step and a viable option when they begin to experience stress related to their own lives and/or work.

Some experienced therapists who have been in treatment earlier in their careers may think of their own therapy as a completed process. However, we conceptualize therapy for the therapist in much the same way we do for our clients—that is, as chapters of therapy in a person's life that correspond to different life stages. For example, one chapter of therapy may be completed and the presenting issues successfully resolved. Yet, life and doing clinical work inevitably present new issues or trigger old ones. It is at these times that therapists should consider opening a new chapter and entering into therapy once again. An experienced supervisor, whose wisdom was valued by younger colleagues, would often ask them if they had sought their own therapy. When some reported that they had not felt the need to, this supervisor would often respond, "Just keep on living." Reinforcing the message of the importance of therapy for counselors normalizes the process of help seeking for therapists in contrast to what Neumann and Gamble (1995) have noted as the reluctance of many therapists to seek treatment and the stigma that some may feel:

> We have noticed, and many of our colleagues in diverse disciplines have confirmed that an alarming number of clinicians are very reluctant to seek personal treatment. Whether this reluctance is due to issues of stigmatization, fears about confidentiality, aversion to assuming a dependent role, or other reasons, varies among clinicians (Guy, 1987; Kilburg, Nathan, & Thoreson, 1986; Mahoney, 1991). Gamble, Pearlman, Lucca, and Allen (1994) found in their survey of licensed psychologists (mean number of years in practice was 15), that nearly 20% of the sample had never been in any type of personal psychotherapy. (p. 346)

Professional Coping Strategies for the Clinician

In addition to the personal self-care strategies discussed above, research has shown that it is also helpful for clinicians to recognize professional strategies that will help them cope with both traumatized clients and the demands of agency-based clinical work. Hunter and Schofield (2006) utilized a qualitative research methodology to explore counselors' professional coping strategies. All of the participants indicated that gaining more experience can help clinicians to feel "less overwhelmed" by their clients' stories (p. 127). It is helpful for supervisors working with new clinicians to normalize their experiences and offer support through good supervision and more training (see next chapter). Therapists should be encouraged to seek continued training opportunities throughout their careers. A number of the clinicians interviewed found that they had to learn to keep their personal and professional lives separate. Another factor identified by many of the therapists in this study was the value of maintaining a positive outlook. Other professional strategies included "creating pre and post-session rituals" and "using within-session coping strategies such as controlled breathing and mental imagery, which helped them to stay focused and sit calmly with the client, despite the challenging nature of the story being told" (Hunter & Schofield, 2006, p. 129).

Some clinicians have found it helpful to take regular holidays, vacations, and time off, or to use an occasional sick day as a "mental health day" when they begin to notice the warning signs of compassion fatigue, secondary traumatization, or burnout. It is important for mental health professionals to take that personal time on a regular basis, yet many dedicated clinicians find it so difficult that they "lose" their unused vacation and/or leave days at the end of the year when a "use it or lose it" policy exists in their workplace. Others have found it helpful to split their workload between settings with large numbers of trauma clients and a different type of setting (Hunter & Schofield, 2006). For example, some clinicians may choose to work part time in trauma programs and then spend the rest of the workweek in a more general outpatient setting, fee-for-service agency, or private practice. Balancing the caseloads of clinicians in trauma work may also be a helpful organizational strategy for agencies to consider.

Doing Social Justice and Anti-Racism Work: Becoming an Advocate

As we discussed above, many mental health professionals come into the field with a strong commitment to social justice issues. Some clinicians have addressed this commitment by becoming involved in advocacy at the local, state, or national level; by lending their expertise to community-based organizations; or by getting involved in national movements like the anti-racism movement. On the other hand, some clinicians are motivated to improve their clients' lives but feel overwhelmed and demoralized by the continued exposure to poverty, homelessness, racism, sexism, and homophobia in the lives of clients. In their research, Hunter and Schofield (2006)[1] found:

> Some counselors discussed their motivation to "make a difference" to their clients' lives or the social context. The sense of advocating for

---

[1]Excerpts from Hunter and Schoefield (2006) in Chapters 15 and 16. Copyright 2006 by Springer. Reprinted by permission.

powerless clients served as a coping function for them through giving them purpose and meaning in their work. (p. 130)

One caution for clinicians: While advocacy is an important and gratifying role for some therapists, it is important that we remember that our primary function is to empower our clients to take charge of their own lives (Boyd-Franklin & Bry, 2000a). When therapists find themselves doing more for their clients than the clients are doing for themselves, it is time to take a step back and wonder if advocacy is counterproductive by stifling the client's self-initiative. A collaborative partnership with our clients that combines some advocacy and more empowerment can be extremely beneficial (Boyd-Franklin & Bry, 2000a).

You Are Not Your Day Job

Some mental health professionals have reported that they feel frustrated in agency settings because organizational mandates and policies prevent them from doing the good work that they have been trained to do. For some, high caseloads and productivity requirements will not allow them to utilize the treatment modalities that they really enjoy, such as evidence-based CBT or long-term psychodynamic therapy, or family or group therapy. Your day job does not have to define or limit your scope of service and professional development. Many of the most satisfied clinicians with whom we have worked have been able to be sustained in the demands of their jobs by opting to incorporate additional components into their work, such as treating one or two clients in evidence-based CBT, running one group, seeing one family per week, or seeing one client in long-term psychodynamic treatment.

Similarly, mental health professionals who have been promoted to supervisory or administrative positions and those who are primarily in teaching or research positions within academia often report that they miss front-line clinical work and the satisfaction of using their clinical skills in direct work with clients. They, too, must also resist feeling constrained by their day jobs. Several examples follow of mental health professionals who were able to renew themselves through expanding beyond a constricting job to include more rewarding and challenging work.

When a social worker was promoted to a supervisory position in his agency and was no longer able to carry a caseload of clients, he decided to do cotherapy with one of his trainees on a family case. This proved beneficial to both the supervisor and the trainee. Each found himself looking forward to this particular case all week. In another situation, a school psychologist was feeling frustrated because she was not able to use her training in evidence-based treatment, as her job as a member of a child study team in a local high school was primarily limited to psychological testing. In the course of that work, however, she identified a group of adolescents who were profoundly depressed and she was able to treat them, utilizing the cognitive-behavioral treatment for depression (Clarke, Lewinsohn, & Hops, 1990; Weersing, Iyengar, Kolko, Birmaher, & Brent, 2006) for which she had received training. This undertaking allowed her to use her clinical skills in the school setting.

A psychologist who had worked exclusively in private practice for a number of years was beginning to feel isolated from colleagues and alone in her work. She spoke to a colleague at a university-based counseling psychology program and offered to conduct a supervisory group for doctoral students. She was able to see the value of her years of clinical work once she had the opportunity to share her knowledge with the eager students. As a consequence of this transformative experience, she felt reenergized not only in her clinical practice but also succeeded in increasing her learning and keeping current on new developments in the field by regularly attending trainings and continuing education programs.

A licensed professional counselor accepted a demanding job as the director of a short-term treatment unit. When no possibility existed there for the long-term psychodynamic therapy that he loved, he registered with a small fee-for-service agency and provided treatment one evening per week. He also furthered his clinical growth and learning and obtained supervision and case consultation experience by starting a peer supervision group of other counselors who met at monthly dinner meetings to discuss challenging cases. As a result of these two proactive efforts, he found that he enjoyed his administrative work more and was able to be more creative in providing direction for his staff.

Two psychology professors at a major university (Boyd-Franklin & Bry, 2000a) who were experienced community psychologists found that they wanted a way to continue to practice community psychology. They created a school- and community-based mental health program in a culturally diverse community. By this act not only did they introduce their students to clients from diverse socioeconomic and ethnic minority groups but they were able to offer a service to clients who were underserved and whose socioeconomic and cultural realities made it unlikely that they would have availed themselves of help at the university-based psychological clinic. Although the professors' primary academic roles involve teaching, research, and administrative work, this program has provided a great deal of gratification for them both and has helped them to continue to "make a difference" by addressing the social justice issues that brought them into the field.

Another social worker who worked with trauma clients full time, specifically with children who were victims of sexual abuse, found the work so draining that not only was she suffering from burnout, she was close to experiencing secondary traumatization. She was single and childless and, without the compensating factor of a rewarding personal life, the end of the workday left her continuing to feel exhausted and overwhelmed. She loved children and decided to volunteer at a local daycare center one evening a week on her way home from work. She discovered that she loved the chance to just enjoy playing with children who had not had the traumatic experiences of her young clients.

An African American graduate student in a research-focused clinical psychology doctoral program was frustrated because she had little opportunity to work with ethnic minority clients during training. She discovered that a licensed psychologist at her church had started a small counseling program. This psychologist offered to supervise the student while she treated several clients at the church's counseling center. Not only was the student able to follow her passion and commitment to working with ethnic minority clients, she increased her cultural competency through this work.

Conclusion

Clinical work can present many challenges for therapists. This chapter has drawn upon the trauma literature to help orient *all* clinicians to the potential effects of vicarious traumatization, compassion fatigue, and burnout. We believe that self-care is an important skill that is often neglected in the training of mental health practitioners. In addition, in the real world today clinicians often find themselves in jobs that do not offer them the opportunity to pursue their passion for a particular form of clinical work. This can sometimes contribute to burnout. The examples above represent clinicians who found creative ways to make a difference and to find value and meaning in an area of their work despite the limitations of their day job. It is our hope that their experiences can help to inspire other clinicians facing similar circumstances.

CHAPTER 16

Supervision, Training, and Organizational Support as Antidotes to Burnout

Introduction

Supervision is often viewed as necessary only for students and early-career mental health professionals. It has been our experience, however, that the privilege of being able to have case consultation or supervision when needed can be a benefit throughout our careers. This chapter explores the challenges of providing supervision that prepares clinicians for the process of doing clinical work in the real world. Given the pressures of productivity requirements, we address the process of group supervision as a vehicle for providing supervision to a larger number of therapists. We encourage clinicians in agencies, where they receive little supervision, to form their own peer supervision groups.

Throughout this chapter, we also explore the role of training and supervision as an "antidote to burnout" for clinicians and supervisors alike (Boyd-Franklin, 2003; Boyd-Franklin & Bry, 2000b). Many therapists and supervisors enter the field with a passion for clinical work. This work, however, can be challenging and demanding. The infusion of new ideas through ongoing training can keep that passion and commitment to the work alive.

At the same time, supervision has been shown to make a major difference for therapists. In their study exploring strategies utilized by counselors in coping with traumatized clients, Hunter and Schofield (2006) reported that clinicians identified the following components of good supervision:

Good supervision involved two main skills: helping the counselor to manage the case effectively by giving advice, direction and reassurance; and affording the counselor the space to debrief from any traumatic incidences or personal responses to the client's story. A good supervisor might limit the number of demanding cases that the supervisee took on and provide him or her with support and variety in their work. (p. 131)

There may also be a difference in the needs of supervisees with different levels of experience and at different stages of their careers. Clinicians in the Hunter and Schofield (2006) study also reported that

less experienced counselors tended to have supervision much more frequently (once a week) than more experienced counselors (once a fortnight or once a month). As the counselors became more experienced their expectations also changed. They felt that they needed less emotional support and encouragement from their supervisor and more practical case discussion and advice about case management. (p. 131)

There is a parallel process in which a good supervisor supports and empowers staff to do excellent work. This allows each clinician to provide a similar process for his or her clients. Too often in our field, good clinicians are promoted to supervisory positions with no training or preparation for the work. Ironically, this is also a parallel process in which academic training often does not prepare clinicians for the challenges of practice in the real world. Productivity demands often curtail the length and quality of clinical work as well as the supervisory process. With these realities in mind, we discuss the ways in which agencies can work to provide an environment in which good supervisors can be developed and the commitment to providing clinical as well as administrative supervision can be maintained.

This chapter also addresses the need for therapists and supervisors alike to be conscious of their own need for support in their work. As indicated above, clinical work can be demanding, particularly when we are working with clients with many real-world problems. In the last chapter, we discussed ways to address the personal needs of the clinician through self-care. Here, we describe the ways in which therapists can be cognizant of their own professional needs and find ways to meet them. It is our belief that isolation is deadly for clinicians as well as clients. Each of us has been fortunate in that we have had the opportunity to work with terrific coworkers, and we each maintain a network of colleagues in the field who continue to support our personal and professional development. This chapter discusses the ways in which clinicians can begin to build those networks in their own lives. This practice is essential for all therapists, especially those who may not have those supports available in their own clinics or agencies or those who may feel isolated in private practice.

The last part of this chapter addresses the need for organizational and administrative support for clinicians. Strategies designed and developed at the Institute for Community Living (ICL), a nonprofit mental health agency in New York City, are discussed. These include empowerment of staff through in-house training opportunities, including case conferences, clinical roundtables, a clinical risk consultation team (CRCT), and the development of a Learning Institute. These strategies are offered here to provide a starting point for clinicians, supervisors, and administrators to explore the process of creating an agencywide culture of support for staff (Blady & Cleek, 2010; Campanelli, 2010; Pappas & Howard, 2009; Wofsy et al., 2009). It is our hope that other clinicians, supervisors, administrators, and directors will be able to utilize aspects of this model in their own agencies.

Empowerment of Clinicians through Supervision

Thus far, this book has focused on the process of empowering clients and families through treatment. Just as empowerment is an extremely important concept in therapy, it also plays a central role in the supervision and training of therapists. As indicated above, we strongly believe that this empowerment process should continue throughout a clinician's career and should not stop once he or she is licensed in his or her discipline. Within this context, empowerment can take the form of enhancing a therapist's use of self, as well as ongoing learning about new models, methods, and modalities of treatment, including evidence-based practices (EBPs). Despite continuing education requirements, many therapists become "stuck" in the approaches that they learned in graduate school and do not continue to expand their knowledge of new approaches. In our experience, the process of learning is invigorating and is clearly an antidote to burnout (Boyd-Franklin, 1989, 2003).

The initial reaction of many mental health providers of all disciplines during their internships and early job positions is often a sense of feeling overwhelmed. Similarly, even more advanced clinicians, as they enter new positions in clinics, hospitals, mental health centers, schools, agencies, and even when they start their own private practices, often reexperience those initial feelings of self-doubt, fears of not being well prepared for real-world realities, and sometimes a sense of being powerless to effect change in their clients' lives. Highly complex cases are a challenge even for experienced therapists. As Boyd-Franklin (1989) has stated:

> For the novice, such common circumstances as initial resistance and suspicion, failure to keep appointments, and inability to follow through on issues can be exceedingly demoralizing and can create a feeling of inadequacy on the part of the therapist.
>
> Many new clinicians (and some "old timers") frequently experience a sense of cognitive dissonance. They may have a great deal of knowledge and training to draw from their educational experiences. . . . They may not, however, have a conceptual framework that allows them to translate this knowledge into effective [clinical] work. . . . One cannot empower others if one feels powerless.
>
> Within this context supervision and training serve a particular role. They provide a supportive environment in which the trainee can feel free to experiment, to acknowledge successes and failures, to risk, and to struggle with the complex tasks of treatment. The task of supervision and training is therefore a gradual empowerment of clinicians. . . . (p. 244)

In our view, this empowerment is brought about by helping clinicians to feel more confident of their skills and by helping them to respond to the demands of the real world. Within this context, the role of the supervisor must be an active and supportive one. As Boyd-Franklin (2003) has emphasized, when a supervisor establishes rapport through a personal, human yet professional connection with the therapist, this models and facilitates a similar bond that the therapist can then create with his or her clients. The best supervisors often model "use of self" for their supervisees and may share their own clinical experiences in the process of establishing a bond with the therapist. Within this context, supervision can provide a supportive container for the clinician.

This parallel process can also apply in other areas. Just as clients and families in the real world often present with feelings of being overwhelmed and powerless to change their circumstances, clinicians often express similar feelings. Boyd-Franklin (1989, 2003) has encouraged supervisors to normalize these feelings. Within this context, supervision becomes a "life raft" for the clinician (p. 245).

Group Supervision

Similarly, group supervision can be an effective learning and training approach, particularly for trainees, interns, and early career clinicians.

This process can be enhanced by the inclusion of experienced clinicians at different levels. It is also an efficient use of the supervisor's time. This is important given the pressures of productivity requirements in the real world. It gives early career clinicians the opportunity to hear about a larger number of cases, learn from their peers' experiences, and increase their exposure to different clinical issues and diagnoses exponentially.

For many supervisors, group supervision allows them to teach general, basic concepts one time rather than in each individual supervision. Similarly, as discussed in the section on case conferences below, this approach can be effective in terms of team building. With the help of the supervisor, members of the supervisory group can begin to see themselves as a team and can support each other and work together. Often groups of trainees can help each other through difficult periods in the training process. This is particularly important in agencies, systems, and organizations in which there may be many demands but not a great deal of support.

Formal and Informal Debriefing

Hunter and Schofield (2006) found that counselors working with traumatized clients appreciated opportunities for both formal and informal debriefing. Many of these therapists valued the option to debrief with their supervisor, even by phone, after a particularly difficult session. The majority of these counselors indicated that they also appreciated the opportunity to debrief informally with other clinicians in their agency.

> Team confidentiality enabled them to talk to one another about their clients, their personal reactions to them, and to feel heard and validated in their work. Most believed that informal debriefing made them better counselors and was an important part of the coping strategies offered by the agencies. (p. 133)

For therapists who do not have supportive colleagues in their agency, or are primarily doing home-based work, or private practice, it is important to develop a supportive network of colleagues in the field who can be available for an informal debriefing when necessary. Some early career professionals, who have found themselves without supervision in their agencies after licensure, have actually contracted with a more senior clinician or supervisor for regular case consultation and supervision outside of their agency setting. As the counselor becomes more experienced, these relationships can be continued on an as-needed consultation basis.

Peer Supervision Groups for Clinical Staff

In many clinics, hospitals, and agencies, experienced and senior staff often receive little direct supervision or case consultation. One of the strategies that can be effective and empowering for these staff has been the development of peer supervision groups initiated and formed by the clinicians themselves. These groups can be lunchtime "brown bag" meetings during which each clinician takes a turn presenting a challenging case and the group then gives input and brainstorms treatment strategies. This approach can counter the isolation that many staff members feel when they are working long hours seeing clients and have little time for interaction with other clinical staff.

It is important that staff see this as an opportunity to empower themselves and enrich their own opportunities for clinical growth and learning. Too often, staff members feel neglected in terms of their own professional growth and development. This is particularly true in difficult times when budget realities lead to cutbacks in these opportunities. Many staff members have the experience of receiving in-depth training during their internships and practicum placements. This often stops abruptly after graduation from their training programs or once they are licensed in their discipline.

The key point here is that it is important for staff to initiate this type of peer group supervision and not to wait for their supervisors or directors to provide it. Many clinicians report that this peer supervisory process validates the fact that they each bring knowledge to the table and that anyone, no matter how experienced, can encounter a difficult client and need this type of input.

With new technology, increased opportunities for support are also available. Clinicians who are in rural or isolated areas have begun reaching out and utilizing Google and Yahoo group technology to create online supervision and support groups. Additionally, there are several listservs that provide a wealth of peer support, information, and case consultation. One such resource is the various listservs on the website for the Association for Contextual Behavioral Science *(http://contextualpsychology.org)* where a wide range of mental health practitioners—from highly experienced clinicians and researchers to new practitioners still working on their degrees—discuss theory, clinical practice, and specific cases. Other similar resources exist, with new ones emerging on a regular basis.

Clinicians in private practice often feel isolated in their work. With this in mind, many therapists and counselors in private practice also form peer supervision groups, which meet regularly to discuss difficult cases. For many of these clinicians, this proactive strategy has added to their learning, kept them engaged in their own professional development, given them a supportive network, and helped them to avoid burnout.

Organizational and Administrative Support for Staff

Hunter and Schofield (2006) have argued that the process of self-care is an ethical responsibility not only of individual clinicians but also of the agencies in which they work:

> Counselors have an ethical responsibility to be self-aware and develop self-coping strategies (Herman, 1992) in order to prevent doing harm in the therapeutic alliance. On the other hand, employers, supervisors, and agencies have a duty to develop preventive coping strategies that will reduce the likelihood of vicarious traumatization and ameliorate its effects (Munroe, 1995). Sexton recommended that agencies implement proactive strategies such as providing specialized training programs, normalizing vicarious traumatization reactions, and offering counselors the opportunity to process the impact of clients' traumatic material. (Sexton, 1999). (p. 123)

Organizational support and the support of coworkers can lessen secondary trauma for clinicians even in stressful situations (Batten & Orsillo, 2002). As indicated above, providing time for ongoing supervision as well as periodic case consultation can be an enormous organizational support for clinicians who are working with clients who may have had traumatic experiences in their lives. Dass-Brailsford (2007) suggests a number of organizational strategies that can support therapists who see large numbers of traumatized clients. These include "lower caseloads of traumatized clients; clear limits on work time; comp time for emergency work over [a] regular 40 hour week; encourag[ing] clinicians to take their vacation, sick and other leave time; work areas that are clean and cheerfully decorated" (p. 307). She emphasizes that the "psychological well-being of counselors should be a priority" (p. 307) for an agency or clinic.

It is important to encourage clinicians to utilize Employee Assistance Programs and other outside opportunities for their own therapy (Dass-Brailsford, 2007). Organizations can provide support for staff through in-service training (Dass-Brailsford, 2007; Neumann & Gamble, 1995). The sections below describe the benefits of different kinds of training opportunities and how these may serve as an "antidote to burnout" (Boyd-Franklin, 1989, 2003).

Staff Support Groups

The intervention of staff support groups is conceptualized differently from group supervision. Support groups provide an ongoing group process to help staff cope with traumatic circumstances and traumatized clients. They are *not* staff trainings or opportunities for supervision, continuing education, or professional development. These groups can provide a rare opportunity for staff to process their own personal feelings about their clients and their work. For staff working in stressful settings with traumatized clients, these support groups can provide a lifeline and a survival mechanism. They can also serve as an organizational strategy to proactively help staff cope with or prevent vicarious or secondary traumatization, compassion fatigue, and burnout. For example, Boyd-Franklin, Steiner, and Boland (1995), in their book on HIV/AIDS, have discussed the value of staff support groups during a time, prior to the development of innovative new medications, when large numbers of clients were dying of AIDS. The toll on the staff personally and professionally from the ongoing experiences of loss, death, and bereavement was enormous. The administrators, in an attempt to provide psychological support for the staff (nurses, doctors, social workers, psychologists, etc.), requested the services of a mental health professional from a nearby community mental health center to provide ongoing staff support groups. Boyd-Franklin et al. (1995) have indicated that while a weekly format for a support group may be ideal, the demands of front-line clinical work and productivity requirements in the real world may not permit this time commitment. These groups can be equally effective even if offered bimonthly or once per month, provided that they are regular and the time is protected for staff.

Once again, the agreements about confidentiality in such groups must be clear (Boyd-Franklin et al., 1995). It may also be helpful to consider how power dynamics might impact feelings of staff safety around disclosure, and to therefore not include supervisors or administrators in the same groups as staff members. It may be difficult for staff to feel safe if those who are evaluating their performance are also present.

Training sites such as internships and externships, as well as academic programs, have found that the use of these support groups, in addition to group supervision, can be effective strategies for new clinicians. These groups can provide beginning therapists with a unique opportunity to process their personal reactions to their clients and to the demands of doing front-line clinical work in the real world.

Organizational Support
through Training Opportunities

Secondary Trauma and Self-Care Workshops

Harris and Fallot (2001) have discussed the importance of agencies providing systematic support for staff to address secondary trauma. Dass-Brailsford (2007) discusses the value of secondary trauma or self-care workshops as a form of organizational support for therapists and counselors. She recommends that these workshops be conducted with a homogeneous group of participants who share similar work. These workshops are particularly effective if they can be offered within a particular agency, because participation can be a strategy for team building and can help to create a "sense of community and support" (p. 299). Because staff members in a particular clinic or agency are more likely to have ongoing relationships with each other, this sense of community and support has the potential to continue over time. If the entire staff of a clinic cannot be released to attend this workshop at the same time, they can be divided into smaller groups so that clinic productivity requirements are not negatively impacted.

From our experience, it is best if an outside trainer or consultant can be brought in to conduct this workshop. If this is not an option given budget cuts, a senior clinician or trusted supervisor might be asked to offer these workshops for clinical staff. This person may be a part of the same agency but on a different unit. It is important that the workshop facilitator be able to create a safe space for participants. In order for this to occur, Dass-Brailsford (2007) emphasizes that confidentiality is essential and participants must agree in the beginning to keep all personal disclosures confidential. She also asserts that different individuals cope with stress in different ways and that they will need to demonstrate mutual respect for each person's reactions. In these workshops, clinicians are taught to identify signs of vicarious traumatization and secondary trauma and these signs and symptoms are subsequently normalized as common reactions to traumatic and stressful clinical material. A large part of the workshop also addresses self-care strategies that are generated by the participants themselves.

Dass-Brailsford (2007) points out that these workshops certainly do not completely negate the effects of working in the trauma field. They can, however, help to inoculate clinicians by making them more aware of the risks of doing clinical work with trauma survivors and the need to develop self-care strategies throughout their careers (Dass-Brailsford, 2007).

In her book, Dass-Brailsford (2007) describes the multilevel benefits to individual clinicians, the organizations or agencies involved, and even the workshop facilitators.

A workplace that confers trust, safety, and support can protect its members from the damaging effects of secondary trauma. A cohesive workplace community in which members constantly remind each other to practice self-care contributes to prevention of secondary trauma. Finally, the act of conducting secondary trauma workshops can be fulfilling for facilitators and remind them to practice their own self-care. (p. 305)

Training and Professional Development as an Antidote to Staff Burnout

Many clinicians and agencies underestimate the value of training as an antidote to burnout (Boyd-Franklin, 2003). Keeping current in advances and best practices in the field can be engaging and empowering for therapists (Smith et al., 2010). Participating in a good training can help clinicians, who may be feeling "stuck" in some of their clinical cases, to have a fresh viewpoint and ideas that can help them to provide even more effective services to their clients. Many agencies have found that offering clinicians administrative or training days each year for continuing education can benefit not only the individual therapist but also the agency as a whole. This is particularly true if clinicians are given the opportunity to come back and share this learning with their colleagues.

In difficult economic times, the option of having a trainer or consultant come in to provide trainings on current advances in the field has been difficult, particularly for some nonprofit agencies. Since many mental health professionals in most disciplines are required to get some continuing education, this strategy can allow more staff to benefit from outside conferences and trainings, particularly if these presentations are institutionalized on a regular basis. More experienced staff can also be invited to offer trainings for others. We have found through our own experiences that this approach can empower individual staff to feel that they have something to offer to their colleagues and sends the message that they can continue to grow throughout their careers. This is an extremely important motivation and strategy for many senior clinicians and supervisors and can provide an antidote to burnout for those working at this level.

Creating an Agency Culture of Support

The last part of this chapter presents a model developed at the Institute for Community Living (ICL) that provides a blueprint for creating an agency culture of support for staff (Blady & Cleek, 2010; Campanelli,

2010; Pappas & Howard, 2009; Wofsy et al., 2009). As mentioned in Chapter 11, the ICL is a New York City-based not-for-profit corporation that assists adults, children, and families impacted by mental illness, and comorbid substance abuse and medical conditions, through a broad array of programs and services. The ICL meets the specialized needs of New Yorkers struggling with mental illness by providing its clients with supportive housing, community support and outreach services, and health care. It also has traditional outpatient clinics that serve a range of children, adolescents, adults, and families. In 2001, Peter Campanelli, the agency CEO, realizing the value of training as an antidote to burnout and the need for an agencywide response to identify and disseminate the most current and innovative best practices in the mental health field to staff, created a Program Design, Evaluation, and Systems Implementation department (PDESI) in addition to a Training and Staff Development office. Both departments began with one staff member and both have gradually grown over the years.

The PDESI department is tasked with identifying and disseminating best practices and evidence-based approaches to staff in an engaging way that contributes to professional development and enhances client services. The department also supports programs in implementing a plan–do–study–act approach wherein interventions are implemented in conjunction with outcome assessment. Review of interventions and client outcomes takes place as a part of this continuous cycle, and helps to inform further development of the intervention itself and provides an opportunity to better understand the work and activities of each program.

For smaller agencies, particularly those that are struggling with decreased funding, it is important to recognize that this strategy need not require the creation of an entire department. Two or more existing senior staff can be recruited and can provide staff training, implementation, and leadership as part of their job description. This is particularly effective if the staff charged with training can collaborate with other agency leaders to become a small team that works together to attend outside trainings, research best practices online, and develop different levels of training for staff throughout the agency.

Best-Practice Trainings as an Empowerment Strategy

Many agencies and clinics find themselves under pressure from funding sources to document that they are providing evidence-based, best-practice interventions. As we have indicated throughout this book, in our experience, most clinicians, supervisors, and administrators in the mental health field enter their disciplines with enthusiasm and a desire to learn and grow. Unfortunately, budget cuts, productivity requirements, and the demands of clinical caseloads often lead to burnout over time. Training in current best-practice interventions, if it is provided by exciting and engaging presenters, can rekindle the desire to learn and grow and can reengage staff in their own professional development. It can also empower staff to feel more effective in their efforts to provide quality care for their clients. In order to accomplish this, the ICL developed an internal Learning Institute and created a three-stage model for sustained best-practice dissemination that provides training and then ongoing consultation and support for clinical staff.

The Learning Institute focuses on three levels of training: (1) exposure at a broad level, (2) acquisition at a finer level of detail, and (3) immersion in the work (Wofsy & Mundy, 2010b). The first level, exposure, consists of large, agencywide trainings. For example, the Learning Institute offers a 10-week, 20-hour course on the core philosophy and strategies in motivational interviewing (MI), an important evidence-based practice (see Chapter 6). The second level, acquisition, involves smaller, specific seminar series that are tailored to the needs of specific groups of clinicians, programs, and units. The focus here is on empowering staff with specific interventions for their client populations. For example, after a large training in the agency on MI, clinical specialists created training modules for staff at different levels to receive ongoing training and case consultation. This process helps to keep staff enthusiasm for the new approaches at a high level and facilitates staff buy-in to the process of learning new innovative best practices in the field. In the third level, immersion, senior clinical specialists provide on-the-ground technical support to foster seamless integration of the new skills.

This level of training is crucial because it allows specific clinicians and programs to request clinical consultation from the trainers and also provides an opportunity to help programs tailor the evidence-based practices to their clients' needs and presenting problems. This third level of training is also important as it can help to address unique technical issues, such as the ongoing support of overnight staff, with best-practice interventions or documentation. This level is often neglected in dissemination efforts and may account for some of the challenges in implementing evidence-based programs in the real world. In this model, the clinical specialists and other senior staff are first trained in a model and then, in turn, provide on-site training and consultation to their own staff. These supports can make the difference between a best practice that is truly adopted by an agency and situations in which trainings occur but the staff becomes frustrated with the process of implementation because it either is ad hoc or never occurs in the first place.

Clinical Risk Consultation Team

In our chapter on risk assessment (Chapter 13), the concept of a clinical risk consultation team (CRCT) was introduced (Blady & Cleek, 2010; Blady et al., 2009; Campanelli, 2010; Pappas & Howard, 2009; Wofsy et al., 2009). In this chapter, we revisit this model with an emphasis on the support that it can provide for clinical staff members working with high-risk clients. Working with high-risk clients can be one of the most stressful aspects of clinical work for many therapists. The definition of at-risk behaviors includes:

> Anytime there is a heightened potential for harm to well-being, func-
> tioning, or stability of an individual. Such behaviors include, but are
> not limited to: self-injurious behavior; suicidal or homicidal ideation,
> intent or behavior; arson; aggressive/assaultive behavior; sexual abuse
> ideation, intent, or behavior; history [of] or current victimization sta-
> tus; uncontrolled, active psychotic symptoms. (Wofsy et al., 2009,
> slide 3)

As discussed in Chapter 13, many clinicians find that they have received little training in risk assessment and crisis intervention strate- gies. Some clinicians feel the need for more organizational support in learning to cope effectively with client crises. With this in mind, a CRCT (Blady & Cleek, 2010; Blady et al., 2009; Campanelli, 2010; Pappas & Howard, 2009; Wofsy et al., 2009) can be convened, as needed, in response to referrals from staff who are feeling challenged by a particu- lar situation or case. It can also provide staff with additional consulta- tion, training support, and administrative backing in their work with at-risk clients.

As illustrated in Chapters 13 and 14, the CRCT has two stand- ing members—a chair and a coordinator. As specific referrals are made, these staff members reach directly out to the referent to get additional information about the situation, and distinctly identify team member- ship for each referral in response to clinician and program requests and agency needs. It is essential that these meetings occur at a regular, pre- dictable time. When possible, it is helpful if the team can meet in the specific clinic or program that is presenting the case. Clearly, in urgent risk assessment situations, such as imminent suicidal or homicidal risk, staff members are encouraged to seek counsel from their supervisor, administrator, consulting psychiatrist, senior clinicians, or emergency room staff to make a determination in terms of the need for hospitaliza- tion or emergency assessment (see Chapter 13). There are many clients, however, who do not meet criteria for acute hospitalization but who are perceived as presenting with ongoing risk. The CRCT provides staff and supervisors with the opportunity to discuss these difficult cases and to support them in working with clients to maintain safety.

In the real world of clinical practice, therapists and counselors must also learn to assess clinical risk in terms of the "degree of likelihood and adverse impact that could result from violent behavior displayed by persons served" (Heckart, as cited in Wofsy et al., 2009). Within this context, clinicians may encounter "precursory events" in which a client presents with behaviors that the counselor believes may be highly predictive of at-risk behaviors. These situations can often persist for long periods of time and, although they can occur in outpatient clinics, they are even more likely in residential programs, day treatment, and school-based programs in which clients are seen for longer periods of time. A collaborative group from the ICL was formed to identify clinical risk identification, intervention, and supervisory strategies to support staff and clients more effectively. This group identified that potential precursory events might include, but are not limited to

> disengagement from treatment or program services; cessation or non-adherence to medication regimens; a sudden change in behavior; onset of serious disturbance in thinking or feeling; recent life change (e.g., recent significant marital or job loss); environmental stressors; anniversaries of traumatic events (e.g., death of family member); and history of performing violent behaviors. (Institute for Community Living, 2008)

Needless to say, clinicians and supervisors faced with these indications of a possible pending crisis often feel concerned and overwhelmed, and are usually left to cope with these types of issues on their own. When this occurs over a period of time, it can result in ongoing stressors, compassion fatigue, and ultimately burnout. The CRCT is a powerful organizational intervention because it conveys an administrative commitment to both the needs of staff and the provision of quality treatment for clients. It validates the "gut feelings" of staff and further assists them with figuring out how to make sense of these feelings and act on them. Follow-up on high-risk cases is facilitated until the risk level goes down. Clients also regularly attend CRCT meetings. Client presence further establishes a network of support for the client and staff member, and provides an opportunity for staff to be exposed to interventions that they might otherwise not have been able to experience.

Experienced clinicians often report that they have a clinical intuition about a particular client in terms of clinical risk, but no systematic outlet for discussing their concerns. Ironically, as indicated above, trainees, externs, and interns are often given more direct supervision on these types of at-risk clients. In our experience, providing ongoing support in the form of a CRCT can be a major part of an antidote to staff burnout. It is also another example in which ongoing training not only helps staff to grow professionally but helps them to feel supported by their administrators in these complex and difficult clinical situations.

Case Conferences and Clinical Roundtables

Two of the most powerful supervisory and training tools that we have at our disposal are the use of case conferences and clinical roundtables. These may even be called "challenging" case conferences in which clinicians at different levels of experience and training can come together to discuss a difficult case. This can be particularly useful to all staff if someone from outside of the unit (e.g., an outside consultant, a senior staff member from another unit, or a guest speaker) is asked to lead the case conference. In order for this model to succeed and result in the influx of new ideas and energy, it is important that all staff feel a sense of safety and that no one assumes the position of having all of the answers. One of the most useful models for this is to have a person prepare a case or write up a brief case summary that can be sent to the group in advance. The person presenting the case can then make a brief presentation to the group, giving the history, current issues, and the areas on which they would appreciate consultation and input. This can be followed by clarifying questions from the group.

The next stage involves brainstorming by the group and often results in helpful observations by different staff members and input on ideas for addressing the current challenges. Members are then asked to summarize the suggestions that have emerged and the future directions that have been clarified. It is particularly helpful if a staff member other than the presenter is asked to take notes and provide the group with a summary of the suggestions that emerge.

We have repeatedly been impressed with the power of this process, not only for individual clinicians but also as a major training tool for staff at all levels of experience. It gives those with experience an excellent opportunity to share that expertise. If senior staff members also present their cases, it conveys a message that learning and clinical consultation is and should be a lifelong process.

Clinical roundtables serve a similar function except that whereas case conferences often occur on a particular unit or in a specific program, clinical roundtables may be agency-wide and may bring together clinicians from different programs. A particularly challenging case can be presented and a panel of senior staff, an outside consultant, or a guest expert can be asked to comment and offer suggestions. This model can also be extremely useful when a new modality or type of treatment is being introduced. The following example illustrates this process.

A counselor and a direct support worker, who work at a residence for persons with intellectual and developmental disabilities, requested a clinical roundtable and presented a newly admitted male client with mild mental retardation who was engaging in unpredictable and, at times, violent behavior toward a specific staff member. Attendees to the roundtable included several therapists from the agency's outpatient mental health clinics, a psychiatric nurse, two social work students, and three other direct support staff from other residences. The presenters were asked to briefly present the client's history, strengths, and difficulties, and articulate one or two specific questions that they would like the roundtable to address. In exploring the client's history, a theory pertaining to a particular staff member's voice triggering the resident's traumatic stress emerged. Concrete intervention ideas included purchasing headphones for the client, contacting past treatment settings to explore the client's trauma history, establishing protocols around the client's arrival back from a day program if that particular staff member was present, and exploring trauma-focused talk therapy or group therapy options. Additionally, a reassessment regarding the client's medication was suggested, as it was unclear at times if the client was responding to internal stimuli. A brief follow-up 3 months later revealed that these interventions, as well as continued support from residential staff, resulted in increased positive relations between the male resident and the staff member.

Use of Consultants

The use of outside consultants has been a well-known intervention in many agencies in the mental health field. In periods of budget cuts, it is often less expensive to invite an outside consultant in to do a specific training than to pay to send staff to a professional training. As noted above, a variation on this might be to pay to send a staff member to a training, who then returns and trains others. Consultants can be particularly useful when an agency is implementing a new program or evidence-based practice. Staff can benefit, not only from the initial training, but also from ongoing supervision and case consultation.

In today's environment, where the pressure for evidence-based practice (EBP) approaches is present in many agencies throughout the country, a consultant can also be utilized to help an agency to develop the tools to evaluate their programs and interventions in order to assure quality services and best practices for our clients.

Conclusion

Supervision, training, and organizational support are some of the most essential antidotes to burnout that mental health services can provide for their therapeutic staff. Supervision can be conducted on an individual, group, or peer basis and can be helpful for beginning and seasoned clinicians alike. Training, whether done through a more formalized agency structure such as a learning institute, or conducted informally by senior therapists, can help clinicians achieve new perspectives on their clients and reinvigorate their work through the learning of new approaches and techniques. The idea of continual learning and growth is as important for staff, clinicians, and agencies, as it is for clients. Through a recognition of this need for ongoing learning, organizations and agencies themselves can proactively support their staff through policies, procedures, and departments that continually evolve and provide a forum for staff to process and address difficult cases. As we have indicated throughout this chapter, each of these interventions can lead to a parallel process by which therapists feel empowered and are therefore able to better empower their clients. These interventions are clearly among the most important investments that an agency can make in their clinical staff.

Concluding Statement

This book has evolved out of our collective experiences as clinicians, supervisors, and administrators and has developed from the process of training therapists and counselors to provide effective treatment and evidence-based practices, to clients in the real world. We have included in this book many of the issues that we feel are essential for clinicians who are new to the field, as well as for those who have several years of experience. One of our main goals throughout has been to empower mental health practitioners and to validate the work that they do on behalf of their clients. With this in mind, we would like to end this book with a story that has provided inspiration for all of us during our collective journey in this field.

Making a Difference: The Starfish Story

When mental health professionals are questioned about why they came into this field, one of the most common responses is that they want to make a difference in the lives of their clients. Many who came into the field with visions of producing change on a macro level are often frustrated when they realize that they are able to see only a small percentage of the clients in their community who need treatment. Others become overwhelmed by the systemic realities such as poverty, homelessness, racism, sexism, and community violence that their clients face on a daily basis. Ultimately, they begin to question whether their work makes a difference.

During times when these thoughts and feelings become overwhelming and we begin to doubt whether our work makes a difference for our clients, we are often reminded of the Starfish Story (adapted from *The Star Thrower* [Eiseley, 2012]), which is paraphrased below:

> A man was walking along the beach early in the morning. The sand, like most mornings, was littered with starfish that had washed up on the shore. If the tide did not carry the starfish back out, they would die in the sun. Up ahead the man saw a little girl who was throwing starfish back in the water. He went up to her and asked, "What are you doing?" She replied, "I am throwing starfish back in the water. If I don't they will die." The man, surprised, replied, "What difference can it possibly make? There are dozens of starfish on the shore." The little girl turned and calmly threw another starfish back in the water and responded, "Well, it made a difference to that one."

Therapists should remember this lesson, particularly when they are faced with the overwhelming societal and systemic issues that they encounter in the real world. Our work makes a difference and can change the lives of our clients and deepen and enrich our own lives as well.

References

Abraham, P. P., Lepisto, B. L., & Schultz, L. (1995). Adolescents' perceptions of process and specialty group therapy. *Psychotherapy, 32,* 70–76.

Abramowitz, J. S., Deacon, B. J., & Whiteside, S. P. (2011). *Exposure therapy for anxiety: Principles and practice.* New York: Guilford Press.

Almeida, R. (2005). Asian Indian families. In M. McGoldrick, J. Giordano, & N. Garcia-Preto (Eds.), *Ethnicity and family therapy* (3rd ed., pp. 377–394). New York: Guilford Press.

American Association of Suicidology. (2005, June 10). *Facts about suicide and depression.* Retrieved September 12, 2006, from *www.suicidology.org/associations/1045/files/Depression.pdf.*

American Psychological Association. (1993). Guidelines for providers of psychological services to ethnic, linguistic, and culturally diverse populations. *American Psychologist, 48,* 45–48.

American Psychological Association. (2003). Guidelines on multicultural education, training, research, practice, and organizational change for psychologists. *American Psychologist, 58,* 377–402.

American Psychological Association Presidential Task Force on Evidence-Based Practice. (2006). Evidence-based practice in psychology. *American Psychologist, 61,* 271–285.

Anthony, W. A. (1993). Recovery from mental illness: The guiding vision of the mental health service system in the 1990's. *Psychosocial Rehabilitation Journal, 16*(4), 11–23.

Aponte, H. J. (1994a). *Bread and spirit: Therapy with the new poor.* New York: Norton.

Aponte, H. J. (1994b). How personal can training get? *Journal of Marital and Family Therapy. 20*(1), 3–15.

Arkowitz, H., & Westra, H. A. (2004). Integrating motivational interviewing and cognitive behavioral therapy in the treatment of depression and anxiety. *Journal of Cognitive Psychotherapy, 18,* 337–350.

345

Arkowitz, H., Westra, H. A., Miller, W. R., & Rollnick, S. (2008). *Motivational interviewing in the treatment of psychological problems*. New York: Guilford Press.

Arnold, D., Calhoun, L. G., Tedeschi, R., & Cann, A. (2005). Vicarious posttraumatic growth in psychotherapy. *Journal of Humanistic Psychology, 45*(2), 239–263.

Assay, T. P., & Lambert, M. J. (1999). The empirical case for the common factors in therapy: Quantitative findings. In M. A. Hubble, B. Duncan, & S. D. Miller (Eds.), *The heart and soul of change: What works in therapy* (pp. 33–56). Washington, DC: American Psychological Association.

Atkinson, D. R., Bui, U., & Mori, S. (2001) Multiculturally sensitive empirically supported treatments: An oxymoron? In J. G. Ponterotto, J. M. Casas, L. A. Suzuki, & C. M. Alexander (Eds.), *Handbook of multicultural counseling* (2nd ed., pp. 542–574). Thousand Oaks, CA: Sage.

Auerhahn, N. C., & Laub, D. (1998). Intergenerational memory of the Holocaust. In Y. Danieli (Ed.), *International handbook of multigenerational legacies of trauma* (pp. 21–41). New York: Plenum Press.

Bachelor, A., & Horvath, A. (1999). The therapeutic relationship. In M. A. Hubble, B. L. Duncan, & S. D. Miller (Eds.), *The heart and soul of change: What works in therapy* (pp. 133–178). Washington, DC: American Psychological Association Press.

Backhaus, K. A. (1984, Nov.–Dec.). Life books: Tool for working with children in placement. *Social Work, 62*, 551–554.

Barlow, D. (Ed.). (2008). *Clinical handbook of psychological disorders: A step-by-step treatment manual* (4th ed.). New York: Guilford Press.

Barlow, D. H. (1996). Health care policy, psychotherapy research, and the future of psychotherapy. *American Psychologist, 51*, 1050–1058.

Barnard, C. (1994). Resiliency: A shift in our perception? *American Journal of Family Therapy, 22*(2), 135–144.

Basset, T., & Stickley, T. (Eds.). (2010). *Voices of experience: Narratives of mental health survivors*. New York: Wiley-Blackwell.

Batista, M. L. (2009). *Rutgers–Somerset Counseling Program: Preventing violence and decreasing risky behaviors among adolescent girls: A training manual*. Unpublished doctoral dissertation, Rutgers University, New Brunswick, NJ.

Batten, S. V., & Orsillo, S. M. (2002). Therapist reactions in the context of collective trauma. *Behavior Therapist, 25*, 36–40.

Beck, A. T. (1964). Thinking and depression: II. Theory and therapy. *Archives of General Psychiatry, 10*, 561–571.

Beck, A. T. (1999). Cognitive aspects of personality disorders and their relation to syndromal disorders: A psychoevolutionary approach. In C. R. Cloninger (Ed.), *Personality and psychopathology* (pp. 411–429). Washington, DC: American Psychiatric Press.

Beck, A. T., Rush, A. J., Shaw, B. E., & Emery, G. (1979). *Cognitive therapy of depression*. New York: Guilford Press.

Beck, J. S. (1995). *Cognitive therapy: Basics and beyond.* New York: Guilford Press.

Beck, J. S. (2005). *Cognitive therapy for challenging problems: What to do when the basics don't work.* New York: Guilford Press.

Beck, J. S. (2011). *Cognitive behavior therapy: Basics and beyond.* New York: Guilford Press.

Berg, I. K. (1994). *Family based services: A solution-focused approach.* New York: Norton.

Berger, R. (2010). EBP: Practitioners in search of evidence. *Journal of Social Work, 10*(2), 175–191.

Bernal, G., & Scharron-del-Rio M. R. (2001). Are empirically supported treatments valid for ethnic minorities? Toward an alternative approach for treatment research. *Cultural Diversity and Ethnic Minority Psychology, 7,* 328–342.

Bien, T. (2010). The four immeasurable minds: Preparing to be present in psychotherapy. In S. F. Hick & T. Bien (Eds.), *Mindfulness and the therapeutic relationship* (pp. 37–54). New York: Guilford Press.

Blady, M., & Cleek, E. N. (2010). *Risky business: Supporting staff in identifying and responding to high clinical risk.* Poster presented at the 2010 National Council for Behavioral Healthcare Conference, San Diego, CA.

Blady, M., Cleek, E. N., & Kamnitzer, D. (2009). *Risky business: Assessment and response to high clinical risk.* Presented at the Annual Association for Community Living Conference, Bolton Landing, NY.

Boscarino, J., Figley, C. R., & Adams, E. (2004). Compassion fatigue following the September 11 terrorist attacks: A study of secondary trauma among New York City social workers. *International Journal of Emergency Mental Health, 6*(20), 57–66.

Bowen, S., Chawla, N., & Marlatt, G. A. (2011). *Mindfulness-based relapse prevention for addictive behaviors: A clinician's guide.* New York: Guilford Press.

Boyd-Franklin, N. (1989). *Black families in therapy: A multisystems approach.* New York: Guilford Press.

Boyd-Franklin, N. (2003). *Black families in therapy: Understanding the African American experience* (2nd ed.). New York: Guilford Press.

Boyd-Franklin, N. (2010). Incorporating spirituality and religion into the treatment of African American clients. *The Counseling Psychologist, 38*(7), 976–1000.

Boyd-Franklin, N., & Bry, B. H. (2000a). *Reaching out in family therapy: Home-based, school, and community interventions.* New York: Guilford Press.

Boyd-Franklin, N., & Bry, B. H. (2000b). Supervision and training. In *Reaching out in family therapy: Home-based, school, and community interventions* (pp. 202–216). New York: Guilford Press.

Boyd-Franklin, N., Franklin, A. J., & Toussaint, P. (2000). *Boys into men: Raising our African American teenage sons.* New York: Plume.

Boyd-Franklin, N., & Lockwood, T. W. (2009). Spirituality and religion:

Implications for psychotherapy with African American families. In F. Walsh (Ed.), *Spirituality resources in family therapy* (2nd ed., pp. 141–155). New York: Guilford Press.

Boyd-Franklin, N., Steiner, G., & Boland, M. (Eds.). (1995). *Children, families, and HIV/AIDS: Psychosocial and therapeutic issues.* New York: Guilford Press.

Bronfenbrenner, V. (1977). Toward an experimental ecology of human development. *American Psychologist, 45,* 513–530.

Brown, L. S. (2006). The neglect of lesbian, gay, bisexual, and transgendered clients. In J. C. Norcross, L. E. Beutler, & R. F. Levant (Eds.), *Evidence-based practices in mental health: Debate and dialogue on fundamental questions* (pp. 346–353). Washington, DC: American Psychological Association.

Brownell, K. D., Marlatt, G. A., Lichtenstein, E., & Wilson, G. T. (1986). Understanding and preventing relapse. *American Psychologist, 41,* 765–782.

Brun, C., & Rapp, R. (2001). Strengths-based case management: Individuals' perspectives on strengths and the case manager relations. *Social Work, 46*(3), 278–288.

Burke, B., Arkowitz, H., & Menchola, M. (2003). The efficacy of motivational interviewing: A meta-analysis of controlled clinical trials. *Journal of Consulting and Clinical Psychology, 71,* 843–861.

Burlingame, G. M., McClendon, D. T., & Alonso, J. (2011). Cohesion in group therapy. In J. C. Norcross (Ed.), *Psychotherapy relationships that work: Evidence-based responsiveness* (2nd ed., pp. 110–131). New York: Oxford University Press.

Burns, B. J., & Hoagwood, K. (2002). *Community treatment for youth: Evidence-based interventions for severe emotional and behavioral disorders.* London: Oxford University Press.

Burns, B. J., Hoagwood K., & Mrazek, P. J. (1999). Effective treatment for mental disorders in children and adolescents. *Clinical Child and Family Psychology Review, 2*(4), 199–254.

Butts, H. F. (2002). The black mask of humanity: Racial/ethnic discrimination and post-traumatic stress disorder. *Journal of the American Academy of Psychiatry and the Law, 30,* 336–339.

Calhoun, G. B., Bartolomucci, C. L., & McLean, B. A. (2005). Building connections: Relational group work with female adolescent offenders. *Women and Therapy, 28*(2), 17–29.

Campanelli, P. C. (2010, April 20). *Supporting staff in identifying and responding to high clinical risk.* Presented by the Institute for Community Living to representatives from the Office of Mental Health.

Carey, B. (2011, June 23). Lives restored: Expert on mental illness reveals her own fight. *New York Times.* Retrieved from *www.nytimes.com/2011/06/23/health/23lives.html?pagewanted=all.*

Carpinello, S. E., Rosenberg, L., Stone, J. L., Schwager, M., & Felton, C. J. (2002). New York State's campaign to implement evidence-based practices for people with serious mental disorders. *Psychiatric Services, 53*(2), 724–729.

Carter, J. A. (2006). Theoretical pluralism and technical eclecticism. In C. D. Goodheart, A. E. Kazdin, & R. J. Sternberg (Eds.), *Evidence-based psychotherapy: Where practice and research meet* (pp. 63–79). Washington, DC: American Psychological Association.

Centers for Disease Control and Prevention. (2006). Fatal injury reports: USA suicide: 2003 official final data. Retrieved September 12, 2006, from *www.cdc.gov/wisqars*.

Chambless, D. L., & Hollon, S. D. (1998). Defining empirically supported therapies. *Journal of Consulting and Clinical Psychology, 66*, 7–18.

Chambless, D. L., Sanderson, W. C., Shoham, V., Johnson, S., Pope, K., Crits-Christoph, P., et al. (1996). An update on empirically validated therapies. *The Clinical Psychologist, 49*, 5–18.

Chaney, E. R., O'Leary, M. R., & Marlatt, G. A. (1978). Skill training with alcoholics. *Journal of Consulting and Clinical Psychology, 46*, 1092–1104.

Chapin, R. K. (2011). *Social policy for effective practice: A strengths approach.* New York: Routledge.

Chorpita, B., Becker, K. D., & Daleiden, E. L. (2007). Understanding the common elements of evidence-based practice. *Journal of American Academy of Child and Adolescent Psychiatry, 46(5)*, 647–652.

Chorpita, B. F., Yim, L. M., Donkervoet, J. C., Arensdorf, A., Amundsen, M. J., McGee, C., et al. (2002). Toward large-scale implementation of empirically supported treatments for children: A review and observations by the Hawaii Empirical Basis to Services Task Force. *Clinical Psychology: Science and Practice, 9*, 165–190.

Clarke, G., Lewinsohn, P., & Hops, H. (1990). *Leader's manual for adolescent groups: Adolescent coping with depression course.* Portland, OR: Kaiser Permanente Center for Health Research. Copies of this manual and the associated workbook may be downloaded from *www.kpchr.org/research/public/acwd/acwd.html*.

Cleek, E. N., Wofsy, M., Boyd-Franklin, N., Mundy, B., & Howell, T. (2012). The Family Empowerment Program: An interdisciplinary approach to working with multi-stressed urban families. *Family Process, 51(2)*, 207–217.

Cohen, J. A, Mannarino, A. P., & Deblinger, E. (2006). *Treating traumatic grief in children and adolescents.* New York: Guilford Press.

Collis, R. (2010). *Your mind is like Google.* Retrieved November 23, 2010, from *adviceonlifeandlove.blogspot.com*.

Colom, F., Vieta, E., & Scott, J. (2006). *Psychoeducation manual for bipolar disorder.* Cambridge, UK: Cambridge University Press.

Comas-Diaz, L. (2006). Cultural variation in the therapeutic relationship. In C. D. Goodheart, A. E. Kazdin, & R. J. Sternberg (Eds.), *Evidence-based psychotherapy: Where practice and research meet* (pp. 81–105). Washington, DC: American Psychological Association.

Comas-Diaz, L., & Padilla, A. A. (1990). Countertransference in working with victims of political repression. *American Journal of Orthopsychiatry, 60(1)*, 125–134.

Connor-Smith, J. K., & Weisz, J. R. (2003). Applying treatment outcome research in clinical practice: Techniques for adapting interventions to the real world. *Child and Adolescent Mental Health, 8,* 3–10.

Connors, G. J., Walitzer, K. S., & Dermen, K. H. (2002). Preparing clients for alcoholism treatment: Effects on treatment participation and outcomes. *Journal of Consulting and Clinical Psychology, 70,* 1161–1169.

Constantine, M. G., Lewis, E. L., Conner, L. C., & Sanchez, D. (2000). Addressing spiritual and religious issues in counseling African Americans: Implications for counselor training and practice. *Counseling and Values, 45,* 28–39.

Corrigan, P. W., Mueser, K. T., Bond, G. R., & Drake, R. E. (2009) *Principles and practice of psychiatric rehabilitation: An empirical approach.* New York: Guilford Press.

Cose, E. (1993). *The rage of the privileged class.* New York: HarperCollins.

Cuijpers, P. (1998). A psychoeducational approach to the treatment of depression: A meta-analysis of Lewinsohn's "coping with depression" course. *Behavior Therapy, 29*(3), 521–533.

Cunningham, M. (2004). Avoiding vicarious traumatization. In N. B. Webb (Ed.), *Mass trauma and violence* (pp. 327–346). New York: Guilford Press.

Curry, S., Marlatt, G. A., & Gordon, J. R. (1987). Abstinence violation effect: Validation of an attributional construct with smoking cessation. *Journal of Consulting and Clinical Psychology, 55,* 145–149.

Danieli, Y. (1998). *International handbook of multigenerational legacies of trauma.* New York: Plenum Press.

Dass-Brailsford, P. (2007). *A practical approach to trauma: Empowering interventions.* Thousand Oaks, CA: Sage.

Dass-Brailsford, P. (2010). *Crisis and disaster counseling: Lessons learned from Hurricane Katrina and other disasters.* Thousand Oaks, CA: Sage.

Davis, M., Eshelman, E. R., & McKay, M. (2008). *The relaxation and stress reduction workbook* (6th ed.). Oakland, CA: New Harbinger.

Deegan, P. (1990). Spirit breaking: When the helping professions hurt. *Humanistic Psychologist, 18*(3), 301–313.

Deegan, P. (1992). The independent living movement and people with psychiatric disabilities: Taking back control over our own lives. *Psychosocial Rehabilitation Journal, 15*(3), 3–19.

DeLeon, P. H., VandenBos, G. R., & Bulatao, E. Q. (1991). Managed mental health care: A history of the federal policy initiative. *Professional Psychology: Research and Practice, 22,* 15–25.

DiClemente, C. C. (1991). Motivational interviewing and the stages of change. In W. R. Miller & S. Rollnick (Eds.), *Motivational interviewing: Preparing people to change addictive behavior.* New York: Guilford Press.

DiClemente, C .C., & Velasquez, M. M. (2002). Motivational interviewing and the stages of change. In W. Miller & S. Rollnick (Eds.), *Motivational interviewing: Preparing people for change* (2nd ed., pp. 201–216). New York: Guilford Press.

DeLucia-Waack, J. L., Gerrity, D. A., Kalodner, C. R., & Riva, M. T. (2004).

Handbook of group counseling and psychotherapy. Thousand Oaks, CA: Sage.

Dies, K. G. (2000). Adolescent development and a model of group psychotherapy: Effective leadership in the new millennium. *Journal of Child and Adolescent Group Therapy, 10*(2), 97–111.

Dies, K. R. (1992). Leadership in adolescent psychotherapy groups: Strategies for effectiveness. *Journal of Child and Adolescent Group Therapy, 2*(3), 149–159.

Dimidjian, S., Hollon, S. D., Dobson, K. S., Schmaling, K. B., Kohenberg, R. J., Addis, M., et al. (2006). Randomized trial of behavioral activation, cognitive therapy, and antidepressant medication in the acute treatment of adults with major depression. *Journal of Consulting and Clinical Psychology, 74*(4), 658–670.

Dimidjian, S., Martell, C. R., Addis, M. E., & Herman-Dunn, R. (2008). Behavioral activation for depression. In D. H. Barlow (Ed.), *Clinical handbook of psychological disorders: A step-by-step treatment manual* (4th ed., pp. 328–364). New York: Guilford Press.

Donley, J. E. (1911). Psychotherapy and re-education. *Journal of Abnormal Psychology, 6,* 1–10.

Drake, R. E., Goldman, H. H., Leff, H. S., Lehman, A. F., Dixon, L., Mueser, K. T., et al. (2001). Implementing evidence-based practices in routine mental health care settings. *Psychiatric Services, 52,* 179–182.

Drake, R. E., Wallach, M. A., & McGovern, M. P. (2005). Future directions in preventing relapse to substance abuse among clients with severe mental illnesses. *Psychiatric Services, 56*(10), 1297–1302.

Duncan, B. L., Miller, S. D., Wampold, B. E., & Hubble, M. A. (Eds.). (2009). *The heart and soul of change.* Washington, DC: American Psychological Association.

Eifert, G. H., & Forsyth, J. P. (2005). *Acceptance and commitment therapy for anxiety disorders: A practitioner's treatment guide to using mindfulness, acceptance, and values-based behavior change strategies.* Oakland, CA: New Harbinger.

Eiseley, L. (2012, February 14). The starfish story. Adapted from *The star thrower.* Retrieved from *www.facebook.com/note.php?note_id=96733027773.*

Elliott, R., Bohart, A. C., Watson, J. C., & Greenberg, L. S. (2010). *Empathy.* In J. C. Norcross (Ed.), *Psychotherapy relationships that work: Evidence-based responsiveness* (2nd ed., pp. 132–152). New York: Oxford University Press. Retrieved from *http://nrepp.samhsa.gov/pdfs/ Norcross_evidence-based_therapy_relationships.pdf* [pp. 13–14].

Elliott, R., Bohart, A. C., Watson, J. C., & Greenberg, L. S. (2011). Empathy. In J. C. Norcross (Ed.), *Psychotherapy relationships that work: Evidence-based responsiveness* (2nd ed., pp. 132–152). New York: Oxford University Press.

Epstein, I. (2011). Reconciling evidence-based practice, evidence-informed practice, and practice-based research: The role of clinical data-mining. *Social Work, 56*(3), 284–289.

Falicov, C. J. (1998). *Latino families in therapy: A guide to multicultural practice*. New York: Guilford Press.

Farber, B. A., & Doolin, E. M. (2010). Positive regard and affirmation. In J. C. Norcross (Ed.), *Psychotherapy relationships that work: Evidence-based therapy relationships* (2nd ed., pp. 168–186). New York: Oxford University Press. Retrieved from *http://nrepp.samhsa.gov/pdfs/Norcross_evidence-based_therapy_relationships.pdf* [pp. 17–18].

Farber, B. A., & Doolin, E. M. (2011). Positive regard and affirmation. In J. C. Norcross (Ed.), *Psychotherapy relationships that work: Evidence-based responsiveness* (2nd ed., pp. 168–186). New York: Oxford University Press.

Figley, C. R. (1995). Compassion fatigue: Toward a new understanding of the costs of caring. In B. H. Stamm (Ed.), *Secondary traumatic stress: Self-care issues for clinical researchers and educators* (2nd ed., pp. 3–28). Lutherville, MD: Sidran Press.

Fishman, D. B. (2009). Case-study knowledge as evidence for guiding practice. *New Jersey Psychologist, 59*(1), 26–28.

Follette, V. M., Palm, K. M., & Hall, M. L. R. (2004). Acceptance, mindfulness, and trauma. In S. Hayes, V. M. Follette, & M. M. Linehan (Eds.), *Mindfulness and acceptance: Expanding the cognitive-behavioral tradition*. New York: Guilford Press.

Follette, V. M., & Pistorello, J. (2007). *Finding life beyond trauma: Using acceptance and commitment therapy to heal from post-traumatic stress and trauma-related problems*. Oakland, CA: New Harbinger.

Franklin, A. J. (2004). *From brotherhood to manhood: How Black men rescue their relationships and dreams from the invisibility syndrome*. Hoboken, NJ: Wiley.

Franklin, A. J., Boyd-Franklin, N., & Kelly, S. (2006). Racism and invisibility: Race-related stress, emotional abuse and psychological trauma for people of color. *Journal of Emotional Abuse, 6*(2/3), 9–30.

Freedman, J. H., & Combs, G. (1996). *Narrative therapy: The social construction of preferred realities*. New York: Norton.

Freeman, A., Schrodt, G. R., Gilson, M., & Ludgate, J. W. (1993). Group cognitive therapy with inpatients. In J. H. Wright, M. E. Thase, A. T. Beck, & J. W. Ludgate (Eds.), *Cognitive therapy with inpatients*. New York: Guilford Press.

Freud, S. (1957). *Introductory lectures on psychoanalysis*. New York: Liveright.

Friedlander, M. L., Escudero, V., Heatherington, L., & Diamond, G. M. (2011). Alliance in couple and family therapy. In J. C. Norcross (Ed.), *Psychotherapy relationships that work: Evidence-based responsiveness* (2nd ed., pp. 92–109). New York: Oxford University Press.

Frierson, R., & Melikian, M. (2002). *Postgraduate medicine online: The practical peer-reviewed journal for primary care physicians*. New York: McGraw-Hill.

Gallagher, D., & Thompson, L. (1982). Treatment of major depressive disorder in older adult outpatients with brief psychotherapies. *Psychotherapy, 19*, 482–490.

Gallup, G., & Newport, F. (2006). *Religion most important to blacks, women and older Americans.* Retrieved from *www.gallup.com/poll/25585/ Religion-Most-Important-Blacks-Women-Older-Americans.aspx.*

Gambrill, E. (2010). Evidence-based practice and the ethics of discretion. *Journal of Social Work, 11*(1), 26–48.

Garcia-Preto, N. (2005). Puerto Rican families. In M. McGoldrick, J. Giordano, & N. Garcia-Preto (Eds.), *Ethnicity and family therapy* (3rd ed., pp. 242–265). New York: Guilford Press.

Garrick, D., & Ewashen, C. (2001). An integrated model for adolescent inpatient group therapy. *Journal of Psychiatric and Mental Health Nursing, 8,* 165–171.

Gaztambide, D. (2011). *Culture, rupture, and the therapeutic relationship with ethnic minority clients: A relational, evidence-based approach to cultural competency.* Unpublished manuscript, Rutgers University, New Brunswick, NJ.

Gehart, D., & McCollum, E. E. (2010). Inviting therapeutic presence: A mindfulness-based approach. In S. F. Hick & T. Bien (Eds.), *Mindfulness and the therapeutic relationship* (pp. 176–194). New York: Guilford Press.

Glodich, A., Allen, J. G., & Arnold, L. (2002). Protocol for a trauma-based psychoeducational group intervention to decrease risk-taking, reenactment, and further violence exposure: Application to the public high school setting. *Journal of Child and Adolescent Group Therapy, 11*(2/3), 87–107.

Godley, M. D., Godley, S. H., Dennis, M. L., Funk, R. R., & Passetti, L. L. (2007). The effect of assertive continuing care on continuing care linkage, adherence and abstinence following residential treatment for adolescents with substance use disorders. *Addiction, 102*(1), 81–93.

Goldstein, E., Stahl, B., Santorelli, S., & Kabat-Zinn, J. (2010). *A mindfulness-based stress reduction workbook.* Oakland, CA: New Harbinger.

Goodheart, C. D. (2006). Evidence, endeavor, and expertise in psychology practice. In C. D. Goodheart, A. E. Kazdin, & R. J. Sternberg. (Eds.), *Evidence-based psychotherapy: Where practice and research meet* (pp. 37–61). Washington, DC: American Psychological Association.

Goodheart, C. D., Kazdin, A. E., & Sternberg, R. J. (Eds.). (2006). *Evidence-based psychotherapy: Where practice and research meet.* Washington, DC: American Psychological Association.

Goodman, R. (1999) The extended version of the Strengths and Difficulties Questionnaire as a guide to child psychiatric cases and consequent burden. *Journal of Child Psychology and Psychiatry, 40,* 791–801.

Gopalan, G., Goldstein, L., Klingenstein, K., Sicher, C., Blake, C., & McKay, M. M. (2010). Engaging families into child mental health treatment: Updates and special considerations. *Journal of the American Academy of Child and Adolescent Psychiatry, 19*(3), 182–196.

Gotham, H. J. (2004). Diffusion of mental health and substance abuse treatments: Development, dissemination, and implementation. *Clinical Psychology: Science and Practice, 11,* 160–176.

Gotham, H. J. (2006). Advancing the implementation of evidence-based practices into clinical practice: How do we get there from here? *Professional Psychology, 37,* 606–613.

Gould, M. S., & Kramer, R.A. (2001). Youth suicide prevention. *Suicide and Life Threatening Behavior, 31,* 6–30.

Haley, J. (1976). *Problem solving therapy.* San Francisco: Jossey-Bass.

Hanh, N. T. (1998). *The heart of the Buddha's teaching: Transforming suffering into peace, joy, and liberation..* Berkeley, CA: Parallax Press.

Harris, M., & Fallot, R. D. (Eds.). (2001). *Using trauma theory to design service systems: New directions for mental health services.* San Francisco, CA: Jossey-Bass.

Harris, R. (2009). *ACT made simple.* Oakland, CA: New Harbinger.

Hartman, A., & Laird, J. (1983). *Family-centered social work practice.* New York: Free Press.

Hartman, C. R. (1995). The nurse-patient relationship and victims of violence. *Research and Theory for Nursing Practice, 9*(2), 175–192.

Hartman, C. R., & Jackson, H. (1994). Rape and the phenomena of countertransference. In J. P. Wilson & J. D. Lindy (Eds.), *Countertransference in the treatment of PTSD* (pp. 206–244). New York: Guilford Press.

Hayes, S. (2006, January 11). *The six core processes of ACT.* Retrieved from http://contextualpsychology.org/the_six_core_processes_of_act.

Hayes, S., Follette, V. M., & Linehan, M. M. (Eds.). (2004). *Mindfulness and acceptance: Expanding the cognitive-behavioral tradition.* New York: Guilford Press.

Hayes, S. C., Barlow, D. H., & Nelson-Gray, R. O. (1999). *The scientist practitioner: Research and accountability in the age of managed care* (2nd ed.). Boston: Allyn & Bacon.

Hayes, S. C., & Smith, S. (2005). *Get out of your mind and into your life: The new acceptance and commitment therapy.* Oakland, CA: New Harbinger.

Hayes, S. C., Strosahl, K. D., & Wilson, K. G. (1999). *Acceptance and commitment therapy: The process and practice of mindful change.* New York: Guilford Press.

Hayes, S. C., Strosahl, K. D., & Wilson, K. G. (2011). *Acceptance and commitment therapy: The process and practice of mindful change* (2nd ed.). New York: Guilford Press.

Henggeler, S. W., & Borduin, C. M. (1990). *Family therapy and beyond: A multisystematic approach to treating the behavior problems of children and adolescents.* Pacific Grove, CA: Brooks/Cole.

Henggeler, S. W., & Santos, A. B. (Eds.). (1997). *Innovative approaches for difficult-to-treat populations.* Washington, DC: American Psychiatric Press.

Henggeler, S. W., Schoenwald, S. K., Borduin, C. M., Rowland, M. D., & Cunningham, P. B. (1998). *Multisystemic treatment of antisocial behavior in children and adolescents.* New York: Guilford Press.

Henggeler, S. W., Schoenwald, S. K., Borduin, C. M., Rowland, M. D., & Cunningham, P. B. (2009). *Multisystemic therapy for antisocial behavior in children and adolescents* (2nd ed.). New York: Guilford Press.

Hernandez, P., Gangsei, D., & Engstrom, D. (2007). Vicarious resilience: A new concept in work with those who survive trauma. *Family Process, 46*(2), 229–241.

Hettema, J., Miller, W. R., & Steele, J. (2005). Motivational interviewing. *Annual Review of Clinical Psychology, 1,* 91–111.

Hick, S. F. (2010). Cultivating therapeutic relationships: The role of mindfulness. In S. F. Hick & T. Bien (Eds.), *Mindfulness and the therapeutic relationship* (pp. 3–18). New York: Guilford Press.

Hick, S. F., & Bien, T. (Eds.). (2010). *Mindfulness and the therapeutic relationship.* New York: Guilford Press.

Hoagwood, K., Burns, B. J., Kiser, L., Ringesien, H., & Schoenwald, S. K. (2001). Evidence-based practice in child and adolescent mental health services. *Psychiatric Services, 52*(9), 1179–1189.

Hoagwood, K., Burns, B. J., & Weisz, J. R. (2002). A profitable conjunction: From science to service in children's mental health. In B. J. Burns & K. Hoagwood (Eds.), *Community treatment for youth: Evidence-based interventions for severe emotional and behavioral disorders* (pp. 327–338). New York: Oxford University Press.

Horvath, A. O., & Bedi, R. P. (2002). The alliance. In J. C. Norcross (Ed.), *Psychotherapy relationships that work: Therapist contributions responsiveness to patients* (pp. 37–70). New York: Oxford University Press.

Horvath, A. O., Del Re, A. C., Flückiger, C., & Symonds, D. (2010). Alliance in individual psychotherapy. In J. C. Norcross (Ed.), *Psychotherapy relationships that work: Evidence-based responsiveness* (2nd ed.). New York: Oxford University Press. Retrieved from *http://nrepp.samhsa.gov/pdfs/Norcross_evidence-based_therapy_relationships.pdf* [pp. 5–6].

Horvath, A. O., Del Re, A. C., Flückiger, C., & Symonds, D. (2011). Alliance in individual psychotherapy. In J. C. Norcross (Ed.). *Psychotherapy relationships that work: Evidence-based responsiveness* (2nd ed., pp. 25–69). New York: Oxford University Press.

Horvath, A. O., & Symonds, B. D. (1991). Relation between working alliance and outcome in psychotherapy: A meta-analysis. *Journal of Counseling Psychology, 38,* 139–149.

Hunter, S. V., & Schofield, M. J. (2006). How counselors cope with traumatized clients: Personal, professional and organizational strategies. *International Journal for Advancement of Counseling, 28*(2), 121–138.

Huppert, J. D., Fabbro, A., & Barlow, D. H. (2006). Evidence-based practice and psychological treatments. In C. D. Goodheart, A. E. Kazdin, & R. J. Sternberg (Eds.), *Evidence-based psychotherapy: Where practice and research meet* (pp. 131–152). Washington, DC: American Psychological Association.

Imber-Black, E. (1988). *Families and larger systems: A family therapist's guide through the labyrinth.* New York: Guilford Press.

Indart, M. (2008). *Effective management of suicidal risk: Current research and practice.* PowerPoint presentation at Rutgers University, New Brunswick, NJ.

Institute for Community Living. (2008, August). *Proceedings from the Clinical Risk Assessment and Intervention Workgroup.* New York, NY.

Institute of Medicine. (2001). *Crossing the quality chasm: A new health system for the 21st century.* Washington, DC: National Academy Press.

Ireys, H. T., Devet, K. A., & Sakwa, D. (2002). Family support and education. In B. J. Burns & K. Hoagwood (Eds.), *Community treatment for youth: Evidence-based interventions for severe emotional and behavioral disorders.* New York: Oxford University Press.

Isaacs, D., & Fitzgerald, D. (1999). Seven alternatives to evidence based medicine. *British Medical Journal, 319,* 1618.

Jarvis, D., & Alexander, L. (2011, March 23). *Partnering with Health Homes and ACOs* [Webinar]. Retrieved from *www.thenationalcouncil.org/cs/recordings_presentations.*

Jenkins, E., & Bell, C. (1994). Violence among inner city high school students and post-traumatic stress disorder. In S. Friedman (Ed.), *Anxiety disorders in African Americans* (pp. 76–88). New York: Springer.

Jensen, P. S., Hoagwood, K. E., & Trickett, E. J. (1999). Ivory towers or earthen trenches? Community collaborations to foster real-world research. *Applied Developmental Science, 3*(4), 206–212.

Jewell, T., Downing, D., & McFarlane, W. (2009). Partnering with families: Multiple family group psychoeducation for schizophrenia. *Journal of Clinical Psychology, 65*(8), 868–878.

Jobes, D. (2006). *Managing suicidal risk: A collaborative approach.* New York: Guilford Press.

Josephs, L. (1996). Women and trauma: A contemporary psychodynamic approach to traumatization for patients in the OB/GYN psychological consultation clinic. *Bulletin of the Menninger Clinic, 60*(1), 22–39.

Kabat-Zinn, J. (1990). *Full catastrophe living: Using the wisdom of your body and mind to face stress, pain, and illness.* New York: Delta.

Kabat-Zinn, J. (2005). *Coming to our senses: Healing ourselves and the world through mindfulness.* New York: Hyperion.

Kazantzis, N., Whittington, C., & Dattilio, F. (2010), Meta-analysis of homework effects in cognitive and behavioral therapy: A replication and extension. *Clinical Psychology: Science and Practice, 17,* 144–156.

Kazdin, A. E. (1997). A model for developing effective treatments: Progression and interplay of theory, research, and practice. *Journal of Clinical Child Psychology, 26*(2), 114–129.

Kazdin, A. E. (2006). Assessment and evaluation in clinical practice. In C. D. Goodheart, A. E. Kazdin, & R. J. Sternberg. (Eds.), *Evidence-based psychotherapy: Where practice and research meet* (pp. 153–177). Washington, DC: American Psychological Association.

Kazdin, A. E. (2008). Evidence-based treatment and practice: New opportunities to bridge clinical research and practice, enhance the knowledge base, and improve patient care. *American Psychologist, 63*(3), 146–159.

Kelly, J. F., & White, W. L. (Eds.). (2011). *Addiction recovery management: Theory, research, and practice.* Totowa, NJ: Humana Press.

Kolden, G. G., Klein, M. H., Wang, C., & Austin, S. B. (2010). Congruence/genuineness. In J. C. Norcross (Ed.), *Psychotherapy relationships that work: Evidence-based therapy relationships.* Retrieved from *http://nrepp.*

samhsa.gov/pdfs/Norcross_evidence-based_therapy_relationships.pdf [pp. 19–20].

Kristeller, J. L., & Hallett, B. (1999). Effects of a meditation-based intervention in the treatment of binge eating. *Journal of Health Psychology, 4,* 357–363.

Lambert, M. J. (1992). Psychotherapy outcome research: Implications for integrative and eclectic therapists. In J. C. Norcross and M.R. Goldfried (Eds.), *Handbook of psychotherapy integration* (pp. 94–129). New York: Basic Books.

Lambert, M. J., & Barley, D. E. (2002). Research summary on the therapeutic relationship and psychotherapy outcome. In J. Norcross (Ed.), *Psychotherapy relationships that work: Therapist contributions and responsiveness to patient needs* (pp. 17–36). New York: Oxford University Press.

Lambert, M. J., Hansen, N. B., Umpress, V., Lunnen, K., Okiishi, J., et. al. (2003). *Administration and scoring manual for the OQ-45.2.* Salt Lake City, UT: American Professional Credentialling Services, LLC.

Lampropoulos, G. K., & Spengler, P. M. (2002). Introduction: Reprioritizing the role of science in a realistic version of the scientist-practitioner model. *Journal of Clinical Psychology, 58,* 1195–1197.

Lee, E. (1997). *Working with Asian Americans: A guide for clinicians.* New York: Guilford Press.

Lee, E., & Mock, M. R. (2005). Asian families. In M. McGoldrick, J. Giordano, & N. Garcia-Preto (Eds.), *Ethnicity and family therapy* (3rd ed., pp. 269–289). New York: Guilford Press.

Lefley, H. P. (2009). *Family psychoeducation for serious mental illness.* New York: Oxford University Press.

Levant, R. F., & Silverstein, L. B. (2006). Treatment as usual. In J. C. Norcross, L. Beutler, & R. F. Levant (Eds.), *Evidence-based practices in mental health: Debate and dialogue on fundamental questions* (pp. 338–345). Washington, DC: American Psychological Association.

Lewinsohn, P. M., Antonuccio, D. O., Breckenridge, J. S., & Teri, L. (1984). *The "Coping with depression" course.* Eugene, OR: Castalia.

Lewinsohn, P. M., Rohde, P., Seeley, J. R., & Baldwin, C. L. (2001). Gender differences in suicide attempts from adolescence to adulthood. *Journal of the American Academy of Child and Adolescent Psychiatry, 40,* 427–434.

Liddle, H. A. (2005). *Troubled teens: Multidimensional family therapy.* New York: Guilford Press.

Liddle, H. A., & Rowe, C. L. (2010). *Adolescent substance abuse: Research and clinical advances.* New York: Guilford Press.

Liddle, H. A., Santisteban, D. A., & Levant, R. F. (Eds.). (2002). *Family psychology: Science-based interventions (decade of behavior).* Washington, DC: American Psychological Association.

Lincoln, C. E., & Mamiya, L. H. (1990). *The black church in the African American experience.* Durham, NC: Duke University Press.

Linehan, M. M. (1993). *Cognitive-behavioral treatment of borderline personality disorder.* New York: Guilford Press.

Linehan, M. M., Armstrong, H. E., Suarez, A., Allmon, D., & Heard, H. L.

(1991). Cognitive-behavioral treatment for chronically parasuicidal borderline patients. *Archives of General Psychiatry, 48,* 1060–1064.

Linehan, M. M., Cochran, B. N., & Kehrer, A. A. (2001). Dialectical behavior therapy for borderline personality disorder. In D. H. Barlow (Ed.), *Clinical handbook of psychological disorders* (3rd ed., pp. 470–522). New York: Guilford Press.

Liu, P., & Chan, C. S. (1996). Lesbian, gay, and bisexual Asian Americans and their families. In J. Laird & R. Green (Eds.), *Lesbians and gays in couples in families: A handbook for therapists* (pp. 137–152). San Francisco: Jossey-Bass.

Ludgate, J. W. (2009). *Cognitive-behavioral therapy and relapse prevention for depression and anxiety.* Sarasota, FL: Professional Resource Press.

Luoma, J., Hayes, S., & Walser, R. (2007). *Learning ACT: An acceptance and commitment therapy skills-training manual for therapists.* Oakland, CA: New Harbinger.

MacLennan, B. W. (2000). The future of adolescent psychotherapy groups in the new millennium. *Journal of Child and Adolescent Group Therapy, 10*(2), 67–75.

MacLennan, B. W., & Dies, K. R. (1992). *Group counseling and psychotherapy with adolescents* (2nd ed.). New York: Columbia University Press.

Madanes, C. (1981). *Strategic family therapy.* San Francisco: Jossey-Bass.

Madsen, W. C. (1999). *Collaborative therapy with multi-stressed families: From old problems to new futures.* New York: Guilford Press.

Madsen, W. C. (2007). *Collaborative therapy with multi-stressed families* (2nd ed.). New York: Guilford Press.

Maris, R. W., Berman, A. L., & Silverman, M. M. (2000). *Comprehensive textbook of suicidology.* New York: Guilford Press.

Marlatt, G. A. (1996). Taxonomy of high-risk situations for alcohol relapse: Evolution and development of a cognitive-behavioral model of relapse. *Addiction, 91*(Suppl.), 37–50.

Marlatt, G. A., Bowen, S., Chawla, N., & Witkiewitz, K. (2008). Mindfulness-based relapse prevention for substance abusers: Therapist training and therapeutic relationships. In S. F. Hick & T. Bien (Eds.), *Mindfulness and the therapeutic relationship* (pp. 107–121). New York: Guilford Press.

Marlatt, G. A., & Donovan, D. M. (Eds.). (2005). *Relapse prevention: Maintenance strategies in the treatment of addictive behaviors* (2nd ed.). New York: Guilford Press.

Marlatt, G. A., & Gordon, J. R. (Eds.). (1985). *Relapse prevention: Maintenance strategies in the treatment of addictive behaviors.* New York: Guilford Press.

Marlatt, G. A., & Witkiewitz, K. (2005). Relapse prevention for alcohol and drug problems. In G. A. Marlatt & D. M. Donovan (Eds.), *Relapse prevention: Maintenance strategies in the treatment of addictive behaviors* (2nd ed., pp. 1–44). New York: Guilford Press.

Masten, A. S. (2001). Ordinary magic: Resilience process in development. *American Psychologist, 56*(3), 227–238.

Masten, A. S., & Coatsworth, J. D. (1998). The development of competence in favorable and unfavorable environments: Lessons learned from successful children. *American Psychologist, 53,* 205–220.

Maxwell, M. J., & Sturm, C. (1994). Countertransference in the treatment of war veterans. In J. P. Wilson & J. D. Lindy (Eds.), *Countertransference in the treatment of PTSD* (pp. 288–307). New York: Guilford Press.

McCann, I. L., & Pearlman, L. A. (1990). Vicarious traumatization: A framework for understanding the psychological effects of working with victims. *Journal of Traumatic Stress, 3*(1), 131–149.

McFarlane, W. R. (2002). *Multifamily groups in the treatment of severe psychiatric disorders.* New York: Guilford Press.

McFarlane, W. R., Dixon, L., Lukens, E., & Lucksted, A. (2003). Family psychoeducation and schizophrenia: A review of the literature. *Journal of Marital and Family Therapy, 29*(2), 223–245.

McGoldrick, M., Giordano, J., & Garcia-Preto, N. (Eds.). (2005). *Ethnicity and family therapy* (3rd ed.). New York: Guilford Press.

McKay, M., & Bannon W. M. (2004). Engaging families in child mental health services. *Child and Adolescent Psychiatric Clinics of North America, 13*(4), 905–921.

McKay, M., & Fanning, P. (2005). *Self-esteem.* Oakland, CA: New Harbinger.

McKay, M. M., Gopalan, G., Franco, L., Kalogerogiannis, K. N., Olshtain-Mann, O., Bannon, W., et al. (2010). It takes a village to deliver and test child and family-focused services. *Research in Social Work Practice, 20*(5), 476–482.

McWilliams, N. (1999). *Psychoanalytic case formulation.* New York: Guilford Press.

McWilliams, N. (2004). *Psychoanalytic psychotherapy: A practitioner's guide.* New York: Guilford Press.

McWilliams, N. (2011). *Psychoanalytic diagnosis: Understanding personality structure in the clinical process* (2nd ed.). New York: Guilford Press.

Meichenbaum, D. (2008). Core tasks of psychotherapy/counseling: What "expert" therapists do and how to use evidence-based principles and interventions to guide clinical practice. Retrieved August 13, 2011, from *www.melissainstitute/org/documents/Meichenbaum-Core_Tasks.pdf.*

Messer, S. B. (2004). Evidence-based practice: Beyond empirically supported treatments. *Professional Psychology: Research and Practice, 35*(6), 580–588.

Messer, S. B. (2006). Patient values and preferences. In J. C. Norcross, L. E. Beutler, & R. F. Levant (Eds.), *Evidence-based practices in mental health: Debate and dialogue on fundamental questions* (pp. 31–55). Washington, DC: American Psychological Association.

Miller, D. B. (1995). Treatment of adolescent interpersonal violence: A cognitive-behavioral group approach. *Journal of Child and Adolescent Group Therapy, 5*(4), 191–200.

Miller, W. R., & Moyers, T. B. (2006). Eight stages in learning motivational interviewing. *Journal of Teaching in the Addictions, 5*(1), 3–17.

Miller, W. R., & Rollnick, S. (1991). *Motivational interviewing: Preparing people to change addictive behavior.* New York: Guilford Press.

Miller, W. R., & Rollnick, S. (2002). *Motivational interviewing: Preparing people for change.* (2nd ed.). New York: Guilford Press.

Miller, W. R., & Rollnick, S. (2009). Ten things motivational interviewing is not. *Behavioral and Cognitive Psychotherapy, 37,* 129–140.

Miller, W. R., & Rollnick, S. (2011). *Strategies for evoking change talk.* Retrieved March 16, 2011, from *www.motivationalinterview.org/ Documents/1%20A%20MI%20Definition%20Principles%20&%20 Approach%20V4%20012911.pdf.*

Miller, W. R., & Rollnick, S. (2013). *Motivational interviewing: Helping people change* (3rd ed.). New York: Guilford Press.

Minuchin, P., Colapinto, J., & Minuchin, S. (2006). *Working with families of the poor* (2nd ed.). New York: Guilford Press.

Minuchin, S. (1974). *Families and family therapy.* Cambridge, MA: Harvard University Press.

Miranda, J., Bernal, G., Lau, A., Kohn, L., Hwang, W. C., & LaFromboise, T. (2005). State of the science on psychological interventions for ethnic minorities. *Annual Review of Clinical Psychology, 1,* 113–142.

Moore, M. (2009). *What is the value of practicing mindfulness meditation?* Retrieved from *www.feltoninstitute.org/articles/Mindfulness%20Meditation%20Paper%20Draft%20two.6.15.09doc.doc.*

Mueser, K. T., Corrigan, P. W., Hilton, D. W., Tanzman, B., Schaub, A., Gingerich, S., et al. (2002). Illness management and recovery: A review of the research. *Psychiatric Services, 53*(10), 1272–1284.

Munroe, J. (1995). Ethical issues associated with secondary trauma in therapists. In B. H. Stamm (Ed.), *Secondary traumatic stress* (2nd ed., pp. 211–229). Baltimore: Sidran Press.

Najavits, L. M. (2002). *Seeking safety: A treatment manual for PTSD and substance abuse.* New York: Guilford Press.

Nath, S. (2005). Pakistani families. In M. McGoldrick, J. Giordano, & N. Garcia-Preto (Eds.), *Ethnicity and family therapy* (3rd ed., pp. 407–420). New York: Guilford Press.

National Alliance on Mental Illness. (2012). *About NAMI.* Retrieved March 12, 2012, from *www.nami.org/Content/NavigationMenu/Inform_Yourself/About_NAMI/About_NAMI.htm.*

National Alliance on Mental Illness New York State—Family Toolkit. (n.d.). Retrieved from *www.naminys.org/family-toolkit.*

Nathan, P. E., & Gorman, J. M. (Eds.). (1998). *A guide to treatments that work.* New York: Oxford University Press.

National Institute of Mental Health (2001, April 9). *Suicide facts and statistics.* Retrieved September 12, 2006, from *http://www.nimh.nih.gov/suicideprevention/suifact.cfm*

Neimeyer, R. A., & Feixas, G. (1990). The role of homework and skill acquisition in the outcome of group cognitive therapy for depression. *Behavior Therapy, 21,* 281–292.

Nemec, P. B., McNamara, S., & Walsh, D. (1992). Direct skills teaching. *Psychosocial Rehabilitation Journal, 16*(1), 12–25.

Neumann, D. A., & Gamble, S. J. (1995). Issues in the professional development of psychotherapists: Countertransference and vicarious traumatization in the new trauma therapist. *Psychotherapy, 32*(2), 341–347.

Nevo, I., & Slonim-Nevo, V. (2011). The myth of evidence-based practice: Towards evidence-informed practice. *British Journal of Social Work, 41*(6), 1176–1197.

New York State Office of Mental Health. (2001, June). *Winds of change: Creating an environment of quality.* Presentation to providers, Brooklyn, NY.

Nichols, M. P. (2009). *The essentials of family therapy* (4th ed.). Boston: Allyn & Bacon.

Nichols, M. P. (2011). *The essentials of family therapy* (5th ed.). Boston: Allyn & Bacon.

Nichols-Goldstein, N. (2001). The essence of effective leadership with adolescent groups: Regression in the service of the ego. *Journal of Child and Adolescent Group Therapy, 11,* 13–17.

Nissen, L. (2001). *Strength-based approaches to work with youth and families: An overview of the literature and web-based resources.* Sacramento: California Institute for Mental Health. Retrieved from *www.cimh.org/contentFiles/Strengths%20based%20Approaches%20L.%20Nissen1.pdf.*

Norcross, J. C. (2002). *Psychotherapy relationships that work: Therapist contributions and responsiveness to patient needs.* New York: Oxford University Press.

Norcross, J. C. (Ed.). (2011a). *Psychotherapy relationships that work: Evidence-based responsiveness* (2nd ed.). New York: Oxford University Press.

Norcross, J. C. (2011b). Purposes, processes, and products of the task force on empirically supported therapy relationships. *Psychotherapy, 38*(4), 345–356.

Norcross, J. C., Beutler, L. E., & Levant, R. F. (Eds.). (2006). *Evidence-based practices in mental health: Debate and dialogue on fundamental questions.* Washington, DC: American Psychological Association.

Norcross, J. C., & Lambert, M. J. (2010). *Evidence-based therapy relationships.* Retrieved from *http://nrepp.samhsa.gov/pdfs/Norcross_evidence-based_therapy_relationships.pdf.*

North Shore Long Island Jewish Healthcare System–Syosset Hospital. (2012). *Decreasing violence in an in-patient behavioral health unit—highlighted in the Annual Maryland Patient Safety Centers Call for Solutions.* Retrieved from *www.marylandpatientsafety.org/html/education/solutions/2012/documents/Decreasing_violence_in_an_in_patient.pdf.*

Olkin, R., & Taliaferro, G. (2006). Evidence-based practices have ignored people with disabilities. In J. C. Norcross, L. E. Beutler, & R. F. Levant (Eds.), *Evidence-based practices in mental health: Debate and dialogue on fundamental questions* (pp. 353–359). Washington, DC: American Psychological Association.

Onken, S. J., Craig, C. M., Ridgway, P., Ralph, R. O., & Cook, J. A. (2007). An analysis of the definitions and elements of recovery: A review of the literature [Special issue]. *Psychiatric Rehabilitation Journal: Mental Health Recovery and System Transformation, 31*(1), 9–22.

Oregon Senate Bill 267 (2005). Information sheet available online at *www.oregon.gov/OCCF/Documents/JCP/L9_SB267_Info_Sheet.pdf?ga=t.*

Orlin, L., & Davis, J. (1993). Assessment and intervention with drug and alcohol abusers in psychiatric settings. In S. L. A. Straussner (Ed.), *Clinical work with substance abusing clients* (pp. 50–68). New York: Guilford Press.

Orlinsky, D. E., & Ronnestad, M. H. (2005). *How therapists develop: A study of therapists' work and professional growth.* Washington, DC: American Psychological Association.

Padesky, C. A., Kuyken, W., & Dudley, R. (2011). *Collaborative case conceptualization: Working effectively with clients in cognitive-behavioral therapy.* New York: Guilford Press.

Pagoto, S. L., Spring, B., Coups, E. J., Mulvaney, S., Coutu, M. F., & Ozakinci, G. (2007). Barriers and facilitators of evidence-based practice perceived by behavioral science health professionals. *Journal of Clinical Psychology, 63,* 695–705.

Pappas, S. V., & Howard, D. (2009, April 24–26). *The Institute for Community Living, Inc., today.* Presented at the ICL Board of Directors Strategic Planning Retreat, New York, NY.

Parson, E. R. (1994). Inner city children of trauma: Urban violence and traumatic stress response syndrome (U-VTS) and therapists' responses. In J. P. Wilson & J. D. Lindy (Eds.), *Countertransference in the treatment of PTSD* (pp. 151–178). New York: Guilford Press.

Pearlman, L. A., & MacIan, P. S. (1995). Vicarious traumatization: An empirical study of the effects of trauma work on trauma therapists. *Professional Psychology: Research Practice, 26*(6), 558–565.

Pearlman, L. A., & Saakvitne, K. W. (1995). Treating therapists with vicarious traumatization and secondary traumatic stress disorders. In C. R. Figley (Ed.), *Compassion fatigue: Coping with secondary traumatic stress disorder in those who treat the traumatized* (pp. 150–177). New York: Brunner/Mazel.

Persons, J. B. (2008). *The case formulation approach to cognitive behavior therapy.* New York: Guilford Press.

Pew Forum on Religion and Public Life. (2009). *A religious portrait of African Americans.* Retrieved from *http://pewforum.org/docs/?DocID=389.*

Pillari, V. (2005). Indian Hindu families. In M. McGoldrick, J. Giordano, & N. Garcia-Preto (Eds.), *Ethnicity and family therapy* (3rd ed., pp. 395–420). New York: Guilford Press.

Pinderhughes, E. (1989). *Understanding race, ethnicity, and power: The key to efficacy in clinical practice.* New York: Free Press.

Pires, S. A. (2002). *Building systems of care: A primer.* Washington, DC: National Technical Assistance Center for Children's Mental Health.

President's New Freedom Commission on Mental Health. (2003). *Achieving the promise: Transforming mental health care in America. Final report.* DHHS Publication No. SMA-03–3832. Rockville, MD: Government Printing Office.

Prochaska, J. O., & DiClemente, C. C. (1982). Transtheoretical therapy: Toward a more integrative model of change. *Psychotherapy: Theory, Research, and Practice, 19,* 276–288.

Prochaska, J. O., DiClemente, C. C., & Norcross, J. C. (1992). In search of how people change: Applications to addictive behaviors. *American Psychologist, 47*(9), 1102–1114.

Ralph, R. O., & Corrigan, P. W. (Eds.). (2005). *Recovery in mental illness: Broadening our understanding of wellness.* Washington, DC: American Psychological Association.

Rapp, C. (1998). *The strengths model: Case management with people suffering from severe and persistent mental illness.* New York: Oxford University Press.

Rathor, S. (2011). *Importance of marriage for Asian Indian women in the U.S.: An exploratory study.* Unpublished doctoral dissertation, Rutgers University, New Brunswick, NJ.

Reed, G. M. (2006). What qualifies as evidence of effective practice?: Clinical expertise. In J. C. Norcross, L. E. Beutler, & R. F. Levant (Eds.), *Evidence-based practices in mental health: Debate and dialogue on the fundamental questions.* Washington, DC: American Psychological Association.

Reed, G. M., & Eisman, E. J. (2006). Uses and misuses of evidence: Managed care, treatment guidelines, and outcomes measurement in professional practice. In C. D. Goodheart, A. E. Kazdin, & R. J. Sternberg (Eds.), *Evidence-based psychotherapy: Where practice and research meet* (pp. 13–35). Washington, DC: American Psychological Association.

Richardson, B., & June, L. (1997). Utilizing and maximizing the resources of the African American church: Strategies and tools for counseling professionals. In C. C. Lee (Ed.), *Multicultural issues in counseling: New approaches to diversity* (2nd ed., pp. 155–170). Alexandria, VA: American Counseling Association.

Riva, M. T., Wachtel, M., & Lasky, G. B. (2004). Effective leadership in group counseling and psychotherapy: Research and practice. In. J. L. DeLucia-Waack, D. A. Gerrity, C. R. Kalodner, & M. T. Riva (Eds.), *Handbook of group counseling and psychotherapy* (pp. 37–48). Thousand Oaks, CA: Sage.

Robin, A. L., & Foster, S. L. (2002). *Negotiating parent–adolescent conflict: A behavioral-family systems approach.* New York: Guilford Press.

Robins, C. J. (2002). Zen principles and mindfulness practice in Dialectical Behavior Therapy. *Cognitive and Behavioral Practice, 9,* 50–57.

Robins, C. J., Schmidt, H., III, & Linehan, M. M. (2004). Dialectical behavior therapy: Synthesizing radical acceptance with skillful means. In S. Hayes, V. M. Follette, & M. M. Linehan (Eds.), *Mindfulness and acceptance: Expanding the cognitive-behavioral tradition* (pp. 30–44). New York: Guilford Press.

Rogers, C. (1951). *Client-centered therapy: Its current practice, implications and theory.* London: Constable.

Rogers, C. (1957). The necessary and sufficient conditions of therapeutic personality change. *Journal of Consulting Psychology, 21,* 95–103. Retrieved from *http://shoreline.edu/dchris/psych236/Documents/Rogers.pdf.*

Rogers, C. (1980). *A way of being.* New York: Houghton Mifflin.

Rudd, M. D. (2006). Suicidality in clinical practice: Anxieties and answers. *Journal of Clinical Psychology, 62,* 157–159.

Rycroft-Malone, J. (2008). Evidence-informed practice: From individual to context. *Journal of Nursing Management, 16,* 404–408.

Saleebey, D. (2000). Power in the people: Strengths and hope. *Advances in Social Work, 1*(2), 127–136.

Salerno, A., Margolies, P., & Cleek, A. (2007, September 11). *Wellness self-management training.* New York: New York State Office of Mental Health & Urban Institute for Behavioral Health.

Salerno, A., Margolies, P., & Cleek, A. (2008a). *Wellness self-management personal workbook.* Albany: New York State Office of Mental Health, WSM Initiative, New York City.

Salerno, A., Margolies, P., & Cleek, A. (2008b). *Wellness self-management training.* Presented at the New York State Office of Mental Health Statewide Initiative, New York.

Salerno, A., Margolies, P., Cleek, A., Pollock, M., Gopalan, G., & Jackson, C. (2011). Best practices: Wellness self-management: An adaptation of the Illness Management and Recovery program in New York State. *Psychiatric Services, 62,* 456–458. (ROPES format described in online supplement [re: Below citation, both the article and the online supplement were cited]: *http://psychservices.psychiatryonline.org/cgi/data/62/5/456/DC1/1.*)

Sanchez-Hucles, J. (1998). Racism: Emotional abusiveness and psychological trauma for ethnic minorities. *Journal of Emotional Abuse, 1,* 69–87.

Shneidman, E. S. (1993). *Suicide as a psychache: A clinical approach to self-destructive behavior.* Northvale, NJ: Aronson.

Schwartz, J. (2011, October 3). *The use of mindfulness in the treatment of obsessive compulsive disorder (OCD).* Retrieved from *http://hope4ocd.com/mindfulness.php.*

Schwartz, J. M., & Beyette, B. (1996). *Brain lock: Free yourself from obsessive compulsive behavior.* New York: HarperCollins.

Schwartz, R. C., & Rogers, J. R. (2004). Suicide assessment and evaluation strategies: A primer for counseling psychologists. *Counseling Psychology Quarterly 17,* 89–97.

Segal, Z. V., Teasdale, J. D., & Williams, J. M. G. (2004). Mindfulness-based cognitive therapy: Theoretical rationale and empirical status. In S. Hayes, V. M. Follette, & M. M. Linehan (Eds.), *Mindfulness and acceptance: Expanding the cognitive-behavioral tradition* (pp. 45–65). New York: Guilford Press.

Segal, Z. V., Williams, J. M. G., & Teasdale, J. D. (2002). *Mindfulness-based cognitive therapy for depression: A new approach to preventing relapse.* New York: Guilford Press.

Segal, Z. V., Williams, M. G., & Teasdale, J. D. (2001). *Mindfulness-based cognitive therapy for depression: A new approach to preventing relapse.* New York: Guilford Press.

Segal, Z. V., Williams, M. G., Teasdale, J. D., & Kabat-Zinn, J. (2012). *Mindfulness-based cognitive therapy for depression: A new approach to preventing relapse* (2nd ed). New York: Guilford Press.

Seligman, M. E. (1990). *Learned optimism.* New York: Knopf.

Seligman, M. E., & Csikszentmihalyi, M. (2000). Positive psychology: An introduction. *American Psychologist, 55*(1), 5–14.

Sexton, T. L., & Alexander, J. F. (2004). *Functional family therapy clinical training manual.* Seattle, WA: FFT Inc.

Shafir, R. (2010). Mindful listening for better outcomes. In S. F. Hick & T. Bien (Eds.), *Mindfulness and the therapeutic relationship* (pp. 215–231). New York: Guilford Press.

Shapiro, S. L., & Izett, C. D. (2010). Meditation: A universal tool for cultivating empathy. In S. F. Hick & T. Bien (Eds.), *Mindfulness and the therapeutic relationship* (pp. 161–175). New York: Guilford Press.

Shapiro, S. L., Schwartz, G. E., & Bonner, G. (1998). Effects of mindfulness-based stress reduction on medical and premedical students. *Journal of Behavioral Medicine, 21*(6), 581–599.

Shea, S. C. (2002). *The practical art of suicide assessment: A guide for mental health professionals and substance abuse counselors.* Hoboken, NJ: Wiley.

Shea, S. C. (2004). The delicate art of eliciting suicidal ideation. *Psychiatric Annals, 34*(5), 385–400.

Shirk, S. R., & Karver, M. (2011). Alliance in child and adolescent psychotherapy. In J. C. Norcross (Ed.), *Psychotherapy relationships that work: Evidence-based therapy relationships.* Retrieved from *http://nrepp.samhsa.gov/pdfs/Norcross_evidence-based_therapy_relationships.pdf* [pp. 7–8].

Siegel, R. D. (2005). Psycho-physiological disorders; embracing pain. In C. K. Gerner, R, D. Siegel, & P. R. Fulton (Eds.), *Mindfulness and psychotherapy* (pp. 173–196). New York: Guilford Press.

Sinason, V. (1991). Psychoanalytic psychotherapy with the severely, profoundly, and multiply handicapped. In R. Szur & S. Miller (Eds.), *Extending horizons: Psychoanalytic psychotherapy with children, adolescents, and families* (pp. 225–242). London: Karnac.

Slade, M. (2009). *Personal recovery and mental illness: A guide for mental health professionals.* New York: Cambridge University Press.

Smith, T., Burgos, J., Dexter, V., Norcott, J., Pappas, S., Shuman, E., et al. (2010). Best practices for improving engagement of clients in clinic care. *Psychiatric Services, 61,* 343–345.

Spring, B. (2007). Evidence-based practice in clinical psychology: What it is, why it matters, what we need to know. *Journal of Clinical Psychology, 63*(7), 611–631.

Staples, L. H. (1990). Powerful ideas about empowerment. *Administration in Social Work, 14*(2), 29–42.

Steinfeld, B. I., Coffman, S. J., & Keyes, J. A. (2009). Implementation of an evidence-based practice in a clinical setting: What happens when you get there? *Professional Psychology: Research and Practice, 40*(4), 410–416.

Straussner, S., & Phillips, N. (Eds.). (2003). *Understanding mass violence.* Boston: Pearson Press.

Straussner, S. L. A. (Ed.). (1993). *Clinical work with substance-abusing clients.* New York: Guilford Press.

Stroul, B. A., & Friedman, R. M. (1986). *A system of care for children and youth with severe emotional disturbances* (Rev. ed.). Washington, DC: Georgetown University Child Development Center, CASSP Technical Assistance Center.

Substance Abuse and Mental Health Services Administration. (2005). *National consensus statement on mental health recovery.* Retrieved from *store. samhsa.gov/shin/content//SMA05–4129/SMA05–4129.pdf.*

Sue, S. (1998). In search of cultural competence in psychotherapy and counseling. *American Psychologist, 53,* 440–448.

Sue, D. W., & Torino, G. C. (2005). Racial-cultural competence: Awareness, knowledge, and skills. In R. T. Carter (Ed.), *Handbook of racial-cultural psychology and counseling: Vol. 2. Training and practice* (pp. 3–18). Hoboken, NJ: Wiley.

Sue, S., & Zane, N. (2006). Ethnic minority populations have been neglected by evidence-based practices. In J. C. Norcross, L. E. Beutler, & R. F. Levant (Eds.), *Evidence-based practices in mental health: Debate and dialogue on fundamental questions* (pp. 329–337). Washington, DC: American Psychological Association.

Szapocznik, J., Hervis, O., & Schwartz, S. (2003). *Therapy manuals for drug addiction: Brief strategic family therapy for adolescent drug abuse.* Bethesda, MD: National Institute on Drug Abuse.

Taylor, R. J., Chatters, L. M., Bullard, K. M., Wallace, J. M., & Jackson, J. S. (2009). Organizational religious behavior among older African Americans: Findings from the National Survey of American Life. *Research on Aging, 31,* 440–462.

Taylor, R. J., Chatters, L. M., & Levin, J. (2004). *Religion in the lives of African Americans: Social, psychological, and health perspectives.* Thousand Oaks, CA: Sage.

Ting, L., Sanders, S., Jacobson, J. M., & Powers, J. R. (2006). Dealing with the aftermath: A qualitative analysis of mental health social workers' reactions after a client suicide. *Social Work, 51*(4), 329–341.

Tosone, C., & Bialkin, L. (2003). Mass violence and secondary trauma. In S. Straussner & N. Phillips (Eds.), *Understanding mass violence* (pp. 157–165). Boston: Pearson Press.

Toth, M. E., Schwartz, R. C., & Kurka, S. T. (2007). Strategies for understanding and assessing suicide risk in psychotherapy. *Annals of the American Psychotherapy Association, 4*(10), 8–18. Retrieved from *http://annalsofpsychotherapy.com/articles/winter07.php?topic=article9.*

Tripanny, R. L., White Kress, V. E., & Wicoxon, S. A. (2004). Preventing vicarious trauma: What counselors should know when working with trauma survivors. *Journal of Counseling and Development, 82,* 31–37.

Turner, P. (2001). Evidence-based practice and physiotherapy in the 1990s. *Physiotherapy Theory and Practice, 17,* 107–121.

Underwood, M., & Dunne-Maxim, K. (1997). *Managing sudden traumatic loss in schools: New Jersey Adolescent Suicide Prevention Project.* New Jersey State Department of Education.

Underwood, M., Fell, F. T., & Spinazzola N. A. (2010). *Lifelines postventions: Responding to suicide and other traumatic death.* Center City, MN: Hazelden.

U.S. Department of Health and Human Services. (1999). *Mental health: A report of the surgeon general.* Rockville, MD: U.S. Department of Health and Human Services, Substance Abuse and Mental Health Services Administration, Center for Mental Health Services, National Institutes of Mental Health. Retrieved March 12, 2012, from *www.surgeongeneral.gov/library/mentalhealth/chapter2/sec10.html.*

U.S. Department of Health and Human Services. (2011). News release: *Affordable Care Act to improve quality of care for people with Medicare.* Retrieved from *www.hhs.gov/news/press/2011pres/03/20110331a.html.*

Videka, L. (2011, March 31). *The future of social work.* Presented at the Institute for Community Living, New York, NY.

Wagner, C., & Ingersoll, K., with Contributors. (2013). *Motivational interviewing in groups.* New York: Guilford Press.

Waldegrave, C. (2005). "Just therapy" with families on low incomes. *Child Welfare League of America, 84*(2), 265–276.

Walsh, F. (1998). *Strengthening family resilience.* New York: Guilford Press.

Walsh, F. (2006). *Strengthening family resilience* (2nd ed.). New York: Guilford Press.

Walsh, F. (Ed.). (2009). *Spiritual resources in family therapy* (2nd ed.). New York: Guilford Press.

Wampold, B. E. (2001). *The great psychotherapy debate: Models, methods, and findings.* Mahwah, NJ: Erlbaum.

Weersing, V. R., Iyengar, S., Kolko, D. J., Birmaher, B., & Brent, D. A. (2006). Effectiveness of cognitive-behavioral therapy for adolescent depression: A benchmarking investigation. *Behavior Therapy, 37,* 36–48.

Weisz, J. R., & Addis, M. E. (2006). The research-practice tango and other choreographic challenges: Using and testing evidence-based psychotherapies in clinical care settings. In C. D. Goodheart, A. E. Kazdin, & R. J. Sternberg (Eds.), *Evidence-based psychotherapy: Where practice and research meet* (pp. 179–206). Washington, DC: American Psychological Association.

Wells, M. G., Burlingame, G. M., Lambert, M. J., Hoag, M. J., & Hope, C. A. (1996). Conceptualization and measurement of patient change during psychotherapy: Development of the Outcome Questionnaire and Youth Outcome Questionnaire. *Psychotherapy: Theory, Research, Practice, Training, 33*(2), 275–283.

References

Westefield, J. S., Range, L. M., Rogers, J. R., Maples, M. R., Bromley, J. L., & Alcorn, J. (2000). Suicide: An overview. *The Counseling Psychologist, 28,* 445–510.

Whaley, A. L., & Davis, K. E. (2007). Cultural competence and evidence-based practice in mental health services: A complementary perspective. *American Psychologist, 62*(6), 563–574.

White, M. (1995). *Re-authorizing lives: Interviews and essays.* Adelaide, South Australia: Dulwich Centre Publications.

White, M., & Epston, D. (1990). *Narrative means to a therapeutic end.* New York: Norton.

White, W., Boyle, M., & Loveland, D. (2005). Recovery from addiction and from mental illness: Shared and contrasting lessons. In R. O. Ralph & P. W. Corrigan (Eds.), *Recovery in mental illness: Broadening our understanding of wellness* (pp. 233–258). Washington, DC: American Psychological Association.

Williams, M. G., Teasdale, J. D., Segal, Z. V., & Kabat-Zinn, J. (2007). *The mindful way through depression: Freeing yourself from chronic unhappiness.* New York: Guilford Press.

Wilson, K. G., & Dufrene, T. (2008). *Mindfulness for two: An acceptance and commitment therapy approach to mindfulness in psychotherapy.* Oakland, CA: New Harbinger.

Wilson, K. G., & Dufrene, T. (2010). *Things might go terribly, horribly, wrong: A guide to life liberated from anxiety.* Oakland, CA: New Harbinger.

Witkiewitz, K., Marlatt, G. A., & Walker, D. (2005). Mindfulness-based relapse prevention for alcohol and substance use disorders. *Journal of Cognitive Psychotherapy, 19,* 211–228.

Wofsy, M. (2006). Is therapy science or art? *ICL Insider.* New York: Institute for Community Living.

Wofsy, M., & Mundy, B. (2010a, June 16). Harm reduction in residential programs. PowerPoint interactive training presented at the Institute for Community Living, Brooklyn, NY.

Wofsy, M., & Mundy, B. (2010b, October). *A 3-tiered approach to evidence-based practice dissemination.* Presented at the New York State Association of Community and Residential Agencies 2010 Annual Conference, Lake George, NY.

Wofsy, M., & Mundy, B. (2011a, January 20). *Group facilitation: Tools, tips, and how-tos.* PowerPoint interactive training presented at the Institute for Community Living, Brooklyn, NY.

Wofsy, M., & Mundy, B. (2011b, March 11). Family engagement part one. Powerpoint interactive training presented at the Institute for Community Living, Brooklyn, NY.

Wofsy, M., Mundy, B., & Tse, J. (2009, October 20). *Introduction to risk assessment and navigation.* PowerPoint interactive training presented at the Institute for Community Living, Brooklyn, NY.

Wolpe, J. (1990). *The practice of behavior therapy* (4th ed). Charlottesville, VA: Pergamon Press.

Worden, J. W. (1991). *Grief counseling and grief therapy: A handbook for the mental health practitioner.* New York: Springer.

Yalom, I. D. (1995). *The theory and practice of group psychotherapy* (4th ed.). New York: Basic Books.

Yalom, I. D., & Leszcz, M. (2005). *Theory and practice of group psychotherapy* (5th ed.). New York: Basic Books.

Young, J. E., Rygh, J. L., Weinberger, A. D., & Beck, A. T. (2008). Cognitive therapy for depression. In D. H. Barlow (Ed.), *Clinical handbook of psychological disorders: A step-by-step treatment manual* (4th ed., pp. 250–305). New York: Guilford Press.

Index